The Cannabis Revolution©

What You Need to Know

Stephen Holt, MD, DSc

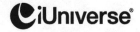

The Cannabis Revolution©
What You Need to Know

Published by the Holt Institute of Medicine (www.hiom.org)

Information from this book can be reproduced in short form only with clear reference to the origin of the work.

Stephen Holt, MD, Holt Institute of Medicine, 25 Amity St., Second Floor, Little Falls, NJ 07424.. E-mail: drholt@hiom.org.

This book may be ordered through booksellers or by contacting: HIOM at 973-256-4660 or 973-256-8057.

iUniverse books may be ordered through booksellers or by contacting:

iUniverse
1663 Liberty Drive
Bloomington, IN 47403
www.iuniverse.com
1-800-Authors (1-800-288-4677)

ISBN: 978-1-4917-7631-5 (sc)
ISBN: 978-1-4917-7633-9 (hc)
ISBN: 978-1-4917-7632-2 (e)

Library of Congress Control Number: 2015916537

Print information available on the last page.

iUniverse rev. date: 3/24/2016

09 16

Contents

CHAPTER 2

CHAPTER 3

CHAPTER 4

MEDICAL CANNABIS...89

CHAPTER 7

CHAPTER 8

CHAPTER 9

CHAPTER 12

Preface

STEPHEN HOLT, MD

Welcome to *The Cannabis Revolution*. The title of this book is an attempt to draw attention to the outcome of recent and rather precipitous legalization of cannabis use in several locations in the United States. Revolutions occur usually in a relatively abrupt manner, and they often present uncertain outcomes. While legalization is now occurring abruptly, it has been suggested by many for about a decade. Many factors have operated in changes of public and political opinions about cannabis use over the past few years, and concerns about its toxicity have been replaced increasingly by perceptions of its safety. The Cannabis Revolution in the United States is a major event for humankind that promises significant medical, economic, social, and political changes or outcomes. Some of these outcomes may exert good influences, and some consequences may be bad. In this book, I hope to at least scratch the surface of the many effects of rapidly increasing cannabis legalization, with a focus on information that may help people engage in the safe and responsible use of cannabis.

Bias has infected literature on the wisdom, or lack thereof, of cannabis use. This book attempts to describe a reasonably balanced account of the medical, social, economic, and political outcomes of the increasing use of cannabis. The subject of cannabis use is hotly debated and misunderstood, but it has protean current and future effects on society. When one peruses books on herbal medicine, it is notable to recognize how few books even mention cannabis. How can this be when millions of Americans use this drug? These writings are designed to help clarify thoughts on cannabis legalization, which is likely to have profound effects on society. It is now time to forget the backbiting or niggling comments about cannabis legalization and face an understanding of the implications of the more widespread use of this drug concoction. Knowledge about cannabis is often quite muddled as a consequence of misinformation.

Cannabis (marijuana) is composed of a diverse collection of biologically active compounds with complex actions and interactions. Of foremost importance are the actions of cannabinoids (phytocannabinoids) that are derived from cannabis on body functions. The body of all vertebrates contains endocannabinoids (molecules that signal) that exert control over many body functions. These controls occur by actions on cannabinoid receptors. The exogenous cannabinoids (phytocannabinoids or cannabis analogues) act on specific cannabinoid receptors (the endocannabinoid receptor systems) that control many body functions. Cannabinoids seem to alter body functions by exerting an "entourage effect." The entourage effect of cannabis involves a process of synergistic and antagonistic effects of cannabinoids. These entourage actions involve the action of terpenoids and other compounds that are derived from the plant Cannabis sativa and other cannabis species. While the complementary actions of terpenoids (essential oils) found in the cannabis plant appear to make a major contribution to the entourage effect, not all compounds that produce the cannabis-entourage effects are identified.

In brief, endocannabinoids work in concert and act by stimulating cannabinoid receptors, thereby controlling many body functions. These circumstances present a complex jigsaw puzzle that is in the process of being constructed as research points the way to an understanding of these intercommunicating systems of complex body controls. These controls are exerted through the endocannabinoid receptor systems. The function of these systems is modified to a variable degree by many factors. Add to these circumstances many circumstances that cause a great degree of variability in the effects of administered cannabinoids, and we have now entered a complex world of mapping cannabinoid activity. This area of science will keep researchers busy for many years.

Following nearly a century of relative inertia, research and clinical activities in medical cannabis use are now proceeding at a frenetic pace. Any author that attempts to provide some contemporary knowledge about cannabis has to face the risk of publishing some material that can be perceived to be rapidly outdated. This book is an attempt to produce current information about marijuana use by sifting and sorting through accurate, misleading, and sometimes-false statements about the medical use of marijuana. Thus, the author has had to insert his own opinions that may differ among some people.

Cannabis use has been embraced rapidly by many people, with some degree of misunderstanding about its safety and responsible use. A modern, widespread perception of cannabis safety has been reinforced by the legalization and decriminalization of its use, together with some degree of both positive and negative propaganda. The complexity of the many ramifications of further marijuana legalization is difficult to characterize, and it involves much future "shifting sand". These dynamic circumstances will occupy politicians and legislative staff for many years to come.

This account of cannabis is based upon my earlier training in therapeutics and clinical pharmacology at the University of Edinburgh, Scotland, and at the Addiction Research Foundation in Ontario, Canada, combined with four decades of medical practice experience. Most of my earlier experience in the medicine of addiction involved research in alcohol use and abuse. I believe that many aspects of alcohol research will be duplicated for use in performing cannabis research in the future. In this book, I have quoted authoritative accounts of the social, political, and medical consequences of cannabis availability and use. However, it is not possible to credit all sources of reporting on cannabis in scientific literature and on the Internet.

The sheer volume of information that I have reviewed leaves me with residual concerns that I have not credited all worthy contributors to the subject of cannabis science. This book may seem to contain a disproportionate amount of material on the negative effects of cannabis use. This situation is due to prohibition of cannabis use for the greater part of the last century, with the result that only approximately one in ten studies in this period of prohibition were designed to examine benefits of cannabis use. One cannot defy the obvious logic that medical benefits of a banned substance are not likely to figure in medical research. The ban on cannabis use and research was upheld with a common, ill-founded belief that it had no medical benefits.

To understand the science of cannabis is to delve into many areas of basic science and clinical experiences, but until relatively recently, much of this information has been incomplete or inadequate or frankly biased. Unfortunately, a significant amount of popular material on cannabis has been subject to zealous reporting and distorted interpretation. In common with any author on the subject of the expanding use of cannabis, I am humbled by the task of trying to create balanced opinions on this subject. I emphasize that the origin of the information in this book is from an eclectic mix of medical information derived from peer-reviewed scientific studies, books, and the evaluation of both zealous and conservative reporting on cannabis. There are many antagonistic viewpoints about cannabis that are matched with positive observational studies reported on the maze of the Internet. When it comes to cannabis reporting, speculation has often been the name of the game. Such speculation is often based on correlated science and not the definition of clear causal associations between cannabis use and adverse or beneficial outcomes.

A short and frank summary of this book is not possible, largely because it is an attempt to represent both sides of arguments about cannabis use and its prevailing or anticipated consequences. I can only scratch the surface of political arguments about cannabis and try to focus on the general effects of cannabis legalization on society. A necessary component of this book is to answer several questions about what to expect from the Cannabis Revolution that I have described and to wade my way through medical applications of this drug mixture that is provided by the revered or occasionally rejected cannabis plant (Cannabis sativa and its related species).

This book differs from other accounts of cannabis use. It is all about a contemporary general-knowledge source of information to tell people what to expect from cannabis use. I am surprised that the rating of sales of books on Amazon.com shows that books about growing cannabis outperform many books on general knowledge about cannabis use. In discussions with book-publishing experts, there is a significant opinion that many people just want to use cannabis with their head in the sand. I predict that this will change as cannabis use starts to mold society. I hope that a large number of readers of this book are parents who can guide their children on the drawbacks of the irresponsible use of cannabis in modern society.

Overall, I support cannabis legalization, but this major step in society has to be analyzed in terms of its good or bad future influences. While writing, I perceived a need to acquire information from people in many walks of life. However, some of the complexities of the science of cannabis interfere with dialogue among many people, including health care workers and politicians. I feel a significant degree of discomfort with the residual, incomplete knowledge that exists in the community about cannabis use. Moreover, I am more concerned to define evidence of a significant lack of education of many politicians and health care workers about cannabis use.

Medical practitioners may expose their practice vulnerabilities when new diseases occur and new public health threats emerge. While it is harsh to define cannabis legalization as a generator of public health problems, a prudent approach is necessary for the responsible use of the psychoactive drug mixture found in Cannabis sativa. The versatile and potent effects of other components of cannabis on body functions require further definition. One puzzling circumstance about the existence of cannabis (marijuana) is to answer the question "Why does this ability of a plant to modify inbuilt controlling systems of body function exist?" Talk or debate about coevolution of man with plants does not really address the reason why.

At the beginning of 2014, twenty US states and the District of

Columbia had medical marijuana legislation, and bills were filed in seventeen states for this purpose. This book asks many questions about the use of cannabis, but as one reads the information, it becomes clear that many of the posed questions may lack a definitive answer. In fact, writing about cannabis use at present in the United States has a lot to do with attempts to answer many unanswerable questions. There remains continuing conflict and emotive reactions about cannabis use among many people.

The partial unleashing of cannabis by recent legislation for medical and recreational use presents clear problems because cannabis lacks standardization that is required by federal government agencies for approval or by some physicians for its use. Furthermore, cannabis remains illegal according to federal law. That said, the relevance of federal law to marijuana use is now challenged as a result of disagreement with the federal government's denial of the medical benefits of cannabis. Moreover, there are no clear guidelines set forth for the monitoring of medical or recreational cannabis use.

There are several areas of continuing uncertainty about the outcome of the use of cannabis that are addressed in these writings. Clearly, the uncertainty of what is being consumed from several sources of cannabis requires definition and reasonable supervision. The characteristics of chemical purity of illicit cannabis remain unclear. Dose/response effects of herbal cannabis often defy measurement with any degree of precision, and toxicity can often be unpredictable. Borrowed science that may be used to predict outcomes of cannabis use are highly suspect, as contemporary patterns and types of cannabis use change. For example, continuous heavy use of modern, high-THC (tetrahydrocannabinol)-containing cannabis seems to result in negative outcomes (e.g., skunk strains, high-THC cannabis) and the precipitation of severe mental disturbances of psychosis. The "suck it and see" mode of administration of cannabis (the autotitration for effect method) is a common but crude way of measuring desired psychoactive effects. The best mode of cannabis delivery of certain types of cannabis remains uncertain, and contraindications for use remain somewhat unclear or doubted.

I have organized the contents of this book to achieve a progressive knowledge about marijuana. Chapter 1 and chapter 2 define the Cannabis Revolution and the expanding use of "drug" components of cannabis, together with an account of different modes of intake. These circumstances are dynamic, and what is stated today may be restated in different terms tomorrow, as a consequence of further research and discovery. Society is beginning to find its way with limited approval of cannabis for recreational use in four states (Colorado, Washington, Alaska, and Oregon) and Washington, DC and the presence of medical legalization in a couple dozen states (including those poised for medical cannabis legalization). The federal government continues to adopt a softening stance on what is now partial, national prohibition of cannabis use, if there is such a status of partial prohibition in what should be a true "United States." The federal government has handed off responsibilities to state governments. *Why would America run the risk of creating conflicting legalization between current state and federal laws?*

Moving through the book, chapters 3 and 4 start to introduce the medical application of cannabis, which is expanded upon in later chapters of the book. Chapter 5 provides some insight into the nutritional use of Cannabis sativa (and other species of cannabis), notably in the form of hemp (cannabis species, e.g., indica). Why the subject of nutrition is often skipped in "cannabis books" is unclear because there has been an increasing tendency to use raw cannabis or hemp in nutritional practice and dietary supplement formulations.

Chapter 6 is a key chapter that describes the operation of the endocannabinoid system and the effects of exogenously administered phytocannabinoids or cannabinoid analogues. This knowledge will be hard to accumulate by some readers, and this is a major reason why I have made the book somewhat repetitive, in order to help and reinforce learning about cannabis science. Chapters 7 through 17 focus on the potential medical use of cannabis and related compounds (extracts or cannabis analogues, used as drugs). There is a variable amount of evidence to support cannabis use in various diseases, and research is rapidly proceeding. Chapter 18 visits the problem of the hidden potaholic in society. This neologism is derived from the use of pot in a surreptitious manner by many young people. Chapter 19 ("The Future") involves a "crystal ball" that lacks complete clarity with attempts to predict the future of cannabis use.

This book echoes many studies on cannabis, and I have tried to avoid bias in reporting. In fact, I have been inclined on occasion to use verbatim statements of other authors to avoid distortion of facts. A characteristic of much marijuana literature is the presence of repeated verbatim statements because conclusions are sometimes equivocal and often not simple in outcome. This is one reason why many arguments prevail and scientists protest the sensationalism that sometimes affects news reporting about cannabis.

In this book, I have attempted to produce a reasonably comprehensive list of references by chapter to create a resource for further study and support for my conclusions. In addition, I have interspersed many references in the body of the writing, especially on subjects that refer to contemporary or key literature. Some of this referencing refers to the Internet. I apologize for any lack of reference to many works on cannabis, but space limitations have challenged my writing skills. The references supplied should allow interested consumers and cannabis health care givers to compare or check my opinions and apply their own interpretation of data, especially when the results of different studies are conflicting.

Individuals with serious diseases that carry a poor prognosis want to believe in the treatments that they are being offered or receiving. Cannabis is finding increasing applications in difficult-to-treat diseases. A strong desire for healing in many patients with recalcitrant disease opens the door to hucksters who want to peddle nostrums or capitalize on patients' fears and wants for disease cures. It is unfortunate that there are a number of promoters of the use of cannabis that exaggerate disease-treatment claims. In particular, cannabis is not a cancer cure, but it has valuable adjunctive cancer-treatment properties. The adjunctive role of cannabis in disease management is increasingly clear in several diseases, but few, if any, cannabis cures exist. Welcome to a significant amount of misinformation about cannabis, especially on the Internet. Cannabis is not an innocuous substance. This situation must precipitate concern, given the frequency of use of cannabis, especially by young people with formative minds. Youngsters have vulnerabilities to disabilities caused by cannabis in later life.

During the writing of this book, the Food and Drug Administration (US) announced that cannabidiol (CBD) is not a dietary supplement. Whether or not this results in a lack of availability of CBD for popular use remains to be seen. This major opinion from the FDA has the likelihood of causing a major change in the current general use of CBD by many people.

Stephen Holt, MD

Sorrento, Florida

Author's Comment

This book possesses certain disadvantages and limitations that are somewhat due to the extensive and sometimes contradictory information on many aspects of the increasing use of cannabis. I perceive my writing as a gateway to general knowledge about cannabis use. Many excellent books on marijuana have appeared over the past decade, with a spurt in publishing in recent times. Gallup polls ten years ago indicated that only one in four people favored medical cannabis legalization, but a subsequent Gallup poll in 2013 indicated that three in five people supported legalization. I have tried to help the reader by placing key information in boxes throughout the text.

Cannabis use and its legalization are emotive subjects as a consequence of some degree of injustice and even bigotry. For many years, the US government has supported a systematic undermining of the value of cannabis in society with some use of twisted logic and a degree of misleading propaganda. Sometimes opinions about cannabis are frank mistruths.

Rational and irrational arguments about cannabis use have led to unavoidable differences of opinion and divisiveness. It has been my ambition to produce a book that is up-to-date and spans a wide range of potential outcomes of the projected widespread use of cannabis in the United States. I think that it is important for authors to disclose their position on marijuana legalization because a lot of opinions expressed about cannabis appear to have been tainted by bias. Moreover, it is easy to reject or deny information that does not support preconceived notions.

Medical cannabis use could be perceived to be a form of alternative and complementary medicine. In a pivotal Special

Article, published in the *New England Journal of Medicine* (1993; 328:246–52), Eisenberg, DM et al. discussed the costs, prevalence, and patterns of use of unconventional medicine in the United States. Over the past twenty years, these aspects of unconventional medicine have expanded to a major degree, resulting in a surprisingly high prevalence of the practice of alternative and complementary medicine. This history is even more eye opening, given the extrapolation of Eisenberg et al. (ibid. 1993) that as long ago as 1990 Americans made an estimated 425 million visits to providers of unconventional therapy. This circumstance exceeded the number of visits to all US primary care physicians (388 million, at that time).

Tens of millions of individuals have used marijuana in recent times, and many of these people consider this agent to be a form of unconventional medical treatment. Despite this situation, knowledge about cannabis use and simply what can be expected from its use are quite deficient in the general population. Furthermore, health care professionals admit deficiencies in their own knowledge about cannabis, and recent studies show an apparent unwillingness to teach cannabis science to doctors or nurses in training.

While alcohol and tobacco use are often noted in a routine physical examination, details of cannabis use are ignored or not documented. Obviously, these circumstances require correction. We can now echo the comments of Eisenberg et al. (ibid. 1993). "The frequency of use of unconventional therapy in the United States is far higher than previously reported. Medical doctors should ask their patients' use of unconventional therapy whenever they obtain a medical history" (*N. Engl. J. Med*, 328 (1993): 246–52). Since marijuana is regarded as unconventional medicine, rocket science is not required to predict the avalanche that will occur with cannabis legalization, in what constitutes part of the Cannabis Revolution.

For supporters of cannabis legalization, such as the author of this book, to produce an account of many of the adverse outcomes of marijuana legalization may seem strange to cannabis protagonists. That said, it has been estimated that prior to five years ago, only one in nine studies were designed to show the benefits of cannabis, but this trend is changing, with more reported positive outcomes of cannabis use. While I support cannabis legalization, there must be vigilance about the ramifications of these evolving circumstances. Note: This book relies heavily on the work of many scientists who are acknowledged in the reference section. References interspersed in the writings are kept to a minimum to avoid a lack of literary flow.

Disclaimer

The author is not recommending cannabis (marijuana) use, and he is not attempting to react against its use. The author presents the facts and his interpretations of cannabis use and science. This book is an attempt to present information on arguments that have been proposed to both support and prevent marijuana use. The author attempts to disclose circumstances where he injects his own opinions. A number of books have provided excellent information on specific aspects of cannabis science, but this book collates information from medical, political, and business sources with a unique mix of knowledge. This knowledge is linked together in a manner that can be understood to a significant degree by the layperson, without boring the medical or scientific reader. The author accepts no responsibility for advice, implied or otherwise, that may be gleaned from this book. The writer discloses his position on his support for the well-planned legalization of marijuana use.

Stephen Holt, MD

Sorrento, Florida

What Is This Book?

A CERTIFICATION PROGRAM

This book is part of a certification program for individuals who wish to counsel on the use of dietary supplements (nutraceuticals) or cannabis related products. This book was written primarily for health enthusiasts, retail store staff, and office staff to improve their knowledge and skills in counseling on the use of cannabis (marijuana). Clinicians seeking basic knowledge on cannabis may benefit from this introductory course. Please note that federal law limits the use of over-the-counter cannabis products to the states of Colorado, Washington, Alaska, and Oregon, as well as Washington, DC, at the time of writing. Recently (2015), the Food and Drug Administration have made it clear that cannabidiol (CBD) cannot be used as a dietary supplement.

This program is complemented by on-site educational resources at specific medical meetings and at the Holt Institute of Medicine (NJ, USA), where training sessions can be scheduled for group learning.

At the end of the book is a certification examination (quiz) that can be detached and mailed to "Quiz," Holt Institute of Medicine, 25 Amity Street, Second Floor, Little Falls, NJ 07424 (Tel: 973-256-4660).

After the answer pages for the examination are completed, detached, and mailed to the above address, an oral examination will be held by telephone or in person with Stephen Holt, MD, or a member of his personal staff. The oral exam will test general knowledge on cannabis.

Upon completion of these requirements, a certificate for a certified cannabis counselor will be issued by the Holt Institute of Medicine. A payment of US $50.00 is required for issuance of a certificate of completion.

Foreword I

CLIFFORD B. CARROLL

The cannabis industry is emerging with rapidity and increasing sophistication. This is happening in many locations, most notably Colorado, Washington state, Oregon, Alaska, and Washington, DC, in the United States, and Uruguay. Small cannabis companies have grown recently into vertically integrated organizations that are often composed of several affiliates. These organizations are conglomerations of cannabis-growing ventures, modern extraction facilities, expert packaging and distribution organizations that specialize in supplying approved dispensaries. These organizations compete with large organizations that sell illicit cannabis of questionable composition and purity. Dr. Holt reminds us of the danger of "fake" or synthetic pot.

Stephen Holt, MD, has been described as a visionary and world leader in natural health care, and he is highly regarded as one of the key innovators in the dietary supplement and functional-food industry. In addition, he is a distinguished clinical pharmacologist. In this book, he uses his vast experience to pave the way for the use of cannabis as both a medicinal agent and recreational drug concoction. While some aspects of this book are conservative, Dr. Holt points to the high value of cannabis use in many social and health applications. This book is unique and different in its approach to the education of health care professionals and the layperson on cannabis science and related issues. It is a must read for millions of people who will use cannabis in the future, as legalization marches forward in the United States.

As a strong supporter of cannabis legalization, I am impressed by Dr. Holt's impartiality in the manner in which he discusses cannabis use in many contexts in the United States. In addition, he touches on certain global implications of cannabis use. Dr. Holt does not proselytize in this book, and he describes the medical, economic, political, and societal aspects of marijuana legalization and its potential widespread use.

Stephen Holt, MD, starts from a position that cannabis legalization is inevitable in the United States. He emphasizes that we should be knowledgeable about its potential outcome on society in general. This book is obviously a must read given the lack of information about cannabis that is obvious in many textbooks of herbal science or medicine.

I applaud this work, which will be seen as a very important contribution to medical and social science.

Clifford B. Carroll

Denver, Colorado

Foreword II

JOHN SALERNO, DO

In the face of current federal prohibition of cannabis, a significant proportion of the US population has postured toward its legalization in a revolutionary manner. Dr. Holt reminds us that revolutions often come with uncertain consequences, but he tells us what we should expect from increasing cannabis use in the present or future. With four states of the Union (at the time of writing) allowing the recreational use of cannabis and a couple of dozen states with legislation to approve its use for medical purposes, there are fundamental changes in the public perception of the safety and potential value of cannabis in modern society. Strong differences of opinion underlie strategies to legalize cannabis, and Dr. Holt faces these issues head-on in a thoughtful and objective manner. After many years of prohibition, cannabis emerges with perceived value and promise for the medical treatment of many diseases. That said, much of the drive for cannabis legalization has resulted from its psychoactive effects, which are used for recreational purposes.

After more than a decade of debates about the decriminalization or legalization of marijuana, society is entering several domains of uncertainty. These domains include the medical, economic, social, and continuing political outcomes surrounding cannabis use. The electorate has not shown landslide support for cannabis legalization, and some residual anxiety exists about the potential negative results of legalization in the short and long term. The presence of cold feet after some degree of legalization is apparent in some states of the Union, but it is difficult to measure. The number-one issue on the minds of many people who contemplate legalization is what to expect? This book tells us about many aspects of what we should expect with cannabis legalization. While scientists, politicians, practicing physicians, and others exhibit varying degrees of ignorance about cannabis use, a pernicious problem exists. How can the average man or woman use cannabis in a responsible manner that will result in safe and efficacious outcomes?

With eloquence and care, Stephen Holt, MD, explores the current and future outcome of the increasing use of cannabis. Dr. Holt is a self-admitted protagonist of cannabis legalization with a wealth of experience and distinction in both alternative and conventional medicine. This book does not hesitate to present issues in a direct manner and incorporate thoughtful opinions that may precipitate debate. That said, the book is logical in the way it reviews scientific, political, and sociobehavioral issues that result from the expanding use of cannabis. While Dr. Holt supports cannabis legalization and decriminalization, he is not afraid to sound bold warnings about the irresponsible use of cannabis, especially by youngsters.

Dr. Holt resists getting too caught up in the never-ending arguments for and against cannabis legalization. In fact, he sees the widespread use of cannabis as inevitable and calls for a proactive approach, with education for everyone about the medical and social consequences of cannabis use. Dr. Holt characterizes the position of cannabis in society using an analogy of Pandora's box where hope remains, but he warns people to be prepared in the circumstance of "the cat being out of the bag."

Cannabis use is a divisive issue in modern society where arguments continue to prevail concerning the potential outcome of its legalization. This book does not ignore this modern contention, but it is written to provide a general knowledge about cannabis science that is portable and understandable by cannabis users and others. When information on cannabis is lumped together, a confusing picture emerges. These writings abolish some of the confusions, but Dr. Holt is not afraid to be frank in his opinions. In this book, Dr. Holt addresses the social, economic, medical, and political outcomes of the expanding use of cannabis, while legislation for the legal use of cannabis (recreational or medical) proceeds with substantial support in many states in the United States.

People have become tired of being told that cannabis use is dangerous and perhaps even evil. In modern times, opinions started to change or at least soften in their criticisms and concerns about cannabis. The modern consumer has learned to view cannabis use as safe, and this has resulted in a coincidental increase (or perhaps causal link) with the greater use of cannabis, especially among young adults. The use of cannabis by children appears to be quite destructive in medical and social outcomes. Unfortunately, it is young people that seem to be particularly vulnerable to several of the documented adverse effects of cannabis, which may persist into adulthood. Some of these effects present uncertain risks of long-term disability. Clearly, time and experience of the increased use of cannabis will reveal the costs and benefits of cannabis legalization in what Dr. Holt calls the "Cannabis Revolution."

John Salerno, DO

Salerno Center, NY, NY

Chapter I

THE CANNABIS REVOLUTION

The Evolving Use of Cannabis

The increasing availability and support for the use of cannabis present important issues of medical, economic, social, legal, and political significance. These challenging events form the basis of the Cannabis Revolution, which has accelerated in its progression in recent times. As cannabis creeps toward the status of national legalization in the United States, many people are attracted by its recreational use and medical treatment applications. As a consequence, a burgeoning cannabis industry is taking shape, but this industry is not always operating like the ethical pharmaceutical or nutraceutical industries. Many people argue that the corporate culture of the cannabis industry will have to change, and consolidation appears to be inevitable. Decisions to legalize or prohibit cannabis (marijuana) use in the United States have triggered endless debates. These arguments are becoming somewhat futile as the United States further evolves with the inevitable legalization and decriminalization of marijuana use. At the time of writing, there has been legalization of cannabis for recreational use in the states of Colorado, Arizona, Oregon, and Washington, as well as Washington, DC. This expanded use of marijuana has emerged with an increasing recognition of the

I

medical benefits of cannabis. These benefits are hard to dismiss and impossible to deny.

Current federal laws regulating cannabis use amount to a circumstance of prohibition. These federal regulations are increasingly perceived as behind the times due to their incorrect definition of cannabis as a drug without medical benefits. President Barack Obama has indicated that legislation and regulation of cannabis use should occur at the state level of government. Accusations have been made that these circumstances are a copout by the federal government. At the time of writing, there are a couple dozen states that have passed legislation for the use of medical marijuana. This circumstance is creating some degree of confusion as each state legalizes cannabis with some differences in legislation and certain parochial restrictions. The absence of consensus opinions on precise indications for the medical applications of cannabis may lead to different future legislation and regulations in some states. At present, there is room for the potential clash of state legislation and federal government policy. Regulatory agencies run by the federal government have found themselves between a rock and a hard place. However, signs are developing that the federal government is backing off or acting like a crocodile with no teeth. A solution to these pending problems would be widespread acceptance of revised federal legislation that could be defined for cannabis legalization. However, this potential approach has been the subject of much disagreement, and it is unlikely to occur.

The former widespread prohibition of cannabis (marijuana) use as a result of the 1937 Marijuana Tax Act has led to an unfortunate lack of scientific studies on the biological actions of the many components of the cannabis plant and their effects on health and well-being. Up until about a decade ago, 90 percent of all cannabis research focused on the negative outcome of cannabis use. Furthermore, a significant number of people have accused regulatory officials of standing in the way of cannabis research, even in recent times. There are some anticipated needs for change in the ever-evolving regulations concerning marijuana use. Political and legal systems will be challenged by some of these changes. Arguably, politicians should not be making unaided medical decisions about indications for cannabis use. That said, widespread concerns exist about the current lack of knowledge about cannabis science among the health care professionals. This situation is compounded by shameful inertia in the planning of medical education on this subject.

The emerging landscape of the use of cannabis presents information overload for many people, including medical professionals. Rapid political reforms have created some degrees of misunderstanding and confusion among the general public. Such misunderstandings could impact the responsible use of herbal cannabis and related products. Therefore, urgent and widespread education is required on how society should apply the psychoactive and medicinal effects of marijuana. This education is necessary to ensure cannabis use in a safe and responsible manner. It is clear that the Internet is playing a role in shaping the use of cannabis, but a significant portion of online information about marijuana is inaccurate, biased, and sometimes incorrect. This situation hampers the broadcast of valid information to help guide the public on the use of cannabis. Moreover, illegal cannabis-like products (synthetic pot) with major toxicity concerns are available for sale on the Internet.

The Cannabis Revolution has mounting support among the general public. For example, the Pew Research Center undertook a survey (March 2013) of the public support for medical cannabis legalization. This survey indicated that 52 percent of the public favored cannabis legalization versus 45 percent against legalization. It is apparent that there have been significant increases in the number of Americans who support marijuana legalization over the past few years, and current estimates are that 58 percent of the population of the United States may favor medical cannabis legalization. While widespread support for medical cannabis use is growing fast, significant reluctance persists not to support the legalization of cannabis for recreational purposes.

Pandora's Box Has Opened

When it comes to the recreational and medical use of cannabis (marijuana), Pandora's box has opened, or is opening, in many locations in the United States. All that remains in the box is hope. Hoping for positive consequences of these circumstances, many people seem to be satisfied with current legislative changes, but some have shown disinterest, and several groups have formed to protest and stop further approvals of its availability. With cannabis legalization, there are changes in the frequency of cannabis use and its selected composition, with preferred types of cannabis that favor the use of high-potency cannabis (rich in THC, tetrahydrcannabinol). One need not be blessed with the talent of a visionary to appreciate that greater strides in legalization and decriminalization of marijuana are around the corner. A principal feature of the hope that remains in Pandora's box is an overriding desire to create circumstances that satisfy the dictum of Hippocrates: "Above all, do no harm." Harmful consequences of cannabis use do exist, even though many people have considered these risks to be low. That said, most young people think that cannabis is quite safe. Moreover, cannabis can contribute in specific circumstances to harm reduction or harm production.

The Revolution

The title of this book describes the global advances of fundamental changes in the acceptance of marijuana use over the past decade and rather precipitous legislation in some places in the United States to accept legalization of its use. Once subject to general prohibition, cannabis consumption has blossomed into circumstances of increasing acceptance and widespread consumption with a dual status (legal or illicit). Depending on where people live in the United States, cannabis is still viewed in a confusing manner as a legal or illicit drug.

Cannabis use is accompanied by a fundamental change in how many people think about this complex natural drug concoction (produced by the plant Cannabis sativa). I reiterate that major factors in its increasing popularity are the perceptions that marijuana is safe or even innocuous. Safety issues remain the basis of occasional ferocious debates among some politicians and scientists, but general opinions of safety have emerged. Perhaps it is more relevant to think about degrees of safety of use that are context specific. Furthermore, the emotional index on cannabis use by consumers is often high, especially for compassionate use in palliative care and for children with severe epilepsy. This book attempts to describe the consequences of the rapidly emerging challenges that are posed by cannabis legalization. Like it or not, the electorate has tilted toward support for "smoking dope."

The DEA's Position on Cannabis

The Drug Enforcement Agency of the United States (DEA) makes it clear that it does not recognize marijuana smoke as a medicine. Their negative opinions focus on smoking cannabis, which they describe as unsafe, and it "has not withstood the rigors of science." The agency has stated that they "will vigorously enforce the CSA (Controlled Substances Act) against individuals and organizations that possess, manufacture or distribute marijuana for recreational use, even if such activities are permitted under state law.".

In the booklet entitled *The DEA Position on Marijuana* (2013), the DEA stresses the lack of a consensus on smoking marijuana as an effective and safe intervention for any disease. While espousing support for ongoing research into the components of marijuana, the DEA take a strong stand against the lobby for legalization of smoked marijuana. The DEA states, "The proposition that smoked marijuana is medicine is, in sum, false-trickery used by those promoting wholesale legalization." These words are provocative and questionable.

There are some signs that the DEA is holding back somewhat in its pursuit or prosecution of what could be considered minor infractions of federal law. Clearly, the DEA is not producing balanced material for the general public on cannabis use in its position manual on marijuana (DEA, ibid. 2013). The position manual of the DEA is written in a staccato format and fails to mention the benefits of cannabis use delivered by methods other than smoking. As one might anticipate, the DEA's position is driven by current draconian federal laws that require revision.

Defensive Positions on Cannabis

The DEA has experienced a great deal of criticism of its actions from supporters of cannabis for both recreational and medical use. There are strong arguments against the DEA's position, which are published in the booklet entitled *The DEA, Four Decades of Impending and Rejecting Science*. This booklet was prepared by the Drug Policy Alliance (www.drugpolicy.org) and MAPS (www. maps.org).

It is clear that political conflicts exist between people with supportive or opposing viewpoints on cannabis legalization. One feature of the antagonist positions adopted by the DEA and the opinions of support from the Drug Policy Alliance is the lack of any balanced dialogue that might be constructive.

The Department of Justice Speaks (Verbatim Quotes)

The US Department of Justice, Office of the Deputy Attorney General, Washington, DC, 20530, June 29, 2011, memorandum For United States Attorneys from James M. Cole, Deputy Attorney General is very relevant to assessing the federal government's present position.

Guidance Regarding the Ogden Memo in Jurisdictions Seeking to Authorize Marijuana for Medical Use (Verbatim)

Over the last several months some of you have requested the Department's assistance in responding to inquiries from State and local governments seeking guidance about the Department's position on enforcement of the Controlled Substances Act (CSA) in jurisdictions that have under consideration, or have implemented, legislation that would sanction and regulate the commercial cultivation and distribution of marijuana purportedly for medical use. Some of these jurisdictions have considered approving the cultivation of large quantities of marijuana, or broadening the regulation and taxation of the substance. You may have seen letters responding to these inquiries by several United States Attorneys. Those letters are entirely consistent with the October 2009 memorandum issued by Deputy Attorney General David Ogden to federal prosecutors in States that have enacted laws authorizing the medical use of marijuana (the "Ogden Memo").

The Department of Justice is committed to the enforcement of the Controlled Substances Act in all States. Congress has determined that marijuana is a dangerous drug and that the illegal distribution and sale of marijuana is a serious crime that provides a significant source of revenue to large scale criminal enterprises, gangs, and cartels. The Ogden memorandum provides guidance to you in deploying your resources to enforce the CSA as part of the exercise of the broad discretion you are given to address federal criminal matters within your districts.

A number of states have enacted some form of legislation relating to the medical use of marijuana. Accordingly, the Ogden Memo reiterated to you that prosecution of significant traffickers of illegal drugs, including marijuana, remains a core priority, but advised that it is likely not an efficient use of federal resources to focus enforcement efforts on individuals with cancer or other serious illnesses who use marijuana as part of a recommended treatment regimen consistent with applicable state law, or their caregivers. The term "caregiver" as used in the memorandum meant just that: individuals providing care to individuals with cancer or other serious illnesses, not commercial operations cultivating, selling or distributing marijuana.

The Department view of the efficient use of limited federal resources as articulated in the Ogden Memorandum has not changed. There has, however, been an increase in the scope of commercial cultivation, sale, distribution and use of marijuana for purported medical purposes. For example, within the past twelve months, several jurisdictions have considered or enacted legislation to authorize multiple large-scale, privately operated industrial marijuana cultivation centers. Some of these planned facilities have revenue projections of millions of dollars based on the planned cultivation of tens of thousands of cannabis plants.

The Ogden Memorandum was never intended to shield such activities from federal enforcement action and prosecution, even where those activities purport to comply with state law. Persons who are in the business of cultivating, selling or distributing marijuana, and those who knowingly facilitate such activities, are in violation of the Controlled Substances Act, regardless of state law. Consistent with resource constraints and the discretion you may exercise in your district, such persons are subject to federal enforcement action, including potential prosecution. State laws or local ordinances are not a defense to civil or criminal enforcement of federal law with respect to such conduct, including enforcement of the CSA. Those who engage in transactions involving the proceeds of such activity may also be in violation of federal money laundering statutes and other federal financial laws.

The Department of Justice is tasked with enforcing existing federal criminal laws in all states, and enforcement of the CSA has long been and remains a core priority.

The above dialogue is taken verbatim from the US Department of Justice, Office of the Deputy Attorney General, August 29, 2013,

Memorandum For All United States Attorneys, from James M. Cole, Deputy Attorney General.

Guidance Regarding Marijuana Enforcement: The Ogden Memorandum (Verbatim)

In October 2009 and June 2011, the Department issued guidance to federal prosecutors concerning marijuana enforcement under the Controlled Substance Act (CSA). This memorandum updates that guidance in light of state ballot initiatives that legalize under state law the possession of small amounts of marijuana and provide for the regulation of marijuana production, processing, and sale. The guidance set forth herein applies to all federal enforcement activity, including civil enforcement and criminal investigations and prosecutions, concerning marijuana in all states.

As the Department noted in its previous guidance, Congress has determined that marijuana is a dangerous drug and that the illegal distribution and sale of marijuana is a serious crime that provides a significant source of revenue to large-scale criminal enterprises, gangs, and cartels. The Department of Justice is committed to enforcement of the CSA consistent with those determinations. The Department is also committed to suing its limited investigative and prosecutorial resources to address the most significant threats in the most effective, consistent, and rational way. In furtherance of those objectives, as several states enacted laws relating to the use of marijuana for medical purposes, the Department in recent years has focused its efforts on certain enforcement priorities that are particularly important to the federal government:

- Preventing the distribution of marijuana to minors;
- Preventing revenue from the sale of marijuana from going to criminal enterprises, gangs, and cartels;

- Preventing the diversion of marijuana from states where it is legal under state law in some form to other states;
- Preventing state-authorized marijuana activity from being used as a cover or pretext for the trafficking of other illegal drugs or other illegal activity;
- Preventing violence and the use of firearms in the cultivation and distribution of marijuana;
- Preventing drugged driving and the exacerbation of other adverse public health consequences associated with marijuana use;
- Preventing the growing of marijuana on public lands and the attendant public safety and environmental dangers posed by marijuana production on public lands; and
- preventing marijuana possession or use on federal property.

These priorities will continue to guide the Department's enforcement of the CSA against marijuana-related conduct. Thus, this memorandum serves as guidance to Department attorneys and law enforcement to focus their enforcement resources and efforts, including prosecution, on persons or organizations whose conduct interferes with any one or more of these priorities, regardless of state law.

Outside of these enforcement priorities, the federal government has traditionally relied on states and local law enforcement agencies to address marijuana activity through enforcement of their own narcotics laws. For example, the Department of justice has not historically devoted resources to prosecuting individuals whose conduct is limited to possession of small amounts of marijuana for personal use on private property. Instead, the Department has left such lower-level or localized activity to state and local authorities and has stepped in to enforce the CSA only when the use, possession, cultivation, or distribution of marijuana has threatened to cause one of the harms identified above.

The enactment of state laws that endeavor to authorize marijuana production, distribution, and possession by establishing a regulatory scheme for these purposes affects this traditional joint federal-state approach to narcotics enforcement. The Department's guidance in this memorandum rests on its expectation that states and local governments that have enacted laws authorizing marijuana-related conduct will implement strong and effective regulatory and enforcement systems that will address the threat those state laws could pose to public safety, public health, and other law enforcement interests. A system adequate to that task must not only contain robust controls and procedures on paper, it must also be effective in practice. Jurisdictions that have implemented systems that provide for regulation of marijuana activity must provide the necessary resources and demonstrate the willingness to enforce their laws and regulations in a manner that ensures they do not undermine federal enforcement priorities.

These enforcement priorities are listed in general terms; each encompasses a variety of conduct that may merit civil or criminal enforcement of the CSA. By way of example only, the Department's interest in preventing the distribution of marijuana to minors would call for enforcement not just when an individual or entity sells or transfers marijuana to a minor, but also when marijuana trafficking takes place near an area associated with minors, when marijuana or marijuana-infused products are marketed in a manner to appeal to minors; or when marijuana is being diverted, directly or indirectly, and purposefully or otherwise to minors must provide the necessary resources and demonstrate the willingness to enforce their laws and regulations in a manner that ensures they do not undermine federal enforcement priorities.

In jurisdictions that have enacted laws legalizing

marijuana in some form and that have also implemented strong and effective regulatory and enforcement systems to control the cultivation, distribution, sale, and possession of marijuana, conduct in compliance with those laws and regulations is less likely to threaten the federal priorities set forth above. Indeed, a robust system may affirmatively address those priorities by, for example, implementing effective measures to prevent diversion of marijuana outside of the regulated system and to other states, prohibiting access to marijuana by minors, and replacing an illicit marijuana trade that funds criminal enterprises with a tightly regulated market in which revenues are tracked and accounted for. In those circumstances, consistent with the traditional allocation of federal-state efforts in this area, enforcement of state law by state and local law enforcement and regulatory bodies should remain the primary means of addressing marijuana-related activity. If state enforcement efforts are not sufficiently robust to protect against the harms set forth above, the federal government may seek to challenge the regulatory structure itself in addition to continuing to bring individual enforcement actions, including criminal prosecutions, focused on those harms.

The Department's previous memoranda specifically addressed the exercise of prosecutorial discretion in states with laws authorizing marijuana cultivation and distribution for medical use. In those contexts, the Department advised that it likely was not an efficient use of federal resources to focus enforcement efforts on seriously ill individuals, or on their individual caregivers. In doing so, the previous guidance drew a distinction between the seriously ill and their caregivers, on the one hand, and large-scale, for-profit commercial enterprises on the other, and advised that the latter continued to be appropriate targets for federal enforcement and prosecution. In drawing this distinction, the Department relied on the common-sense judgment that the size of a marijuana operation was a reasonable proxy for assessing whether marijuana trafficking implicates the federal enforcement priorities set forth above.

As explained above, however, both the existence of a strong and effective state regulatory system, and an operation's compliance with such a system, may allay the threat that an operation's size poses to federal enforcement interests. Accordingly, in exercising prosecutorial discretion, prosecutors should not consider the size or commercial nature of a marijuana operation alone as a proxy for assessing whether marijuana trafficking implicates the Department's enforcement priorities listed above. Rather, prosecutors should continue to review marijuana cases on a case-by-case basis and weigh all available information and evidence including, but not limited to, whether the operation is demonstrably in compliance with a strong and effective state regulatory system. A marijuana operation's large scale or for-profit nature may be a relevant consideration for assessing the extent to which it undermines a particular federal enforcement priority. The primary question in all cases—and in all jurisdiction—should be whether the conduct at issue implicates one or more of the enforcement priorities listed above.

Is the Federal Government in a Legal Bind?

On the one hand, some federal government institutions report promising or putative benefits of cannabis on health, but on the other hand the federal government sits on legislation that seems to deny such benefits. Furthermore, the federal government sits on a key patent that espouses important health benefits of cannabis. This patent relates to cannabis-induced neuroprotection, neurogenesis, and antioxidant effects, which was filed as a result of research performed by the National Institutes of Health. Moreover, the National Cancer Institute (a division of the federal government's National Institutes of Health) has announced that cannabis may have benefits in the treatment of certain cancers. This opinion has been echoed by the Institute of Medicine.

Other federal agencies have had to admit certain benefits of cannabis treatment in the treatment of other diseases. Some legal experts claim that this position of the federal government on cannabis legislation is both hypocritical and indefensible. To view medical cannabis as an outlawed issue or to fail to have legislation in place to legalize medical cannabis use has been described often as quite irresponsible behavior on the part of governments, both state and federal. The federal government should perhaps remove itself from a necessity to speak with a forked tongue on cannabis use. On these issues there is a clear need to poop rather than just sit on the potty.

Cannabis Use

The National Survey on Drug Use and Health (NSDUH) of 2009 indicated that 104 million Americans age twelve years and older reported the use of marijuana on one or more occasions. In this survey, 42 percent of all individuals reported a prior use of cannabis. It is useful to ponder the reasons why people use cannabis. Some of the principal reasons for cannabis use are summarized in table 1.

Table 1. Common reasons for cannabis use:

- for recreational purposes to achieve a "high"
- self-medication of pain, insomnia, and stress with cannabis
- psychological relief and distraction from disease symptoms (e.g., improved tolerability of pain)
- a popular modern recommendation for alternate medical treatments, reinforced by a growing perception of cannabis safety Episodic escape from unpleasant experiences associated with the presence of disease or stressful life events
- medical indications for use

Many studies or observations of the use of marijuana on a

parochial or national level have been performed. Of course, the impact of widespread cannabis use on society is yet to be realized in many locations in the United States. The National Survey on Drug Abuse and Health (NSDAH) of 2010 estimated the annual use of illicit cannabis accounted for about 76.8 percent of all illicit drug use. In this and other epidemiological studies, cannabis consumption was most prevalent in teenagers and young adults (age range, eighteen to twenty-five years).

The Monitoring of the Future Survey found that in 2011 there was common use of cannabis, especially in older teenagers (twelfth graders). Table 2 shows the 2011 data on use in school children.

Table 2. Percentage current and past year use of cannabis by schoolchildren in 2011 (Monitoring the Future Survey 2011)

School Grade	Past Year Use	Current Use (2011)
8th	12.5 percent	7.2 percent
10th	28.8 percent	17.6 percent
12th	32.8 percent	20.6 percent

To place a simple interpretation on the above data indicates that one in three to five twelfth graders had used marijuana in the past year (table 2, data reported in 2011). The high prevalence of marijuana use in young people is a worrisome circumstance, and this burden is likely to increase with further legalization of cannabis for recreational use and perhaps medical use. Recent studies imply that medical cannabis diverted from adult use is a common source for young users. The prevention of cannabis use in underage individuals (younger than eighteen or twenty-one years) has been woefully inadequate. Moreover, considerable concern exists about the potential for the escalating use of synthetic cannabis (cannabis mimics), especially by young people. Synthetic pot has high toxicity and increasing use as an illicit drug.

Marijuana use seems to be increasing attendances at hospital emergency departments. For example in 2012, cannabis use was a factor in 376,000 emergency department visits in the United States. In addition, there is need to recognize that increasing use of synthetic cannabis mimics is more likely than regular herbal cannabis to precipitate a hospital attendance for overdosing or toxicity.

Toward the Responsible Use of Cannabis

Along with a mounting self-reliance to use marijuana comes some degree of vague interpretations of poorly defined guidelines adopted by the general public for its use. Arguably, many physicians use vague cannabis-monitoring guidelines or even fail to monitor its use. For example, there is limited agreement on dosage requirements for the creation of a high or even for the management of certain diseases. This circumstance is due to unpredictable dose-response relationships and other factors. Cannabis dosing by smoking is a moving target, as tolerance to its use develops often quite rapidly (a couple of weeks). Components of cannabis (the exocannabinoids: phytocannabinoids or cannabis-derived drugs or mimics) appear to have activity at wide ranges of dosage administration, and they sometimes produce paradoxical effects. These paradoxical effects are characterized by opposite effects on body function at different dosages.

Knowledge about safe and effective dosing of cannabis is improving slowly as experience of its use increases and the effects of specific components of cannabis are clarified. In other words, the optimum dosages of cannabis required for desired medical benefits are still often unclear, even when using preparations that have been standardized for their cannabinoid content. Reasonably careful use of auto-titration methods of dosage assessment is often quite valuable. In this situation, cannabis is used with increasing dosage to gain an effect. While this works well with smoking cannabis, it has problems in gauging doses from cannabis edibles because of slow and unpredictable absorption. Dosage requirements of cannabis or its components seem to differ significantly in the potential therapy of various diseases. There is a need for public education to reach a level where ideally most people can enjoy the safe use of marijuana, with a realistic recognition of its disadvantages and limitations. This is one of the main reasons why I wrote this book!

Cannabis Receptors

In brief, cannabis interacts with a well-organized system of fascinating body receptors that respond with a complex array of biological responses. These receptors constitute a major feature of the endocannabinoid system of the body. This endocannabinoid system also includes synthesizing and degrading mechanisms of endocannabinoids. These mechanisms play a role in the duration and quality of effects of endocannabinoids on cannabinoid receptors. The cannabinoid receptors are referred to as CB-1 and CB-2 receptors (and perhaps other receptors—e.g., CB-3 receptors). The active biological components of cannabis include cannabinoids and other compounds (e.g., terpenoids found in essential oils). Terpenoids can trigger or modulate the functions of endocannabinoid system by receptor interactions (direct or indirect).

This system of cannabinoid receptors is ubiquitous in the brain and body of humans. In brief, the CB-1 receptors are most common in the central nervous system CNS, and CB-2 receptors are ubiquitous in the immune system of the body. These matters are addressed in more detail later in this book. Ubiquity of cannabis receptors breeds many different effects of cannabinoids on body function and structure. While there is a call for public education on cannabis, many physicians and health care givers admit a lack of knowledge about the outcomes of cannabis use, and few have direct clinical experience with cannabis use.

Despite the widespread use of cannabis, few medical schools teach about the use of this drug, but this situation may be changing. Evidence exists in academic research studies that individuals responsible for educational planning in medical schools have often grossly neglected teaching about cannabis science and use. Moreover, some of these individuals have made biased and archaic statements about the lack of need and value of education about cannabis.

Education about Cannabis: A Key Initiative

To encourage safe and effective use of cannabis, there is a need to make the public aware of the many physical, psychological, medical, and social consequences of marijuana use. This book is an attempt to bridge the gap in general knowledge about cannabis (marijuana and hemp) and its derivatives. While the book does not claim to contain unique messages about cannabis, it is a contemporary attempt to provide balanced opinion and information concerning the public health implications of the consumption of this plant that has complex effects on humankind.

Clearly, it is now more important to educate about cannabis use than continue the debates concerning its legalization in an endless manner. Some politicians have turned a deaf ear to the need for public education on cannabis while they continue to wallow in their ignorance. Education about the consequences of cannabis use is particularly important for our younger generations who appear increasingly attracted and vulnerable to its use. Early onset of cannabis use in adolescents is a predictor of several problems in later life, and it tends to carry a poor prognosis for future health. Moreover, I have emphasized that education on the subject of substance abuse and drug dependence is noticeably inadequate in instructional programs at all levels of education.

Continuing Vigilance for Safety

While I am a protagonist of the legalization of marijuana, I emphasize that the last thing that modern society in the United States needs is cannabis availability without appropriate degrees of follow-up observations or reasonable vigilance of its use, especially in teenagers. This vigilance should be aimed at protecting public safety. It is reassuring that state governments in Colorado and Washington have set up panels of medical experts to monitor many key outcomes of cannabis legalization for recreational use. The future of the expansion of cannabis use means that we should try to prepare society for both negative and positive events or outcomes that could result from cannabis legalization. This book describes some of the known disadvantages and limitations of cannabis use. To hold these opinions is to risk much criticism from some cannabis activists or supporters, but it is important for individuals to understand the outcomes of cannabis use, using their own powers of objectivity.

There is a dearth of definitive data on cannabis use. For every report of a negative event related to marijuana is a report denying an association. Refuting claims of adverse events due to cannabis are particularly important to support general safety claims that are used to support cannabis legalization. For example, a reasonable national consensus exists that cannabis use makes significant contributions to motor vehicle accidents. That said, a recent federal government report posted on February 9, 2015, by the National Traffic Safety Administration, indicated that car accidents in Virginia Beach, Virginia (during a twenty-month period ending in 2012) showed that in a random sample of three thousand accident-involved drivers, there was no evidence that marijuana presence in the body made an individual more prone to accidents.

Addressing Risks

A tendency has arisen to keep pushing statements about the universal safety and innocuous nature of cannabis, but this situation is counterproductive when it comes to the safe use of this plant. There is a common perception that cannabis is a low-risk substance, but universal safety is not present with any drug use (vide infra). In recent times increasing perceptions of cannabis safety have driven its increasing use, especially among young people. When it comes to cannabis consumption, degrees of criminality are a major function of state laws in specific geographic locations or the initiatives of law enforcement to support federal or state laws. It seems that the amount of cannabis possessed by an individual is often assumed to be a measure of the likelihood of the individual to deal the plant.

Cannabis products should not contain harmful ingredients that have been added (e.g., adulterants such as synthetic cannabinoids) or contaminants (e.g., microbial toxins or organisms). Spraying miscellaneous, nonspecific plant material with chemicals that mimic the effects of cannabis (synthetic pot) for use in smoking is a growing public health problem. Cannabis needs to be prepared for consumption with good cultivation and quality-control standards. It should be labeled appropriately, and this practice has been shown to reduce accidental exposure of children to cannabis use. These circumstances are only possible if legal and approved forms of cannabis are used by the general public or if dispensaries focus on the sale of quality products that are labeled in a responsible manner.

The need to have quality control of cannabis products disqualifies the use of much illicit or illegal material, where these guidelines for safe use are most often ignored. It may also question the home cultivation of cannabis when good growing practices are not applied. That said, there is no real consensus on "good growing practices for the home," especially among the average consumer who may wish to grow his or her own plants. The role of safe fertilizers or other chemical growing aids is underexplored and relatively unregulated. Guidance on growing cannabis that is published on the Internet can be quite confusing and sometimes misleading.

A Note on Taxation and Cannabis Use

Taxation of cannabis has major implications for its general use. Some studies in Holland (Europe), where use of cannabis has gained national acceptance, show a consumer preference for whole herbal cannabis rather than officially approved types of cannabis or cannabis analogues (pharmaceuticals) or extracts. Economics seem to play a role in shaping these consumer opinions, decisions, and activities. There is an increasing trend for street cannabis to be cheaper than approved medical cannabis, largely due to taxation of the latter.

One factor working against the selection of legal cannabis preparations is the fact that there is sometimes greater effect of the psychoactive properties of marijuana from illicit sources, as a consequence of selective growing or hybridization of high THC-containing (delta-9-tetrahydrocannabinol) strains of cannabis (skunk-like strains). I believe that the taxation levied on approved cannabis use will continue to shape sales channels of supply or distribution in the future. The markup of cannabis materials or analogues by the dietary supplement, "cannabis," and pharmaceutical industries has led to product sales that are often beyond the financial reach of many people. The cost of legalized cannabis is out of control in the United States, just like the cost of many pharmaceuticals.

Cannabis and Coevolution

Perhaps one of the most puzzling features of cannabis is to explain why vertebrate animals, including humankind, have a complex system of controls that are influenced profoundly by collection of natural drugs found in a plant. While evolutionary theories (co-evolution of man and cannabis) are conjured up to explain the controlling actions of cannabis on body functions, the reasons for the existence of such elaborate endocannabinoid controls of the body remain an unsolved mystery.

Other plants can exhibit intimate controls on body functions but not to the degree and complexity of cannabis. Examples include poppies (opium) and peppers (capsicum). In the late Victorian era, cannabis was compounded often with plant extracts of opium and capsicum. This trilogy of compounds caused effects on human endogenous cannabinoid systems, opioid receptors (endorphin receptors), and vanilloid receptors (capsaicin receptors).

Much evidence has been presented that endocannabinoid deficiency may be responsible for several disease manifestations (concepts proposed by the celebrated expert Ethan B. Russo). There are several disorders that have been related to endocannabinoid dysregulation or deficiency, including irritable bowel syndrome, fibromyalgia, and migraine. One link among such diseases is the presence of what has been termed "functional symptomatology." "Functional" disorders have been hypothesized to be explained, to some degree, by alterations in the endocannabinoid system of body controls, or as part of an endocannabinoid deficiency syndrome (see later, theories of Ethan B. Russo and others).

Awareness of Cannabis Risks

There is no doubt that public awareness and education about the risks or negative outcomes of cannabis use tend to reduce cannabis intake. Epidemiological (population) surveys in the year 1979 indicated that marijuana was believed to pose major risks to approximately 35 percent of high school seniors. Eight years later, major risk was perceived to be present in 75 percent of school seniors. Coincidental with this recognition or perception of high risks of marijuana use, there was a fall in the use of the drug from 10.7 percent to 2.9 percent by teenagers (in the period 1978 to 1989). This reduction in cannabis use was erased with subsequent perceptions of the low risk or "safety" of cannabis use. There is a problem with arbitrary opinions or perceptions about the safety of cannabis because cannabis is not universally safe, and high-risk groups are present in society (e.g., adolescents, individuals with heart disease, or children in utero). These days, the overall use of cannabis in otherwise healthy people is perceived to be generally safe, but cannabis has not been shown to be "generally recognized as safe" (GRAS) by specific regulatory definitions.

Recent research has indicated that smoking high potency "skunk-like cannabis" can damage the corpus callosum of the brain. This structure plays a vital role in communication between the two brain hemispheres and it contains a high concentration of cannabinoid receptors (delta-9-THC) (Rigucci S et al Effect of high-potency cannabis on corpus callosum microstructure, Psychological Medicine, 2015; 1 DOI: 10.1017/S0332917 15002342).

The results of this high potency cannabis research suggest that the greater intake of high potency cannabis the greater the neurological damage may be. This study concludes that the frequency and potency of the cannabis used may be an important predictor of a risk of mental disease induced by cannabis intake. Moreover, recent studies in Denmark have drawn attention to very high concentrations of THC in skunk cannabis that is increasing in availability in several European countries (data from Aarhus University). Danish Cannabis appears to be stronger than ever. The concentration of the euphoriant THC in cannabis has tripled in the space of 20 years ("Science Daily, 19 November, 2015).

Important: Definition of Terms

It is unfortunate that a significant amount of information about cannabis and its related products is confused by the use of loose or inaccurate terminology. With simplification, it is useful to consider four main types of cannabis: (1) Cannabis sativa in its classic forms of whole herbal cannabis (marijuana), often grown for its THC content (skunk) but also produced for a high CBD content (e.g., Charlotte's Web); (2) extracted hashish and hash oil composed of extracted resins, usually concentrated for THC content; (3) pharmaceutical-grade synthetic biopharmaceutical agents containing tetrahydrocannabinol (THC) analogues or other synthesized cannabinoids and cannabinoids, extracted in standardized forms from herbal sources; and (4) dangerous synthetic forms of psychoactive compounds with cannabinoid-like effects. These latter compounds are not classic cannabinoids, and they are illegal.

In brief, *marijuana* and *cannabis* are terms that refer to a greenish-gray mixture of dried, shredded flowers, buds, stems, and leaves of the plant of the genus and species Cannabis sativa (or sometimes other species of the family of plants, known as Cannabinaceae). Other species of cannabis include Cannabis ruderalis and indica. As mentioned earlier, cannabis is a term that is often used interchangeably with other words (marijuana and marihuana) or a variety of popular or slang names. That said, the word "cannabis" can be used to refer to the whole class of "weeds" that fall into the botanical group of Cannabinaceae. This group of plants includes *hemp*.

Hashish or *hashish oil* refers to the resinous secretions of the cannabis plant. Hashish occurs in solid forms or oils of varying thickness (viscosity). These resinous secretions can be collected and dried from specific parts of the cannabis plant. They are often subject to some degree of compression to form solids, and they are used in smoking. Different types of processing of hashish oil involve the use of solvents or more efficient carbon dioxide extraction techniques. Tetrahydrocannabinol or cannabidiol predominant forms of hashish can be produced and they are increasingly used in vaporization.

Marijuana (cannabis) has many uses, including ceremonial and religious activity. However, the two common uses of cannabis are for recreational consumption to achieve a high (euphoric feeling) and consumption for a variety of medical purposes (e.g., appetite stimulation, pain control, potential cancer treatment, etc.). The most revered and well-known component of cannabis for the production of recreational highs is THC, but other cannabinoids present in cannabis have wide-ranging, nonpsychoactive effects or mild psychoactive effects. Such effects may be of medicinal value in selected circumstances. In the United States, cannabinoids without psychoactive effects are no longer permitted to be used in dietary supplements (e.g., cannabidiol [CBD] present in hemp oil). These compounds (cannabinoids) are potentially powerful biological-response modifiers (e.g., cannabidiol). Cannabidiol (CBD) can act to reduce the psychoactive effects of THC. In simple terms, cannabinoids can be considered to be examples of nature's drugs.

Beyond some confusion in terminology, it is apparent that there are many potential medicinal components of marijuana or hemp (cannabis). A class of compounds known as terpenoids found in cannabis essential oils can modify the actions of cannabinoids. As mentioned earlier, this modification of the effects of cannabinoids is part of what is known as an entourage effect of cannabis (collaborative effects of cannabis components, synergistic or antagonistic). Cannabinoids that are nonpsychoactive appeared formerly to be able to be used as dietary supplements (nutraceuticals), provided that they were of hemp origin and marketed and sold in compliance with the conditions set forth in the US Dietary Supplement Health and Education Act (DSHEA, 1994). The DSHEA (1994) refers to dietary supplements as substances that are not food and not drugs. These circumstances concerning CBD availability do not exist currently, but they have been challenged by the FDA recently in all states of the Union. The general use of cannabinoids (other than THC) is rejected with the argument that all cannabis material is considered to be a Class 1 substance (illegal). This situation is debated, but supplements containing cannabidiol are still widely available for purchase without current signs of regulatory interference.

What does this circumstance really mean when it comes to cannabis use? Products that contain significant amounts of THC (greater than 0.3 percent concentration of THC) have to be reserved for medical-prescription use (except in Colorado, Washington,

Alaska, Oregon and Washington DC, where recreational cannabis is available, at the time of writing). However, I repeat (for clarity) that there is a widespread opinion that nutraceuticals or dietary supplements derived from cannabis (hemp) without psychoactive effects (devoid of significant THC concentration) have been formerly made available for sale as a dietary supplement. New terminology has been applied to dietary supplements containing cannabis components that are not psychoactive. This term is "cannaceutical," but like the word nutraceutical, it has no regulatory meaning. In brief, CBD is not a legal dietary supplement.

Dietary supplements derived from cannabis plants most often involve the sale of hemp-derived compounds (e.g., hemp oil, which contains cannabidiol [CBD] in varying amount). There are many hybrids among different cannabis species of plant, with different cannabinoid contents. To emphasize the main difference between hemp and cannabis or marijuana is the general recognition of higher concentrations of THC in cannabis (marijuana) versus hemp. In summary, the THC content of cannabis is responsible for the psychoactive effects, and it should be noted with clarity that hemp oil tends to contain more cannabidiol (CBD) with little THC (less than 0.3 percent).

It is unfortunate that several terms that describe cannabis-derived products are used in a synonymous manner. Unfortunately, the terms are not always synonyms, and active components vary from preparation to preparation. Synonyms in use include cannabis, marijuana, marihuana, pot, shit, reefer, buds, grass, weed, dope, ganja, herb, boom, Mary Jane, Sinsemilla, hash, hash oil, blow, blunt, green, Indian hemp, kilobricks, skunk, Thai sticks, etc. These different terms do not result in a clear definition of the contents of the cannabis. What's next in this newfound world of cannabis neologisms?

Differences between Hemp and Marijuana (Cannabis)

Cannabis refers to the genus of plants that produce both hemp (often indica) and marijuana (often sativa). It is sometimes confusing for people that the sativa species of cannabis may be classified sometimes as hemp. There may be many types of the cannabis plant, but as noted earlier, these plants can be different in their composition and structure due to special plant-breeding techniques. Composition and structure determine their use as hemp or marijuana. To reiterate, there are three common species of cannabis, known as sativa, indica, and ruderalis. C. ruderalis has the lowest levels of THC (delta-9-tetrahydrocannabinol). C. sativa grown for "high feelings" (cannabis or marijuana) tends to have higher levels of THC than CBD (cannabidiol), and C. indica has higher levels of CBD than THC.

Using a process of artificial selection, different varieties of plant are used for different purposes (e.g., medicine, industrial purposes, and food). Industrial hemp is derived from C. indica, and it invariably contains low levels of THC (<0.3 percent but usually no greater than 1–4 percent). The hemp form of C. indica is artificially selected to grow as a tall plant, which is used for industrial purposes (hemp oil or fiber). In brief, C. sativa produces short, bushy plants that are used for marijuana (buds, leaves, and flowers), and hemp comes from tall plants with fibrous stalks and few flowers. The fibrous components of hemp can be used to make rope and cloth. Thus hemp looks different from plants used for marijuana.

More on Distinguishing Hemp from Cannabis

As already mentioned, hemp can be often distinguished from marijuana (often referred to as cannabis) by its physical appearance, and it is used primarily for industrial purposes, as a consequence of the physical and chemical properties of its seeds (oil) and fiber. Hemp fibers are used as rope, paper, and canvas, and hemp-seed oil is used sometimes as a component of varnish and paint. As noted earlier, industrial types of hemp often contain less that 0.3 percent of THC, and they are devoid of significant psychoactive effects. In contrast, marijuana (cannabis) often contains 5–20 percent of THC (as high as 30 percent THC), and it alters central nervous system function, often resulting in a high. As noted earlier, the maximum amount of THC defined as allowable in hemp-based dietary supplements is 0.3 percent.

Hemp oil has been used to alleviate symptoms and signs of

several diseases. In what is called an "ethereal form" of oil, hemp can be used for anti-inflammatory actions and antiallergic properties. The presence of the cannabinoids CBD and CBN (cannabidiol and cannabinol, respectively) account for several other beneficial health effects of hemp. Moreover, ethereal oil of hemp contains a number of bioactive terpenoids such as myrcene, caryophyllene, pinene, alpha humulene, allo-aromadendrene, bisabolol, and so forth. These chemicals are examples of monoterpenoids, sesquiterpenoids, and terpene oxides. As noted earlier, terpenes are believed to collaborators in the entourage effect of cannabis.

Industrial hemp production in the United States is allowable under the Farm Bill signed by President Obama in the early part of 2014. This bill contains amendments that legalize hemp for research purposes (www.votehemp.com/FarmBill). These introduced farm bills (2013 and 2014) to separate hemp from marijuana in the Controlled Substances Act, and they give state governments the rights to regulate hemp growing and product production under state Laws.

Classifying Cannabinoids by Origin

To memorize each action or putative actions of the various (one hundred or more) phytocannabinoids in cannabis is a monumental task. Some cannabinoids have few if any biological actions because they are metabolic end products. A simple way to classify cannabinoids is by their origin.

Table 3. Cannabinoids in a simple classification by origin

Cannabinoid Type	Comments
Plant	Also known as phytocannabinoids, found mainly in seeds, flowers, leaves, and stems. Variation in content by strain of cannabis or species (sativa and indica).

Endogenous (from within)	The two main examples are (1) arachidonoylethanolamine or anandamide (AE) and (2) arachidonoylglycerol (2-AG). AE and 2-AG exert "tonicity" in control of body functions, and they are manipulated by inhibiting their breakdown (hydrolase dependent degradation). The inhibited enzymes are FAAH or MAGL for AE and 2-AG, respectively.
Purified	Naturally occurring phytocannabinoids (e.g., CBD and THC) mixed with ballast components comprise Sativex. Sativex is a pharmaceutical with a proprietary mixture of CBD and THC.
Synthetic	Drugs are best termed "analogues" that can be synthesized. Examples include CB-1 agonists (CPP-55, ACPA), CB-2 agonists JWH–133, NMP7, and AM1241, CB-1/CB-2 nonselective agonists (CP55, 940), adjumelic acid (AJA), Nabilone, Dronabinol, and others.
Synthetic pot (misnamed as cannabinoids)	Note: synthetic cannabinoids are sometimes misclassified and go by the common name "synthetic pot." These forms of cannabis are not phytocannabinoids, but they have an ability to mimic some cannabinoid effects (e.g., mimic THC). They are potentially dangerous and toxic. They are a major public health risk in children and teenagers and should receive more research and stringent controls.

Recently (2015), the United Nations renewed warning to Colorado, Washington, and Uruguay that cannabis legalization does not conform with international drug treaties (www.theguardian.com/society/2015, reported by Alan Travis). The International Control Narcotics Board report of the UN (INCB) reinforces the notion that limiting the use of narcotics to medical or scientific use is a necessary component that underpins international drug control framework.

Colorado retail stores (dispensaries) opened on January 1, 2014, and in their first year of operation they sold seventeen tons of recreational marijuana. However, sales of medicinal pot amounted to approximately fifty tons (posted online at www.cannabisnews.com by Daniel Wallis February 28, 2015). Add this to the estimated 40 percent of total sales as illicit cannabis.

Conclusion

The Cannabis Revolution has emerged over a period of a decade or so. It was heralded (starting in January 2014) by recent legalization for recreational use in two states and for medical use in two dozen states. Currently, there are four states with recreational legalization of cannabis (Colorado, Washington, Oregon and Alaska), as well as Washington DC. These events have forced a need for education on the benefits or risks of cannabis use. Much misunderstanding of cannabis use and science has been produced by biased reporting. The medical, social, political, and economic outcomes of increasing cannabis use are legion.

Chapter 2

DIFFERENT MODES OF CANNABIS INTAKE

Beware of "Synthetic Cannabis": Synthetic Pot

Many agencies of state and federal governments have undertaken the initiative to ban "synthetic pot" use. This threat, primarily to youngsters, has not been addressed in a timely or aggressive manner. The use of synthetic pot is a growing and serious public health concern. A variety of herbal mixtures with various salts and other chemical additives constitute a group of products that are considered, often inaccurately, to be forms of synthetic marijuana or cannabis. These herbal mixtures often contain mixed plants with no specific biological actions that are sprayed with chemicals that mimic the effects of THC, which is found in whole herbal cannabis (but these chemicals are not cannabinoids). There are a number of names that have emerged to label this type of synthetic pot, which is not to be confused with synthetic analogues of cannabis that are drugs (e.g., Marinol or dronabinol, etc., [pharmaceuticals]). Names to label this synthetic pot include K2, spice, Yucatan weed, moon rocks, and so forth. While these and similar substances are touted and sold as safe and legal, they are neither. These substances are sold sometimes as disguised household items, such as bath salts. Despite this situation of danger to the public, efforts to identify these drug concoctions and regulate their use remains problematic. In a deceptive manner, synthetic marijuana preparations are often labeled "not for human consumption," but they are frequently sold as both "edibles" or "additives" to smoking mixtures.

It is very difficult to know or even guess the many components of various forms of synthetic pot. Although mind-altering actions of these preparations exist, I emphasize that these effects are not due to any specific content of THC, unless there has been intentional mixing with true herbal cannabis. Synthetic pot has frequent and unpleasant reactions in the cannabis novice. In some cases, these chemicals are much more potent in their psychoactive properties than regular herbal cannabis, and some are in development as putative cannabis analogues (drug research). Use of synthetic pot has resulted in a number of emergency hospital attendances where recipients of synthetic pot have presented with acute symptoms of psychosis, altered mental status, and abnormal mental behavior. Other adverse effects reported after the use of synthetic forms of pot include seizures, hallucinations, and a variety of negative psychological reactions (confusion, fear, and anxiety, etc.).

Medical literature makes it clear that synthetic pot, or what may be considered compounds that can be erroneously considered to be natural cannabis or cannabis derivatives or (marijuana) substitutes, are dangerous. They must be avoided. It is unfortunate that synthetic marijuana (pot or cannabis) has been labeled incorrectly in common language. As mentioned earlier, these preparations of synthetic pot are not legal and are often toxic. In brief, synthetic pot is an underestimated and growing public health concern among teenagers, and its low cost drives its sale.

Aspects of the Law in the United States

The Drug Enforcement Agency (DEA) treats marijuana (cannabis) as a Category 1 drug (under the Controlled Substances Act). Of course, the DEA adopts the federal government's stance on marijuana (cannabis) by defining the characteristics of a schedule I drug as:

"Schedule I drugs are classified as having a high potential for abuse, no currently accepted medical use in treatment in the United States, and a lack of accepted safety for use of the drug or other substances under medical supervision." (Drug Enforcement Administration: Drug Fact Sheet, www.justice.gov)

To describe marijuana, using current guidelines of the DEA, causes a lot of negative reaction from the protagonists for its legalization and some degree of unnecessary confusion among consumers. The magnitude of these emotive reactions is apparent in detailed accounts of "How to Spark a Cannabis Revolution" (www.thecannabisgeek.com). This advice on revolution stems, in part, from perceptions about the failure of alcohol prohibition, which is now associated with a modern and growing perception of the failure of marijuana prohibition.

Changes in state law in 2012 that legalized recreational cannabis use in Colorado and Washington conflict with existing federal law that describes the illegal sale and distribution of cannabis to be a criminal act. In addition, any person who grows more than one hundred cannabis plants without official authorization can be sentenced to a minimum of five years in prison. However, the federal government does not appear to be actively pursuing certain acts of noncompliance with federal law in states where legalization has been undertaken. There is a welcome trend in the federal government to back off on prohibition, but federal legislation that defines marijuana as illegal remains intact. Law enforcement seems to be appropriately tolerant to cannabis use in the clear presence of medical necessity for cannabis use, confirmed by a physician. That said, reports exist of elderly people with medical needs who face up to ten years in prison as a consequence of state and federal law enforcers raiding homes where cannabis was being cultivated in 2012. This outrageous circumstance exists in Washington state, where marijuana has been legalized for both recreational and medical use (www.cannabisnews.com/Feb.13, 2015).

This apparent conflicting set of legal circumstances has been somewhat clarified by the Department of Justice (DOJ). The DOJ has provided a definition of important residual areas of law enforcement under the existing federal law that is contained within the Controlled Substances Act. Table 4 lists an adapted and repeated summary (late 2014) of many of the most important areas of potential federal prosecution and priorities for control of cannabis use, at the time of writing.

Table 4. Priorities for controls of cannabis use adopted by the federal government

These priorities listed below are designed to promote the responsible use of marijuana, and they are argued to be of different degrees of importance. Methods to control cannabis use in teenagers are very important initiatives that have not received adequate attention. (Found in the Ogden memorandum and documented earlier.)

- distribution of cannabis to minors
- transfer of cannabis from states of legalization to those of nonlegalization
- support of criminal activity from sales of cannabis
- using state-legalized cannabis as a cover for other illegal drug sales
- elimination of guns and violence in the growing and distribution of cannabis
- prevention of the use of public land for cannabis growing
- elimination of cannabis use or possession on federal property
- prevention of driving under the influence of cannabis

In February 2015 the Food and Drug Administration (FDA) issued warning letters to seven companies that are selling cannabidiol-(CBD)-containing products. It has been anticipated that the FDA would take some action against CBD nutraceutical product marketing and its advertising, especially if it is based on medical claims. The Dietary Supplement and Health Education Act (DSHEA 1994) makes it clear that disease prevention or treatment claims are not allowed to be used in the description or sales of dietary supplements. In the event that this occurs, the agent in question becomes classified as a drug or an adulterated drug if it has a therapeutic or medicinal claim.

The warning letters could be considered good news for the purveyors of cannabis because the letters did not advise the cessation of CBD product sales. However, the letters did make it clear that medical claims associated with CBD products would not be tolerated. *Marijuana Business Daily* (March 10, 2015) reports that this action may be the "first shot across the bow" of nutraceutical marijuana sales. Moreover, it is speculated that these actions by the FDA may signal larger policy changes at the federal government level.

Laboratory analyses by the FDA of several alleged CBD-containing products show that some of them do not contain any CBD. The amounts of CBD in the products seem to be subtherapeutic with CBD concentrations ranging from 0 to 2.6 percent (with THC concentration compliance of less than 0.3 percent and most of the CBD concentrations in about 0.3 to 0.5 percent range). Thus, the arguments are redundant to some degree. What is forgotten is that hemp foods were in the food chain prior to 1994 and are considered by some to be dietary supplements under DSHEA (1994) regulations. In May 2015, the Food and Drug Administration released statements that CBD (cannabidiol) is not to be viewed as a dietary supplement. This has caused major upheaval for some purveyors of CBD who sell this compound often mixed with hemp oil.

Reducing Harm with Cannabis Use

Robert Melamede, MD, of Colorado and others have emphasized that endocannabinoids play an important role in controlling all systems of the body. In fact, the endocannabinoid system promotes the harmony of body functions and maintains body homeostasis. These findings support the hypothesis that humans and animals use the endocannabinoid system as part of a harm reduction program (Melamede, R., *Harm Reduction Journal*, 2, 17, 2005).

Therefore, phytocannabinoids (cannabis plant derived exocannabinoids) and some of their analogues may have activity for harm reduction. Many scientists subscribe to the notion that there is major social benefit when drug use policies are helpful to drug users, rather than when they are focused on punitive measures. As mentioned earlier, an important conceptual overview provided by R. Melamede and others is that the endocannabinoid system is one of nature's methods of maintaining homeostasis (Melamede, R., ibid. 2005). This circumstance is relevant to antiaging where endocannabinoids can protect against some of the undesirable biochemical changes that determine the aging process. That said, a number of scientists have suggested that cannabis causes harm to users and others. Much contention prevails.

Perspectives on the Harm Caused by Substance Abuse

Cannabis use has been described by some protagonists of its legalization to be harmless. Emerging data show this to be a shaky general opinion, and safety of cannabis use is context specific. UK studies of individual harm to drug users were reported recently in the *Lancet* (2010). This article assessed the effects of different drugs on harm by assessing criteria such as dependence, death rates, and impaired mental function ("Drug Harms in the UK," *Lancet*, Nov. 1, 2010). In addition, this study investigated "harm to others" as assessed by parameters such as crime rates and adverse environmental consequences.

In brief, it was found in this "Drug Harm Study" (ibid. 2010) that alcohol was the most harmful drug overall. On the one hand, the most harmful drugs to users were specified as crack cocaine, heroin, and methamphetamine. On the other hand alcohol, heroin, and crack appeared to be the most harmful illicit drugs to others. Cannabis had a harm score that ranked it in eighth place in front of liquid ecstasy (GHB). These studies give a macro-view of the impact of the use of various drugs on well-being and indicate that the results of cannabis use do involve some limited harm to both users and others. There is a paradox here. Cannabis is described as valuable in harm reduction, but it has implications for causing harm (in some circumstances).

Cannabis: Intake and Modes of Delivery

Components of cannabis are most often delivered by smoking, but cannabis can be consumed in oils, dispensed with carrier substances, eaten in foods and candies, imbibed in cannabis beverages, used in volatile preparations, and sometimes administered in standard pill or elixir forms. Unusual and uncommon modes of human delivery occur by the rectum and even by insertion into the vagina. This latter route of administration has no advantages and should be avoided. Rectal delivery of cannabis will partially bypass the normal metabolism of the drug by the liver (first-pass metabolic effect) and result in the absorption of higher amounts of active ingredients (e.g., THC), especially if they are in the hemisuccinate form. Injected marijuana or its derivatives are to be considered highly dangerous, at least because many injected fluids made from illicit herbal cannabis have uncertain contents and a high rate of contamination with toxins.

Vaporizing Cannabis: An Increasingly Preferred Method

The use of vaporization of cannabis has provided what has been described as a convenient, popular, safe, and effective way of delivering cannabis. A large number of physicians and cannabis experts have endorsed vaporization as a healthier option than smoking. Vaporizers heat cannabis at lower temperatures than smoking to result in a much lower production of carcinogens and other toxic irritants that are found in cannabis smoke. In other words, heating cannabis without combustion results in an inhalant that contains active cannabinoids without excessive amounts of potentially harmful products of combustion.

Landmark studies on the comparisons of toxic burdens from tobacco smoking and cannabis smoking show that smoking marijuana results in a substantially greater burden of the delivery of tar and carbon monoxide than the smoking of tobacco products. These observations occurred in a manner that was independent of tetrahydrocannabinol (THC) content of the smoked cannabis. While cannabis is associated with airways irritation and bronchitis, the link between marijuana smoking and lung cancer remains arguable but highly likely.

Vaporization is an efficient delivery method for THC, with findings that vaporizers can often deliver about 46 percent of THC into vapor. In comparative studies, smoking a marijuana joint was less efficient, by delivering less than 25 percent of the THC. A large international survey on forms of administration of cannabis showed that herbal, nonpharmaceutical cannabis products received a higher "appreciation" score by study participants than approved drug products (pharmaceuticals) containing cannabinoids (Hazekamp, A. et al., *Journal of Psychoactive Drugs*, 45, 3, 199–210, 2013). In these surveys, vaporization has a high ranking for the absence of intolerable side effects. Other advantages of inhaled vaporized cannabis include the ability of the person to titrate the dosage with small puffs that do not require intense inhalation. Finally, vaporization may present some cost advantages because of its efficiency of the concentrated delivery of cannabinoids.

The avoidance of lung damage from smoking cannabis was recently taken into account in the New York State medical cannabis legislation that recommends against cannabis smoking, with some unofficial and tangential endorsement of edibles and vaporization. Vaping has become increasingly popular in recent times, and there are many devices available, some of which have gained acceptance by regulatory officials in Canada and Europe. Most cannabis "vapers" (users) prefer cordless, portable devices, but there are large tabletop models for the real enthusiast. The principles of preparing cannabis material for vaporization are reasonably standard, but they are not standardized for the delivery of different dosages of cannabinoids. Please note that the author is not promoting the use of vaporization of cannabis, which is illegal in many US states.

The key steps to preparation for vaporization are shown in table 5, with important disclaimer statements to conform with local laws.

Table 5. Key steps in the preparation and use of a portable vaporizing device for marijuana

The directions are rough guidelines only, and individuals must check with all safety instructions. Not to be done outside the approved jurisdiction of medical or recreational use of cannabis. Information is freely available on the Internet. That said, the author is highly motivated to propose only safe and legal cannabis use in a responsible manner.

- Cannabis is ground to powder.
- The powder is placed in a heating chamber of a vaporizer.
- Devices should not be shared.

This brief overview of vaporization techniques can be supplemented by reference to the website www.VapeCritic. com. The vaporization market is growing in an exponential manner (www.slate.com/articles/technology/2014/07vaporizers).

Vaping on the Rise: Edibles Present Problems

Recent reports (December 2014) from the CDC indicate that the use of e-cigarettes and various vaporization methods for tobacco are on the rise, especially in teenagers. Coincidental with this situation is the greater use of vaporizing methods for cannabis administration. There are several proposed advantages of vaping both tobacco and cannabis, but the safety and efficacy of this mode of delivery is still under investigation. As noted earlier, the health advantages of the vaporized delivery of cannabis compared with smoking are apparent, with the production of smaller amounts of toxic chemicals such as carbon monoxide, polycyclic hydrocarbons, and tar. The speed of onset of psychoactive effects of cannabis may be faster with cannabis smoking, but some studies disagree with this conclusion (in favor of vaping). As noted, both smoking and vaporization are able to be self-titrated for effects, which are significant advantages in cannabis use.

The use of vaporization does not necessarily eliminate unwanted toxic products derived from cannabis. The amounts of cannabinoids released by vaporization increase with increasing temperature of the vaporization process. Temperatures of vaporization are often about 180°C–195°C, but higher vaporization temperatures increase the release of cannabinoids and some toxic products.

Much controversy surrounds the use of edible marijuana preparations, particularly in young people. Cannabis edibles are viewed as a particular risk for children. The possibility of accidental ingestion by children and the childhood attractions of cannabis cookies and candies (jollies) are circumstances of residual concern. These events in children have resulted in adverse medical outcomes with attendances at emergency rooms in hospitals, despite the safety rhetoric from the suppliers. Edibles have been used in pranks on unsuspecting individuals, such as schoolteachers. Cannabis education in children is a public health priority, especially in locations of approved recreational use of cannabis. A significant proportion of children who have taken cannabis edibles acquire them from a parent, with or without permission. Giving pot to kids is nefarious behavior.

The dosage of cannabis that is eaten (or consumed) often determines the intensity of the acute effects of its bioactive components (THC). As mentioned earlier, variable metabolism of orally absorbed cannabis occurs in the liver (referred to as first-pass metabolic effects). Therefore, there is great variation from one person to another (interindividual variation) in the outcome of smoking cannabis or ingesting cannabis edibles. There are no clear guidelines on how much cannabis is safe to eat, and regulations of dosing are still being investigated and developed in jurisdictions that permit both the medical and recreational use of cannabis. There are many factors that can affect the absorption of THC and other bioactive components of marijuana, even including the foodstuff in which it is delivered! Unfortunately, the amount of cannabis that is used in edibles is often a best guess when it comes to cannabinoid dosing, and delays in achieving a cannabis high from cannabis edibles can result in repeated consumption because of delayed absorption that delays onset of psychoactive effects. This situation carries a greater risk of overdose or toxicity.

An Overview of Consuming Cannabis

As mentioned earlier, there are several common ways to deliver cannabis, which include by inhalation, by oral, and by topical means. The most popular method of cannabis delivery is by "cigarette" smoking (blunts or joints). The modes of consumption are summarized in table 6.

Table 6. Modes of delivery of cannabis (adapted from the Internet)

Delivery Method	Comment
Vaporization	Vaporization is becoming a preferred method for cannabis use compared with smoking. This is because vaporization is reported to be healthier than smoking and its use is easier to disguise. Vaporizers can be used with cannabis concentrates in oil or wax forms that can be added to herbal mixtures or contained within cartridges.
Smoking	Smoking is often undertaken by the use of rolling papers, but smoking devices may be preferred (e.g., hand pipes, bongs, water pipes, hookahs). Some devices are designed to allegedly filter out harmful constituents.
Dabbing	Involves the vaporization of high concentrations of cannabinoids. These concentrates are placed on a heated metal object (e.g., a heated nail) that produces a vapor, which is collected into a glass globe for inhalation.
Tinctures	These liquid extracts of cannabis are rapidly absorbed and may be administered with reasonable controls against overdosing. They are usually given in "dropper amounts," which contain the cannabis concentrate in alcohol, glycerol, coconut oil, olive oil, and/or vinegar.

Oils	This delivery system is intermediate in its timing of effects between standard edibles and tinctures. Solvents are used to dissolve the concentrate, which is then evaporated to produce a thick substance (heavy oil) for subsequent use. Both high THC and high CBD oils are available for consumption.
Edibles	"Edibles" is a term used to describe all foods that are fortified with cannabis. The time of onset of edibles in producing a psychoactive effect is quite variable and often delayed. Foods are often made with simple infusion of fat-loving substances containing cannabis, (e.g., olive oil, butter, etc.). Some consumers have shown a preference for alternative oral delivery methods including juicing and selective incorporation of cannabis flowers in baking.
Topical Delivery	Topical delivery remains localized, and its THC content is not absorbed to a degree that can cause a high. Topicals have found uses as pain-control agents for arthritis and muscle pain, as well as therapeutic preparations for eczema, psoriasis, acne, and pruritus. Recent product development includes beauty-care products with lotions, soap, and even combinations with essential oils to develop aromatherapy treatments.
Other Methods	Several alternative oral delivery systems have been popularized for marijuana consumption, including capsules, tablets, delayed-release formulations, and a variety of beverages (e.g., tea, soda, and cola).

Different Cannabinoid Drugs

Cannabinoid analogues (drugs) can be classified simply into (1) cannabinoid receptor agonists, (2) cannabinoid receptor antagonists, and (3) compounds that interfere with the inactivation of endocannabinoids. Interference with endocannabinoid inactivation by the use of enzyme inhibitors makes these latter compounds indirect agonists that work by increasing the availability of endocannabinoids at cannabinoid receptors (e.g., FAAH and MAGDL). Table 7 provides a summary of the actions of several cannabinoid drugs.

Table 7. Main types of cannabinoid drugs with comments on their actions

Note most of these drugs are not available for prescription usage. This area of cannabis research is complex and sometimes quite confusing. Rimonabant (a cannabis receptor antagonist) has been withdrawn from use.

Cannabinoid Drug	Comment
Cannabinoid receptor agonists	Classical, nonclassical, amino-alkyindole, and eicosanoid cannabinoid agonists have been distinguished for classification: (1) Classical receptor agonists include delta-9-THC, delta-8-THC, cannabinol and cannabinoid analogues, e.g., HU-210 (11-hydroxy-delta-8-THC-demethylheptyl). (2) Nonclassical cannabinoids are bicyclic or tricyclic compounds derived from delta-9-THC, e.g., CP55, 940 which is more potent than delta-9-THC. (3) Amino-alkylindoles, e.g., WIN 55, 212-2 and JWH-015 tend to have prominent CB-2 receptor agonist effects. (4) Eicosanoids are related to the endocannabinoid anandamide. Chemical modification of anandamide produces a range of CB-1 selective agonists.

Inhibitors of anandamide inactivation	This inhibitory effect works to increase the concentration of endocannabinoids that are available to interact with CB-receptors. Examples are AM404 and VDM11. AM404 inhibits anandamide transport and amplifies its effects. VDM11 produces similar effects to AM404.
Cannabinoid receptor antagonists	SR141716A (rimonabant) and SR144528 are potent CB-1 and CB-2 receptor antagonists. Many studies show that SR141716A acts on CB-1 receptors and produce effects that are opposite to those of cannabinoid receptor agonists.

Ajumelic Acid (CT3): An Example of Required Research

Ajumelic acid (CT3) is a drug that is being investigated in the treatment of several conditions. The drug is a modification metabolite of THC with CB-1 receptor stimulating activity. It seems to be distinguished by its ability to reduce pain without causing psychoactive effects. As noted, research with ajulemic acid shows that there is a potential separation of psychoactive and analgesic effects of an analogue of THC in humans. Research shows that ajulemic acid (CT3) may be useful in a variety of conditions, including cancer management, inflammatory disease, abnormal lipid metabolism, and multiple sclerosis. It has specific antifibrotic activity, which has led to studies in fibrotic disease (e.g., cystic fibrosis and scleroderma). The work required to show benefit in all of these conditions illustrates the scope of the enormous challenge of developing cannabis-related drugs (analogues) for therapeutic indications.

A proprietary form of ajulemic acid is available in clinical trials as the drug Resunab. This drug works on CB2 receptors. Its mechanism of action involves reduction in the synthesis of proinflammatory eicosanoids (e.g., PGE2 and LTB4), with an increase in anti-inflammatory eicosanoids (e.g., PGJ2 and LXA4).

A Note on Different Effects of Cannabinoids

Table 8. Factors that may result in differences of the perceived outcome of scientific or general information about cannabis use

Many factors may explain the different reported effects and outcomes of the use of whole cannabis or its derivatives (extracts and synthetic drug analogues). Some of these factors that cause differences in observations of the effects of cannabis are summarized in table 8.

- dosage and types of cannabinoids or extracts used in various studies
- length of exposure to cannabis
- specific receptor targeting
- species differences in effects of cannabis; also, effects of age and gender
- different modes of delivery of cannabis
- design of experiments in animals and humans
- difference in interpretations of outcome measures
- the health and nutritional status of the individual who is studied in clinical research projects
- bias of investigators who hold different opinions on legalization of cannabis

Perhaps one of the most important issues with the use of illicit cannabis is not knowing what is delivered as a consequence of nonstandardized delivery methods, compounded by uncertainty of product contents. Rough guidelines of cannabis strength can be gauged by knowing the type of cannabis that is consumed. These days, skunk types of cannabis are favored for use because of their high THC content (approximately 20 percent THC). When I was a teenager in the 1960s, the highest THC cannabis available was about 4 percent.

Marijuana Availability and Negative Health Outcomes

While we have witnessed the global occurrence of cannabis dependence or addiction, it has been argued by some that unequivocal evidence of damage to health by cannabis has not been documented in the United States. This apparent and somewhat misleading perception of the innocuous nature of cannabis survives, and this perception is increasing. I am concerned that this situation could contribute to irresponsible use of cannabis. Driving the perception of the safety of cannabis use drives the greater use of cannabis. This situation has colored political opinions in recent times, but one may question whether or not some political opinions that guide votes on legalization for marijuana use are fully informed opinions.

Perhaps we can learn lessons from comparisons of earlier experiences with cannabis use in different countries (societies). For example, in the 1930s in India, addiction and long-term use of potent cannabis was more common than in the United States. At that time, evidence of health damage was reported in 42 percent of a sample of Indian chronic cannabis users. This prevalence of adverse health effects of marijuana was not experienced in the 1930s in the United States, but cannabis was banned in the United States in 1937 (under the Marijuana Tax Act, 1937).

It may be logical to believe that the increase in cannabis use in recent times in the United States could lead to a higher incidence of negative manifestations of chronic cannabis use. This would be a situation more like that encountered earlier in India. That said, more recent examinations of disease profiles resulting from cannabis use in countries with widespread acceptance of marijuana (e.g., the Netherlands, Europe) have not shown such a marked prevalence of negative health effects of cannabis, such as those encountered eighty years ago in India. Placing cannabis use into a retrospective scope is difficult.

Cannabis and Positive Health Outcomes

Researchers in Israel have put cannabis interventions into a clinical perspective, with observations made in increasing numbers of patients who describe the occurrence of significant health benefits with cannabis use. In a recent study in Israel, patients with an age range of sixty-nine to 101 years received medical cannabis by various modes of delivery for several medical conditions, including pain, lack of appetite, body wasting, and quality of life. The positive outcomes of cannabis related treatments in this latter study are listed in table 9.

Table 9. Positive outcomes of cannabis use in an elderly group of nursing home residents (adapted from *Science Daily*, www.sciencedailyonline.com)

One of the most notable outcomes of this study was the ability of cannabis-treated patients to lower intake of several drugs used in the treatment of their medical disorders (e.g., reductions in mood stabilizers and pain relievers). These valuable drug-sparing effects of cannabis require further confirmation and have great therapeutic potential.

- assistance with increase in body weight
- improvements in quality-of-life measures
- reduction of muscle spasms
- decrease in pain
- increased sleeping times
- decrease in nightmares
- reductions in flashbacks in cases of PTSD
- reduction in the need for overall medication (drug) use

Cannabis: Key Characteristics at a Glance—A Revision

At this stage, I believe that it is valuable to summarize key facts about marijuana use to reinforce learning. These facts are summarized below in table 10.

Table 10. Key characteristics of cannabis, hemp, and derivatives (modified from data at www.drugs.com/illicit/cannabis)

- Cannabis sativa, indica, and ruderalis are species of the Cannabinaceae family of plants.
- Cannabis contains cannabinoids, the most common of which are delta-9-tetrahydrocannabinol (delta-9-THC) and cannabidiol (CBD).
- Dried leaves and tops of the cannabis plant are often referred to as marijuana. In popular language, marijuana and cannabis are terms used interchangeably.
- Resinous secretions of the plant are called hashish or hashish oil.
- The most common ways to take cannabis are by smoking, vaporization, or eating (edibles).
- Cannabis is a schedule I drug under the Controlled Substances Act (no medical use) according to the federal government, but it has been allowed for medical use in two dozen states of the United States (at the time of writing).
- Cannabis containing THC causes altered states of consciousness and a high, with impaired memory, coordination, and concentration.
- Cannabis is used in several medical conditions, with reports of variable benefits (e.g., cancer, glaucoma, HIV/AIDS, muscle spasms, epilepsy, pain control, nausea, vomiting, and wasting syndromes [severe weight loss], etc.).
- CBD oil (realm oil) has been given "orphan drug" status by the FDA for treatment of Dravet's Syndrome (epilepsy in childhood). CBD oil is often derived from the strain of a plant called "Charlotte's Web." As of July 2014, about one dozen states have approved the use of CBD oil in research, particularly for epilepsy. Strong arguments exist that CBD is a dietary supplement. A majority of Americans support legalization of cannabis—52 percent for (pro) and 45 percent against (con).

Conclusion

There are few general accounts that compare and contrast the modes of use of cannabis in published books. Statements that cannabis is a miracle, panacea drug concoction have to be tempered by realistic viewpoints. The mode of consumption of cannabis has major effects on outcomes of its use. Cannabis has promising medical use, but caution must be applied to secure the responsible use of this drug mixture. Readers must understand that cannabis use is restricted by federal and state law in many locations in the United States. The author advises that individuals check the legal status of cannabis for medical or recreational use in various locations in the United States, with the knowledge that only Alaska, Oregon, Colorado, Washington state, and Washington, DC, allow the recreational use of cannabis.

Chapter 3

THE EXPANDING USE OF CANNABIS

Milestones in Cannabis Knowledge

It is not possible to credit all the contributors to the growing knowledge about cannabis, nor is it possible for the author to credit all major findings of the thousands of scientists who are currently gearing up their activity in cannabis research. However, it is relevant to present a brief historical sketch of cannabis use, which has been a topic of discussion by many authors. This sketch will permit an understanding of the evolution of cannabis use in society that has culminated in modern applications of this plant. Arguments prevail about the first documented use of cannabis by humans, but ancient Chinese writings, about five thousand years ago, refer to its use for treating constipation, rheumatic pains, malaria, and assistance with childbirth. Other historical Chinese records imply that cannabis was mixed with wine and administered as an anesthetic during surgery.

Spread of the use of cannabis as medicine occurred in Europe in the nineteenth century. This export of cannabis from the east to the west, through intervening continents, was reinforced by the work of an Irish physician (W. B. O'Shaughnessy). While working in India, this physician documented favorable observations of cannabis use for several diseases or disorders. These early medical

51

applications included its use as an anticonvulsant, antiemetic, hypnotic, and antispasmodic. These findings popularized the application of cannabis for a variety of medical disorders in British medicine. Interests in cannabis therapies peaked in the late Victorian period. It was publication of the favorable medicinal usage of cannabis in the 1840s that led to expanded use of cannabis products in Europe and the United States.

The late part of the nineteenth century witnessed an unleashing of many remedies containing cannabis in both Europe and North America. Many of these remedies were produced by compounding pharmacy and contained feel-good substances such as opium. The common use of cannabis as a home remedy in the late 1800s was replaced in the early twentieth century by the common sale of cannabis products that had been produced by poor standards of manufacturing. Some decline in the use of cannabis occurred at this time, because the treatment may have been worse than the disease, at least from the symptomatic point of view. This situation was followed, in the late 1920s, by the outlawing of cannabis use as a consequence of a consensus opinion developed through the 1925 Convention on the Production and Distribution of Dangerous Drugs. However, the prescription of marijuana (cannabis) for medical needs survived in many areas in Europe and the United States, and law enforcement sometimes turned a blind eye to cannabis use.

Final prohibition of cannabis use was made under the 1971 Misuse of Drugs Act, but both the illicit and medical use of marijuana had been compromised greatly by the Marijuana Tax Act of 1937. It is apparent that research and medical cannabis use was prohibited from 1937 onward, resulting in gaps in our knowledge about this valuable mixture of natural drugs. Special parochial recommendations for the compassionate use of marijuana in the United States emerged in the periods of 1976 to 1992, but this use was considered to be a loophole in the law according to several influential bodies of opinion. It has been reported that marijuana use was modest in the United States prior to 1930, except among Mexican laborers who were domiciled mainly in southwest states. However, illicit use of marijuana spread widely in the United States from the 1930s onward, but valid information on the prevalence of its use remained poorly defined. Obviously, any questions posed to marijuana users would be highly influenced by desires for nondisclosure because of the serious legal consequences of marijuana use.

Table 11 contains a potted history of marijuana law in the United States, presented in part by Dr. David Allen.

Table 11. A history of principal events in the United States that shaped the history of marijuana use to a major degree (adapted from David B. Allen's "A History of Marijuana Law in the United States," http://cannabisdigest.ca/history-marijuana-law-use, June 1, 2014)

- **1937:** Marijuana Tax Act Passes. Harry Anslinger and the Federal Bureau of Narcotics, in the period 1937–39, prosecuted more than three thousand doctors who were American Medical Association (AMA) members for what were considered to be illegal prescriptions of marijuana. This resulted in the AMA removing cannabis from the national pharmacopoeia.
- **1938:** The La Guardia Report indicated, "the catastrophic effects of marijuana smoking are unfounded."
- **1939:** The great crackdown on US physicians results in the arrest of about three thousand physicians for prescribing marijuana.
- **1949:** Only three physicians arrested for prescribing marijuana.
- **1967:** Marijuana Tax Act found to be unconstitutional (Judge Timothy Leary).
- **1970:** Under the Richard Nixon era, cannabis is listed as a schedule I drug with no bona fide medical use.
- **1972:** The Schafer Report recommends decriminalizing of "simple possession."
- **Today:** Cannabis legalization for medical use in a couple dozen states and legalization for recreational use in Colorado and Washington state (January 2014), and Oregon, Alaska, and Washington, DC (2015).

David B. Allen, MD, has produced excellent reporting on cannabis use on the website www.cannabisdigest.ca. A revealing comment has been made by Dr. Allen concerning the aphorisms of Harry Anslinger. Dr. Allen states: "Harry Anslinger knew that the key to keeping his miserable bureaucratic job was to prevent any scientist from disproving his disinformation" (David B. Allen, ibid. June 1, 2014).

Mechoulam Wakes the Sleeping Giant

Deserving of the title Father of Cannabis Research, Dr. Raphael Mechoulam, from Israel, started his groundbreaking studies on marijuana approximately fifty years ago. In the early 1960s, Dr. Mechoulam determined the structure of cannabidiol (CBD) and discovered the presence of delta-9-tetrahydrocannabinol (THC). It was recognized that THC was the psychoactive ingredient of marijuana, and further scientific studies cast light on the presence of cannabinoid receptors and the endocannabinoid pathways (systems) in the body. It was Dr. Mechoulam who woke the sleeping giant of marijuana.

Dr. R. Mechoulam and other researchers continued to isolate many compounds from the cannabis plant. These days it is known that at least 480 natural substances are present in cannabis, and more than sixty (up to one hundred) of these compounds are cannabinoids and their metabolites. These mixtures of cannabinoids are unique to the cannabis plant, and they work together, in an entourage effect, with a degree of synergy that appears to be superior to their effects when they are used in an isolated manner. Table 12 shows many natural components of cannabis, present in varying amounts. This information is subject to much further review in this book.

Table 12. Some natural substances in cannabis (modified from CNN Health, Sanjay Gupta, MD, 2014)

Delta 9 tetrahydrocannabinol
Cannabigerols (CBG)
Cannabichromenes (CBC)
Other Cannabidiols (CBD)
Other Tetrahydrocannabinols (THC)
Cannabinol (CBN) and cannabinodiol (CBDL)
Other cannabinoids (such as cannabicyclol [CBL], cannabielsoin [CBE], cannabitriol [CBT] and other miscellaneous types)
Other constituents of the cannabis plant are nitrogenous compounds (27 known), amino acids (18), proteins (3), glycoproteins (6), enzymes (2), sugars and related compounds (34, hydrocarbons (50), simple alcohols (7), aldehydes (13), ketones (13), simple acids (21), fatty acids (22), simple esters (12), lactones (1), steroids (11), terpenes (120), noncannabinoid phenols (25), flavonoids (21), vitamins (1), pigments (2), and other elements (9).

An inspection of the components of cannabis listed in table 11 shows how complex it is to isolate and characterize different biologically active substances from the marijuana plant. Moreover, some of the cannabinoids are metabolic end products or artifacts, produced by measurement techniques. More research is needed to define the actions of cannabinoids and further postulate or demonstrate how they work in a synergistic, antagonistic, or cooperative manner. As mentioned earlier, drugs made from individual components of marijuana (e.g., Marinol, pure synthetic THC) do not have the same wide-ranging effects on the body in comparison with whole herbal cannabis, with its entourage actions.

Several scientists have focused on the entourage effect, where it is recognized that the real thing (herbal marijuana) outperforms single or simple groups of isolated components of marijuana on a changing variety of body functions. When it comes to prescribed forms of THC, many patients tend to prefer the effects or perceived benefits of the whole herbal preparation of cannabis. To explore an analogous circumstance in general health management, there have been many discussions of reductionism in nutrition, where isolated or limited mixtures of nutrients (e.g., as found in some dietary supplements) are not perceived to be as effective as whole food sources of mixed vitamins or botanicals. A similar circumstance holds true for the effects of cannabis. The single drug/single receptor approach to disease has a demonstrated therapeutic inadequacy in a variety of circumstances.

The Cannabis High

The most common reason for cannabis use is to achieve psychoactive effects that amount to the high feelings. Many descriptions of the status of being high with cannabis exist in popular and medical literature. Table 13 summarizes key characteristics of the high status that is achievable with THC-containing cannabis and some cannabis analogues (drugs and synthetic pot).

Table 13. The variable outcomes and aspects of a marijuana high

• The "giggles" or a relaxed feeling	• Lack of concentration
• Euphoria	• Disruption of short-term memory
• Flow of ideas	• Impaired cognitive function
• Hallucinations, usually mild	• Music appreciation
• Sensation of "time expansion"	• Sensitivity to stimuli
• Lightheadedness, floating sensations	• Appetite increase and food interest
• Variable sexual arousal or dampening	• Aggression or passivism

The sociobehavioral effects of cannabis are quite variable. Important contributions to the psychological effects of marijuana have been referred to as the "set and setting" circumstances. In brief, individuals can magnify their mood with cannabis. If they are feeling down, they can develop amplified downer feelings. Reverse effects can sometimes occur if mood is depressed. However, these effects are not predictable. Other factors operate on changes in psychological status, such as dosage, personality, concomitant drug use, and several physiological variables.

The Whitey: A Bad Trip

It is stated often that overdose deaths do not occur from cannabis or delta-9-tetrahydrocannibol (THC). This situation is explained by its low acute toxicity and low density of cannabinoid receptors in the brain stem, where vital body functions are often controlled. On the other hand, long-term heavy use of cannabis has negative sequelae that are sometimes claimed to be uncertain in their causal association with cannabis consumption. Excessive intake of cannabis can result in nausea, vomiting, increased heart rate, mood changes, sedation, impaired coordination, and occasional hallucinations. Chronic effects of cannabis on memory, IQ, and brain morphology (structure) are hotly debated.

There is an uncommon circumstance of cannabis overdose that results in severe and complex influences that is termed a "whitey" or "bad trip" or "negative ride." With the whitey, the victim develops several unpleasant physical and psychological effects, including nausea, vomiting, anxiety, sometimes together with a paranoid or catatonic state. Cardiorespiratory symptoms sometimes occur with effects of sedation or excess periods of energy. The whitey experience is infrequently associated with hallucinations and acute mental breakdown that is fortunately reversible. If this experience occurs, individuals are advised to seek urgent medical care, but symptoms are often temporary, and they resolve spontaneously. The afflicted person with the whitey should be placed in a safe environment and monitored.

Cannabis and Coffee and Alcohol

Cannabis smokers have learned that coffee drinking can result in an extension of a cannabis high. The same may be true of caffeinated energy drinks. Experiments in animals seem to suggest that memory problems resulting from THC consumption may actually be made worse by caffeine. Surveys have shown common mixing of caffeine intake with cannabis use in college students. This circumstance of memory reduction could result in decreased intellectual performance. Another concern is that THC-containing beverages may be laced with caffeine, resulting in uncertain effects on cognition. Mixing energy drinks or other caffeinated drinks with cannabis is not a good idea.

The reason for these caffeine/cannabis reactions rests in the knowledge that caffeine and cannabis alter dopamine neurotransmitter functions, notably in the thalamus and striatum of the brain. It appears likely that caffeine may influence the response of CB-1 receptors to THC, but mechanisms of these effects remain uncertain. It is clear that combined alcohol and cannabis consumption may compound each other's adverse central nervous system effects.

The Dopamine Reward System

Research conducted by NIDA (National Institute on Drug Abuse) in laboratory animals indicates that stimulation of glutamate neurons in the brain (dorsal raphe nucleus) results in activation of dopamine-containing neurons. These neurons play a role in the brain's reward system. Dopamine and glutamate are neurotransmitters with specific effects (table 14).

Table 14. Actions of dopamine and glutamate. Glutamate is commonly considered to be excitatory, and dopamine is referred to in a popular manner as the pleasure neurotransmitter. A number of drugs of abuse increase brain dopamine concentrations. Cannabis promotes dopamine availability.

Substance	Actions
Glutamate	• neural communication
	• memory formation
	• learning
dopamine	• emotion
	• motivation
	• control of movement
	• feelings of pleasure

The researchers at NIDA who were involved in these studies have presented evidence that there is a reward pathway in the brain that is initiated in the dorsal raphe nucleus and ends with the activation of the dopamine reward system. This study is particularly important because it casts light on the control of motivation, which can be replaced by an antimotivational syndrome in some cannabis users. Again, the cannabis paradox appears.

The Responsible Use of Cannabis

Many institutions, researchers, and agencies are still developing guidelines for the responsible use of cannabis, but the recreational cannabis user often has a lukewarm feeling about these efforts. As stated repeatedly, the prohibition of cannabis use has not worked, resulting in its status as the most widely abused illicit drug on a global basis. Medical experts and others have stressed the value of taking standardized preparations of marijuana that are produced with good growing and manufacturing practices (GMP). However, in places where cannabis has been used in a relatively unencumbered manner for years (e.g., a decade in Holland), surveys show that there is a tendency for people to actually prefer street sources of the drug. This preference has been driven by several factors, including economics. The high cost of legal marijuana is driven by both taxation and high margin on its sale. A secondary contribution to cannabis use involves the selection of high-THC-containing cannabis (e.g., skunk). This skunk-like type of cannabis is called "Made in England." The UK is the principal source of skunk.

The notions that cannabis is the cat out of the bag and that Pandora's box is open are reasonable assumptions in modern society in the United States. I have no doubt that with future vigilance and inevitable further political legislation, the legal landscape of cannabis use may have to change. At present, we have a difficult circumstance where there is no consensus on the clinical recommendations for the monitoring of individuals taking medical cannabis. Furthermore, health care practitioners who can monitor medical cannabis intake in an accomplished manner are in the minority. Despite the residual arguments on the ability of cannabis to induce tolerance or result in drug dependence and drug abuse, it is clear that marijuana should be made available to the public with some warnings and precautions for its use. Appropriate labeling has helped to prevent childhood use of cannabis. At present, this responsible disclosure is not always made on labels of cannabis product sold in legalized states. I submit, again, that at the time of writing, this is a neglected area that must be addressed, especially in the zones of the recreational use of cannabis. This is important from a public health perspective, and the responsibility for this activity now rests with state governments.

Forward-looking individuals have discussed preventive-medicine strategies to address some of the anticipated problems of the more widespread use of cannabis. In fact, post-legalization monitoring strategies have been put in place (to an inadequate degree) in Washington state, Colorado, Alaska, Oregon, and Washington, DC. Primary prevention of cannabis use has not worked with prohibition. This situation could have been anticipated as a consequence of the precedent set by the failure of alcohol prohibition. Secondary prevention of cannabis-related problems would involve the early diagnosis of cannabis abuse or dependence and intervention with treatment. This should occur at a time when prognosis for recovery remains favorable. This approach has been suggested for different types of drug abuse (notably alcohol), and it has some potential merit in attempting to reduce the prevalence of cannabis use in problematic circumstances. Literature on prevention of alcohol abuse supports this contention. (Holt, S., Skinner, H.A., Israel, Y., "Identification of alcohol abuse, II, Clinical and laboratory indicators," *Canadian Medical Association Journal* 124, no. 10 (1981): 1279–94. Holt, S., Skinner, H.A., "Confronting Alcoholism," *Canadian Medical Association Journal* 51 (1990): 8–9. Holt, S., "Tackling the alcohol problem: the case for secondary prevention," *Journal of the South Carolina Medical Association* 85, no. 12 (1989): 582–4.)

It seems important to construct a valid series of measures of physical and sociobehavioral consequences of cannabis abuse that can be placed into screening instruments that have a high level of diagnostic discrimination for the identification of cannabis abuse. The concept of the occult cannabis abuser is not as well defined as the occult alcohol abuser, but a growth in the prevalence of the hidden marijuana abuser can be anticipated, especially with the increasing recreational use of cannabis. For example, the use of cannabis with a vaporizer is seen as a major advantage by users to disguise cannabis use compared with smoking. Despite the spread of legalization of cannabis use, the users may still feel stigmatized by a substantial part of society. Use detection is required in children.

While many people ponder the future of the widespread availability of cannabis in the United States, it seems quite reasonable to present several precautions and warnings for cannabis use (especially in children and adolescents). Increasing knowledge about the health-challenging consequences of cannabis use in adults and teenagers will help in the self-identification and self-intervention for cannabis-related physical and medical disorders (hopefully before they become established). Vigilance over cannabis use will be improved if circumstances that present potential danger are identified by both health care workers and individuals who opt for the cannabis lifestyle. This situation can only be achieved if education on cannabis use is increased.

A list of medical circumstances that present a higher risk/benefit ratio of marijuana use are detailed below (table 15), (derived from "Information used for Healthcare Professionals, Cannabis and the Cannabinoids," *Health Canada*, Feb. 2013, senior author: Hanan Abramovici). This document is one of the best sources of general medical information that has been relied upon for content when writing parts of this book (Abramovici, ibid. 2013). Childhood (adolescent) use of cannabis must be controlled because of the magnified adverse effects of the drug on mental health and persistent developmental problems in these younger age groups.

Table 15. Medical circumstances creating a high risk/benefit ratio for cannabis use (modified from Abramovici et al., ibid. 2013)

- **Cardiorespiratory disease can be exacerbated by cannabis smoking.** The cardiovascular consequence of cannabis use involves the precipitation of tachycardia and low or high blood pressure. Cannabis use may result coronary artery spasm and myocardial infarction in susceptible individuals. Asthma may be made worse (or better) by cannabis smoking. Smoking cannabis may also result in aggravation of chronic obstructive airways disease and chest infections. Arguably, cannabis causes bullous lung disease.

- **Cannabis is best avoided in individuals with severe renal or hepatic disease.** Chronic hepatitis C combined with cannabis use appears to often result in worsening of hepatic steatosis (or fibrosis), but some opinions differ.

- **The presence of psychiatric disorders** such as psychotic reactions or a family history of such disorders (e.g., schizophrenia) are often viewed as a contraindication to cannabis use. However, cannabis has been used in psychiatric illness with variable benefits (e.g., CBD use in schizophrenia).

- While cannabis has shown some promise in the **treatment of substance abuse,** involving alcohol or other drugs, its use in these circumstances has to be carefully monitored. Cannabis is a gateway drug in some individuals, with a contribution to graduation from soft to hard drugs.

- **Patients with major depression, mania, and significant mood disturbance** should be monitored with care when they use cannabis. There is sometimes a compounded risk of suicide.

- **Cannabis is potentially dangerous in pregnancy, and it may be associated with birth defects.** Women of childbearing age should be taking an effective contraceptive when using cannabis, and its use should be avoided completely in pregnancy, with breastfeeding and in women planning pregnancy.

- **Cannabis has drug interaction potential,** and it is especially important to exercise caution if sedative, hypnotic, or other psychoactive drugs are consumed with cannabis.

Any individual who takes cannabis for the first time should seek reasonable supervision, even if such supervision involves adult, non-health care workers. There are many circumstances where warnings about cannabis use should be made as a consequence of the presence of the psychoactive cannabinoid, THC. One may infer the nature of many of these warnings, because cannabis may cause memory impairment, cognitive decline, altered mood or perceptions, poor judgment, decreased controls of impulsive behavior, and so forth. Special guidelines for the use of cannabis that act as warnings include discussions about dosing, the precipitation of anxiety or psychosis, motor vehicle accidents, occupational hazards, use in pregnancy or lactation, and effects on fertility. Excellence in cannabis labeling practices is required, and this is an important public health initiative that can prevent cannabis exposure in children. Cartoonlike labeling attracts kids! These items are summarized in table 16 below and will be covered in greater detail in subsequent sections of this book.

Table 16. A summary of the principal warnings that may be considered for individuals who wish to engage in the responsible use of cannabis

I think that this list of warnings can be given to a cannabis user with obvious benefits.

Warning	Comment
Dosing	Gauging the dosage of cannabinoids from smoking is notoriously difficult, and it is dependent on smoking methods. Cannabis users are advised to smoke or use vaporized cannabis in a slow incremental manner while they attempt to monitor effects on themselves (the self-titration paradigm). The effects of cannabis edibles usually have an onset greater than thirty minutes or longer following their consumption (up to two hours). Rapid or slow gastric emptying may alter peak blood concentrations of ingested cannabinoids. It may be easier to overdose on edibles as a consequence of delayed onset of actions, which results in many adverse symptoms and signs (e.g., cardiovascular responses or severe psychological changes, etc.).
Psychosis and Anxiety	It is strongly advised that a person who develops a psychotic or a severe emotional reaction (excessive anxiety or panic attacks) to cannabis use should attend an emergency medical facility. The features of psychosis include disorganized behavior, suicidal thoughts, loss of contact with reality, hallucinations, memory loss, delusions, and so forth.
Motor Vehicle Use and Occupational Hazards	Mental alertness and coordination are impaired by cannabis use for variable periods of time, sometimes up to twenty-four hours in duration. Alcohol and cannabis use act to fragment many functions of the brain when intoxication by the drug is present. Individuals who continue to deny that cannabis causes fatalities must consider motor vehicle and occupational accidents as potential causes of death (which may be secondary occurrences following cannabis use).

Pregnancy and Lactation	Cannabinoids are able to be detected in maternal milk, and they are absorbed by the neonate. It appears that maternal endocannabinoids affect fertilization, implantation of the embryo, oviductal transport, and both fetal and placental development. Some evidence of long-term damage to the fetus by cannabis exists. This is manifest as childhood learning and developmental problems.

This section of the book is very important for the cannabis user and health care giver who have a joint responsibility for safe drug use. The information provided is relevant to all contexts of the use of cannabis, including recreational and medical applications. Also, it has relevance to the use of cannabis-based pharmaceuticals that are approved for medical use (or close to approval in the United States). Common examples of these substances (drugs) include nabilone (Cesamet), nabiximols (Sativex), and dronabinol (Marinol).

Much information on the adverse effects of cannabis ingestion comes from its recreational use, but the side effects of cannabis drugs (analogues) are beginning to be encountered and monitored increasingly in clinical trials. However, these trials tend to permit only short-term observations of drug effects. There is much less information available on the long-term effects of cannabis use. An analysis of adverse effects of cannabinoids used in medicinal compounds indicates the potential occurrence of psychiatric problems, mixed problems with brain function, gastrointestinal disorders, cardiorespiratory problems, and so forth. Mixed drug use is often encountered in association with taking cannabis. Therefore, it is sometimes difficult to separate problems caused by cannabis per se from problems caused by the concomitant use of alcohol, tobacco, and other illicit drugs. A popular gateway jump is from cannabis to cocaine.

Stephen Holt, MD, DSc

Medical School Teaching about Cannabis

In the presence of increased use of cannabis and a large body of published research, it is argued that most doctors of medicine have a poor general knowledge about this substance. What is the root cause of this ignorance? For many years, cannabis has not been on the medical radar screen because of long-standing prohibition. However, long-standing prohibition did not stop significant usage of cannabis. Recent studies involving a survey of 157 American medical schools showed variable acceptance of the science of the endocannabinoid system and its relevance to medical education. This survey revealed that not one school that was surveyed taught science of the endocannabinoid system in an organized course (www.cannabisdigest.ca/survey-endocannabinoid-system-medical schools/). Fortunately, these circumstances are changing.

The researchers performing this survey on medical education encountered much resistance in deriving data from university staff (administration and teachers) due to reluctance to answer questions and suspicions about the intent of the questions. This raises support for obvious conclusions that there is not only widespread lack of knowledge on cannabis by practicing physicians, but the medical doctors of the future may remain somewhat ignorant on the subject without extra structured education. This is a very serious problem in medical education, given the common and increasing use of cannabis.

Fortunately, an increasing number of teaching seminars on cannabis science have been developed in recent times. However, there is a lack of knowledge about cannabis among many sectors of the public. This situation has been somewhat matched with prevailing medical ignorance about this important subject. At the end of this book is a cannabis quiz to help reinforce learning. Do we have a significant number of uninformed physicians with the granted authority of issuing medical cannabis prescriptions or recommending cards for medical use in states where medical marijuana is legalized? Unfortunately, yes! This situation has to change.

Should Cannabis Be Sold or Prescribed with Warnings?

It is clear that cannabis poses a number of areas of potential health concerns, as do many over-the-counter or prescription drugs or herbal products. These days, consumers of medicine are exposed to long lists of warnings for use and potential side effects of drugs, but such warnings are notably absent from many marijuana products sold in legal dispensaries in Colorado, Washington state, Alaska, Oregon, and Washington, DC. In my recent trips to several Colorado dispensaries, I heard a constant message about the benefits of cannabis from salespeople. While this is to be expected, any requests that I made about recommendations for the safe use of cannabis resulted in frequent jaw dropping.

Regulatory bodies demand that potentially adverse circumstances of pharmaceutical treatments should be disclosed to the general public. While a responsibility exists with health care practitioners to promote the safe use of medication, the patient has to accept some responsibility for deriving knowledge about the potential adverse effects of medication that he or she uses. I trust that much of the information provided in this book helps with the responsible and safe use of cannabis.

There is an emerging but inadequate attempt in pharmacies and cannabis-dispensing sites to disclose potential adverse effects of cannabis, but, as noted earlier, disclosures are sometimes incomplete. Table 17 summarizes adverse effects of cannabis and warnings to be taken into account with its use. However, cannabinoids are considered to be relatively safe when used for specific conditions at average recommended dosages, even though dosages of many marijuana preparations are not clear. In brief, cannabis can affect almost every organ system in the body (table 17).

Table 17. Risks and warnings about cannabis use

Arguments prevail about the prevalence and severity of adverse effects associated with marijuana (cannabis) use. Modified from information provided by Mayo Clinic online. Evidence to support correlated or associated disorders is highly variable. It is clear that correlated occurrences of problems are not evidence of direct causal links, which can only be shown by prospective/longitudinal research studies.

Effects on the Body	Comment
Allergies including rashes, asthma, nasal congestion	Avoidance is necessary with history of allergies to the Cannabaceae family of plants.
Dizziness	Most often caused by THC in cannabis.
Lowering of blood-alcohol levels	Variable effect of CBD.
Increased risk of bleeding	Interaction with anticoagulants and caution in individuals with disorders of bleeding.
Altered blood-glucose levels, lowering blood glucose	May affect diabetic control, requires medical supervision.
Low blood pressure	Results in dizziness and potential for loss of consciousness (fainting).
Alters actions of cytochrome P450 enzyme systems that metabolize drugs	Blood levels of certain drugs may increase. Metabolic drug interactions.
Alters estrogen metabolism	May need monitoring and recognition of potential interactions with hormone-replacement therapies.
Caution in immune deficiency	May contribute to diminished immune function but may in some circumstances boost or assist immune function.

Contribution to enhanced or reduced actions of other drugs (e.g., barbiturates, antipsychotic medications, CNS depressants, p-glycoprotein-regulated drugs)	Drug interactions variable, may contribute to drug side effects.
Caution in individuals with a present or past history of addictions or drug abuse	Marijuana may cause psychological and physical dependence (addiction). Evidence exists that it is gateway drug that can promote the use of hard drugs in susceptible individuals (e.g., cocaine).
Eye problems	While cannabis has been used to treat glaucoma (high pressure in the eye), it can sometimes increase eye pressure. Pink and dry eyes with altered vision are common in marijuana smokers. This is the appearance of being "banged up."
Caution for use in seizure disorders or in individuals taking antiseizure medication	Marijuana may treat seizures, but it can also precipitate seizures in certain circumstances.
Cardiovascular disease: cautions	Marijuana may cause tachycardia, abnormal heartbeats (arrhythmias), disrupted blood flow to organs and the extremities, coronary artery spasm, heart attack, and it can contribute to cardiac failure.
Cautions for use in individuals with ADHD and learning disabilities	Cannabis causes problems with learning, attentiveness, memory, organizational skills, and other mental tasks. Cannabis may improve or sometimes exacerbate ADHD.
May worsen several skin conditions	May cause hives, rashes, mouth irritations, and increase or decrease pruritus (itching).

Digestive disorders	Cannabis may cause dental problems, halitosis, foul tastes, burning or swelling of the tongue, diarrhea, dry mouth (exacerbating tooth decay), indigestion, nausea, abdominal pain, and vomiting.
Caution in presence of arthritis or musculoskeletal disorders	Marijuana may have adverse effects on bone structure as a result of long-term administration. It can contribute to falls and injuries, cause muscle pain, cause twitching, abnormal coordination, and restlessness.
Drowsiness, sedation, status of being "stoned"	Obvious avoidance of driving and operating machinery necessary. May contribute to workplace and recreational accidents.
General, nonspecific symptoms	May cause disorientation, behavioral disturbances, headaches, excessive fatigue, reduced attention span, and so forth.
Pregnancy, breastfeeding, or intentions to become pregnant	Complete abstinence from cannabis is required in pregnancy and during breastfeeding. Associations described with some fetal abnormalities and low birth weight or other developmental disorders.
Lung disease	Claims that cannabis smoking is not a cause of lung disease are questioned. While cannabis has been used to treat asthma, smoking may precipitate bronchoconstriction (asthma). Marijuana smoking often results in coughing and extra phlegm production (irritant bronchitis). An increased prevalence of lung cancer in cannabis smokers is hypothesized and likely, but it is not confirmed. Cannabis smokers are often tobacco smokers.

Mental illness	The possibility of exacerbating or precipitating abnormal psychiatric status is a significant problem (e.g., psychosis).
Miscellaneous potential problems with cannabis use	Street cannabis-derived substances are very dangerous if injected. Marijuana may be associated with burning sensations in different parts of the body, arteritis, changes in erectile function, changes in overall quality of life, confusion, other mental aberrations, and alterations in body weight.

Cannabis Use Disorder

There have been debates about the precise definition of cannabis use disorder (CUD). While CUD and cannabis dependence may have similarities, they may require different types of treatment interventions. In brief, cannabis dependence syndrome has a succinct description provided by the World Health Organization, summarized as "reported use of cannabinoids that typically includes a strong desire to take the drug, difficulties in controlling its use, persistent use despite harmful consequences, a higher priority given to drug use than to other activities and obligations, increased tolerance, and sometimes a physical withdrawal state." (1CD/10/description)

In contrast, the characteristics described for making the diagnosis of CUD include complex clinical descriptions that are summarized in the Diagnostic Criteria of the American Psychiatric Association (APA). While these APA criteria for CUD are of great importance to clinicians in health care, they are useful for providing some insight for patients into problems that can develop. However, it is *not* advisable for individuals to make a self-diagnosis of CUD because recognizing this disorder by the afflicted individual is often inaccurate. All illicit substance abusers are inclined to use the mental dynamisms of denial, projection, and rationalization. It is known that an accurate diagnosis of CUD requires assessment by a qualified health care giver. In the absence of such an individual, special questionnaires or computer-assisted interrogation may be valuable in diagnosis. (Holt, S., et al, "Computer assessment of lifestyle in a gastroenterology clinic," *Digestive Diseases and Sciences* 37, no. 7 (1987): 993–996.)

The characteristics of CUD proposed by the APA are defined in some detail with a description of anticipated consequences. A diagnosis of cannabis use disorder permits some disease-outcome predictions that result from long-term heavy cannabis use. These predictions include a high probability of disinhibition, resulting in abnormal behavior with intoxication, impaired vehicle operations, poor impulse control, risk-taking behavior, and irresponsible actions. Other predicted problems with a medium probability of occurrence include academic or vocational failures linked to impaired memory and motivation, cognitive problems, occasional severe adverse effects such as psychosis precipitation, tendencies for social withdrawal, child neglect, denial, projection and rationalization, together with a tendency for poor self-care habits.

Assessments for Cannabis Use Disorders

Several screening methods and diagnostic instruments have been applied in the detection of CUD. That said, many individuals who are heavy consumers of cannabis do not often present themselves for help or interventions for excessive cannabis use. The characteristics of CUD often involve an active avoidance of any form of medical intervention. Clearly, cannabis use disorders remain underdiagnosed and somewhat occult. While detection of alcohol problems is sometimes foremost in the minds of clinicians, this is not often the case with marijuana. As repeatedly stressed throughout this book, adolescents who use cannabis have greater risks of future disabilities than adult-onset users. The inference is that assertive attempts must be made to identify and intervene in the young (underage) person who uses cannabis. These methods of secondary prevention in youngsters must be supported by appropriate public health planning with effective interventions.

Jan Bashford, writing from the National Cannabis Prevention and Information Center in Australia, has proposed several important clinical issues and research initiatives that require further study. These issues are summarized in table 18. The scientific review constructed by Jan Bashford has permitted the identification of several research initiatives that are required to further advance the validation and overall value of screening diagnostic methods and assessment tactics for cannabis use. These initiatives are listed below (adapted from J. Bashford online, retrieved 2014). The following approaches may reduce harm from cannabis use.

Table 18. Clinical practice recommendations that may assist in harm reduction (adapted from Bashford, J., www.ncpic/staticpdfs/backgroundpapers.com)

- definition of the practical applications of tools for cannabis screening and assessment
- assessment of validity of diagnostic or detection tools
- applications of screening in high-risk groups
- impact of screening and assessment methods on interventions
- routine screening for cannabis use in young people (adolescents and teenagers)
- sound preintervention assessment for cannabis use problems
- early or brief interventions applied with preclinical cannabis problems or risky patterns of use
- the detection of comorbid and psychiatric disorders of major importance in cannabis use assessments
- the formation of therapeutic alliances, a key role in cannabis use problems

The legalization of cannabis for medical and recreational purposes has stimulated opinions that recommendations for harm reduction of cannabis are outdated and superfluous. However, I believe that the reader should be exposed to opinions about cannabis use, even if such opinions are perceived to be superfluous or dated. In my opinion, harm reduction by avoidance of cannabis is a high priority for some users of cannabis, especially youngsters and individuals at high risks of heavy, chronic cannabis use.

Medicinal and Street Cannabis

Standards for the use of prescription-grade cannabis are still evolving in many countries, but they have been present in several European countries for about a decade, most notably in the Netherlands. The government in the Netherlands (Holland) passed legislation in 2003 for medical-grade cannabis to be dispensed in pharmacies, and law enforcement in Holland has shown tolerance for cannabis use for about ten years or so. With recent legalization of cannabis (recreational and medical) in Colorado, Washington state, Alaska, Oregon, and Washington, DC, many people are attempting to forecast the challenges and problems that will occur with greater amounts of cannabis intake and its more widespread use. It is believed that much can be learned from some of the outcomes or problems that have been experienced with the long-term apparent legalization of cannabis in places such as the Netherlands.

While the Dutch Office of Medicinal Cannabis (OMC) supervises the production of cannabis plant material to produce products with pharmaceutical standards, Holland has an intricate chain of channels of distribution of illicit cannabis, most often found in coffeeshops. As mentioned, the illicit use of cannabis is well tolerated by law enforcement and regulatory affairs in the Netherlands. Herbal cannabis comes in many varieties for recreational and medicinal uses in Holland, and a large tourist industry for cannabis use exists.

Inevitably, users of cannabis (marijuana) in Holland have compared the price and perceived qualities of coffeeshop versus OMC (regulated) types of cannabis. From studies of the experiences of the users of both types of cannabis (street forms and OMC-approved cannabis), it has been concluded often by the user that coffeeshop cannabis is more attractive for recreational and even medicinal use, largely due to its cheaper prices and perceived effects. This situation of a preference for illicit cannabis use could occur in the United States as certain states gear up taxation policies for cannabis and the illicit market focuses on improving the quality or enhancing the psychoactive effects of cannabis.

Studies show that users of herbal cannabis in Holland may not perceive a clear difference between OMC-approved and coffee shop types of herbal marijuana. Consumers of cannabis may even conclude that cheaper material (herbal street cannabis) has the best quality with an economic advantage. Of course, the reality is that street cannabis does not have the production quality and standardization of OMC-approved cannabis products. Clearly, the performance of the street cannabis due to its THC content is an attractive attribute because most consumers are looking for a high.

Overall, the assessment of the quality of cannabis products by reasonably stringent oversight and testing by the OMC in Holland does not seem to be foremost in the mind of many Dutch consumers of cannabis. Nor does it seem to impress them. There is no doubt that the maintenance of quality standards in medicinal cannabis involves repeated analytic testing, which is an expensive but safe pathway for approved cannabis use, compared with street or coffeeshop cannabis. Thus, perceptions, selections, and choices by consumers may favor a move in the future to support the sale of illicit cannabis in the United States This seems likely to occur at the expense of sales of government or institutionally approved cannabis products, which are arguably too expensive.

It is clear in Holland that comparisons of the contents between street cannabis and available medicinal (OMC-approved) cannabis show that there is a public health risk with the sale of unregulated cannabis. This risk involves the common contamination of herbal cannabis (street drug, herbal cannabis) with pesticides, fungicides, heavy metals, infectious organisms, or deliberate adulterants. A range of deliberate adulterants may show up in street cannabis, such as different herbal mixtures or spiking agents that can enhance the acute psychological reactions of marijuana (e.g.,

K-2, spice, etc.) and other compounds. These compounds are described inaccurately as synthetic cannabinoids. These spiking substances are often toxic, especially for the uninitiated user. They are *not* naturally occurring phytocannabinoids.

Obviously, the informed consumer would be expected to select government-approved sources of cannabis, which would be anticipated to be safer than street cannabis, but studies of the active biological components of cannabis (cannabinoids) are quite similar, or as potent, in street and regulated forms of whole cannabis. Therefore, the perceived or actual effectiveness of cannabis may be indistinguishable between the pharmaceutical-controlled varieties of cannabis and its cousins, the street forms. I believe that this information on differences between cannabis of different origins is highly relevant in assisting consumers to make safe and informed choices that will serve to enhance public safety.

Some users of cannabis are alarmed by the use of gamma radiation in the necessary sterilization of cannabis, but studies of microbial contamination of street types of herbal cannabis show potential contamination with intestinal bacteria and fungi (Penicillium, Cladosporum, and Aspergillus). Certain of these microbes can produce dangerous exotoxins and mycotoxins (e.g., Aflatoxin, Ochratoxin A and B, and Sterigmatocystin). Gamma radiation used for the sterilization of cannabis is generally perceived as safe and necessary.

Aflatoxins are potent carcinogens, and other fungal toxins may be responsible for neurological toxicity of some street forms of cannabis. The microbial content of nonsterilized cannabis is highly problematic in patients who have immune deficiency (e.g., HIV or AIDS) because of their increased susceptibility to opportunistic infections in states of immune deficiency. Moreover, microbial agents such as Aspergillus make significant contributions to illness from opportunistic lung infection in immunodeficient individuals. A number of clinical observations imply that medical application of cannabis that originates from uncontrolled or illegal sources appears to be a significant health risk. This health risk would expect to be magnified in people who consume large amounts of street (uncontrolled) cannabis on a regular basis. Thus, there is a real dose-dependent health risk of certain types of street cannabis, especially those types that are spiked with synthetic pot or contaminated with microorganisms or toxins.

Cannabis and Opioid Use and Abuse

The past decade has witnessed an alarming increase in fatalities from opiate overdose. Over this period the Centers for Disease Control and Prevention reports a five-fold increase in deaths from opiate overdose in females and a three-fold increase in males. The magnitude of this problem is large, thereby creating major public health concerns. For several years, the number of deaths in women from opioid overdosing has exceeded the number of fatalities from motor vehicle injuries. Recent data shows that the states with legalization of medical marijuana (cannabis) appear to have lower death rates from oxycodone, opioid drugs, morphine-like compounds, and heroin. This association may be causal.

An important clinical proposal is that cannabis can provide effective pain relief without the need to rely heavily on opioids and similar drugs. At least, cannabis can reduce the required dosage of analgesics for pain relief because of its synergistic effects with opioids. The real danger with opioid overdosing is suppression of breathing, which is very uncommon with marijuana use. As mentioned earlier, this is perhaps due, in part, to the lower density of cannabinoid receptors in the brain stem, where breathing and vital body functions are controlled.

The Cannabis (THC) Sequence of Effects

There is an important sequence of events when THC gets into the brain. This sequence is illustrated below:

Entrance of THC to the brain>	Euphoria "Reward system Stimulation">	Dopamine release cause "pleasure">
Relaxation commonly > but several other effects may occur, e.g. heightened sensory perception	Euphoria subsides > individual may be sleepy with a depressed mood.	In some cases anxiety, fear, distrust or pain may occur.

Coincidental with the above progression of events is reduced ability to form memories or engage in mental agility, which may be compromised in combination with learning disabilities. The above noted effects are a consequence of THC content of marijuana.

Hash Oil (Hashish)

Hashish is a word derived from Arabic that means "grass," but this assertion has been disputed. It is made efficiently from purified preparations of glandular hairs of the cannabis plant, called trichomes. These trichomes are mixed with varying amounts of flowers and leaves to produce "good smokeable pot." The resulting plant material is separated often by mechanical means, using a sieve or iced water, and it forms a powder that is called kief. Compression and heating of kief results in the production of solid or heavy (thick) liquid forms of hashish. Hashish and tobacco are often smoked together.

Solvent extraction of resins can be produced using alcohol or hexane in which the fat-loving substances (lipophilic material) can be made soluble. Various methods of further extraction involve processes of evaporation to produce hash oil (also known as "honey oil"). The manufacturing processes used in the production of hashish or hash oil are potentially quite dangerous when flammable materials are used. These production processes have caused accidents and explosions that have resulted in serious injury or death.

The major reason for hash or hash oil production is to concentrate tetrahydrocannabinol (THC), in order to produce a potent preparation with strong psychoactive properties Many variations in the source of material and techniques of preparation can be used. Thus, hash preparations have varying potencies, with THC contents up to 90 percent. Unfortunately, adulterants are sometimes added to hash, resulting in high risks of toxicity.

In common with cannabis, hashish use affects memory, judgment, learning, and attentiveness (table 19). It seems that hashish is recognized to have some different and often more pronounced effects than regular cannabis, probably because of its increased content of THC.

Table 19. Effects of hashish or hash oil use, which may sometimes occur more often with greater severity than with the use of regular, whole, herbal cannabis

• Anxiety	• Panic attacks
• Disorientation	• Emotional reactions
• Learning problems	• Poor attention span
• Psychotic reactions	• Fatigue
• Paranoia	• Poor coordination
• Loss of motivation	• Lung disorders
• Confusion	• Distorted body perceptions

Hash is arguably not safe, and it is illegal in many locations in the United States. Hashish and hash oil are consumed in a variety of ways (different delivery methods), including smoking, dabbing, vaporization, and eating. Hash oil is administered often by dabbing oil material onto a hot surface, which forms a vapor that can be directed through a water pipe into the recipient's lungs. The author makes no recommendations to use hash in any form.

Cannabinoid-like Substances in Other Plants?

Cannabinoids are discussed most often as though they are exclusive to the genus of Cannabis plants. However, compounds with cannabinoid-like effects are present in other plants. Alkamides (alkylamides) are found in species of Echinacea (purpurea, angustifolia, and pallida), and they can interact with CB-2 receptors (cannabinoid receptors). Moreover, catechins (found in Camellia sinensis) and yangonin (present in Kava kava) can interact with human cannabinoid receptors. Other plant sources of cannabinoid-like compounds are present in Acmella oleracea and Radula marginata. The effects of these noncannabis types of compounds with cannabinoid-like activity are not fully understood or characterized.

Stephen Holt, MD, DSc

Today's Cannabis Is Different from Yesterday's

There is an increasing trend to develop strains of recreational cannabis with a high THC content and low content of CBD. Therefore, it has been proposed that modern cannabis (high THC, low CBD) of today is fundamentally different in its psychoactive effects than cannabis used thirty or more years ago. The significance of this difference in composition is that CBD counteracts some of the psychoactive effects of cannabis (THC). This may result in more balanced effects on the central nervous system. In simple terms, high THC/low CBD forms of cannabis are an apple, and the reverse composition is an orange, when it comes to psychoactive effects.

Some opinions have questioned this modern circumstance of much more potent THC-containing Cannabis sativa plants because early use of female plants (sinsemilla) with high THC concentrations has been recorded. However, some studies in the United States implied that herbal cannabis had a content of 3.4 percent THC and 0.3 percent CBD in 1993, which contrasts with cannabis measured in 2008 with a content of 8.8 percent THC and low CBD (0.4 percent). Other studies have confirmed these types of differences. That said, a popular variety of cannabis with high THC (about 20 percent THC concentration) is called skunk, which often carries a label stating "Made in England." As the name suggests, this type of cannabis has a smell resembling the discharge from a skunk. Toil as we may to make generalized statements on the effects of cannabis use, uncertainty about cannabis composition (cannabinoid content) that is consumed still clouds the picture. This circumstance is not readily avoided even by controlled growing environments and availability of different seeds, especially in homegrown cannabis produce.

Recent studies have claimed to refute some of the evidence that modern cannabis preparations are more potent than cannabis that was used ten to twenty years ago. That said, street cannabis samples that were analyzed in the 1970s and 1980s tended to average about 2–4 percent concentrations of THC. In contrast, modern street types of cannabis that satisfy the habits of recreational users may contain about 14–20 percent concentration of THC. The consequences of general and chronic exposure to higher dosages of THC are not fully understood, but it is generally believed that exposure to THC is greater with contemporary forms of street marijuana.

In the inexperienced user, higher concentrations of THC can result in a greater prevalence of acute adverse reactions. There appear to have been several regional trends in the United States that show a rise in emergency department visits for medical circumstances related to cannabis use, especially overdosing problems in young people. As implied earlier, greater risks for cannabis addiction seem to occur in individuals who consume large amounts of cannabis on a frequent and continuous basis and those who use hashish or synthetic pot. This situation is recognized in Colorado, which has developed recently new legislation to regulate hash use.

Cannabis Legalization and the Black Market

Evidence is mounting that cannabis legalization in the United States has started to damage the black market for cannabis produced in several countries, most notably Mexico and Central America. In these locations, economic influences in the United States have altered profits that can result from cannabis cultivation. It is estimated that the wholesale price of Mexican cannabis has decreased in the past five years by up to 75 percent.

There is clear evidence that American users of cannabis are now buying much more American-grown Cannabis, with a result that Mexican and Central American growers and their drug cartels are feeling the pinch. Studies issued previously by the RAND corporation and the Mexican Competeveness Institute both show that cartel income can be reduced to about one-third as a consequence of American legalization of pot.

Thus, legalization appears to be exerting some favorable effects, at least in cutting down on drug smuggling. Perhaps this success of emerging markets in legal jurisdictions in the United States will prove attractive to foreign drug cartels that could look for participation in the legalized cannabis-growing industry in the United States.

Concerns about the Cannabis Industry

There are signs that all is not well within the rapidly emerging cannabis industry in the United States. A large number of private or public companies are establishing themselves in the industry with positive involvement of investors and good intentions. Several stock market analysts have written about the financial complexities of the cannabis business, and there are concerns about the quality and potential safety of some available dietary supplement products (e.g., CBD-containing substances) that are produced from hemp using poor manufacturing methods. These concerns have emerged against a background of some complaints about specific hemp products that have caused sickness (Martin A. Lee, Director, Project CBD at www.projectcbd.org with publication on Oct. 14, 2014, of "Hemp Hustlers" article).

The quality-assurance procedures placed into the manufacture of dietary supplements (e.g., hemp oil) have been questioned. Some products may be potentially quite toxic due to residual presence of solvents (e.g., hexane), and some have been found to contain an array of toxic heavy metals (e.g., silver, nickel, selenium, molybdenum, and arsenic). Of some concern is the lack of consistency of cannabinoid contents of certain products (especially edibles). In addition, there are some examples of commercially available hemp oil containing as much as 2.5 percent THC (upper limit allowed is 0.3 percent).

To add to these contentions, there have been discussions about poor moral and ethical behavior with financial corruption among executives of a number of small cannabis operations in the United States. No doubt, these overall problems will be dealt with in a process of closer vigilance of cannabis production and sale. These situations create a new task for several state governments. That said, there are excellent manufacturers of cannabis products (e.g., G. W. Pharmaceuticals Ltd., England, UK).

Medicinal Benefits of Cannabis

Favorable opinions on the health benefits of cannabis have recently triggered the escalating medicinal use of cannabis. This situation has been reinforced by favorable reports of the clinical outcome of the treatment of many diseases, even though many of these reports involve anecdotal experiences. Media reports describe thought leaders who have changed their minds about the value of cannabis as a medicinal agent. Most notable among this group is the positive opinion about medical marijuana expressed by the chief medical correspondent of CNN, Dr. Sanjay Gupta. Dr. Gupta has highlighted the fact that until recently only approximately 6 percent of studies examined the health benefits of cannabis. In comparison, there is a much larger amount of research on its adverse effects. This situation has created skewed opinions that influence circumstances in the evaluation of the outcomes of cannabis use.

The health benefits of marijuana use have been summarized in an excellent manner by J. Welsh and K. Loria (www.businessinsider.com/healthbenefits-of-medicalmarijuana-2014). These disease-state or condition-specific applications of cannabis are listed in table 20 below.

Table 20. A list of some of the principal health benefits or positive effects of cannabis (adapted from Welsh, J., Loria, K., www.businessinsider.com)

Disease/Disorder	
• glaucoma relief • lung disorders	• anxiety relief • pain relief / antinausea effects
• epilepsy control	• Alzheimer's disease
• antimetastatic effect	• pain in multiple sclerosis
• hepatitis C benefit	• PTSD
• inflammatory bowel disease	• post-stroke protection
• arthritis • metabolic support	• brain trauma, concussions, anchronic traumatic encephalopathy
• autoimmune disease	• sleep disturbances
• Parkinson's disease	• positive effect on creativity but negative effect on short-term memory

Stephen Holt, MD, DSc

Medicinal Futures of Cannabis

Most people acknowledge that the writing is on the wall concerning the use of herbal cannabis, which is here to stay in the United States. That said, medical cannabis use and further research on new cannabis drugs have produced encouraging results and some concerns. Cannabis contains a highly complex collection of different chemicals with diverse clinical effects. This knowledge has been used to support the preferential use of cannabis (marijuana) in its more natural (whole herbal) form rather than when it is taken as isolated components of the plant (e.g., THC or its analogues or CBD, available alone in certain pharmaceuticals). It appears that the inevitable development of many regulatory-approved pharmaceutical-types of cannabinoid products will occur within five to ten years. Protagonists of cannabis use argue that its safety and effectiveness have been substantiated in a variety of medical or recreational circumstances, but no pharmaceutical agent is completely without adverse effects, especially if used inappropriately. The pundits who gloss over safety issues are misleading the public because, at present, we cannot define many of the potential outcomes of the widespread use of cannabis in society, especially with its long-term use.

Thoughtful physicians and regulators have proposed that the ideal scientific and regulatory approaches to cannabis use should stress that it is shown to be safe and effective for each of the indications for which it is considered to have potential benefit. The emerging legislation that governs marijuana availability makes these prudent approaches in approval processes appear impractical or of diminished importance, and they are claimed by some to be increasingly redundant. These circumstances have generated much disagreement, especially among scientists and physicians.

Several scholarly articles have appeared on the future of cannabis as medicine. These articles argue that cannabis is much safer than many commonly available medications. Furthermore, cannabis use has been considered to be relatively safe in comparison with the adverse effects of chronic alcohol intake. However, there is inherent fallacy in using examples of "worse" substances of potential abuse (e.g., alcohol) to justify cannabis use itself. It is the outcome of the use of cannabis itself that is the real issue to be examined in risk/benefit assessments.

A review of general comments about marijuana is justified at this stage in this book to facilitate learning. Modern trends to pharmaceuticalize cannabis have not tended to result in the development of drugs that can outperform the complex actions of intact, whole, herbal marijuana. As noted earlier, such differences are dependent to a major degree on the content of various cannabinoids and other compounds that account for the overall entourage effects of herbal cannabis. As mentioned previously, the entourage effect means, in simple terms, that the many natural components of cannabis work best together (synergy) (Gupta, S., "Medical marijuana and the entourage effect," CNN Health, March 11, 2014).

Many scientists and physicians express their confidence that herbal marijuana use is now well established with adequate justification. In addition, it is predicted that pharmaceutical discoveries of the actions of cannabinoids will lead to the development of a range of drugs with diverse, beneficial, therapeutic applications. That said, there is some residual doubt that these cannabinoid pharmaceuticals will be able to have the same degree of applicability, effectiveness, and safety that has been experienced with whole herbal cannabis. While a current public perception of the superior effects of cannabis smoking often exists, the downside risks are the vascular and pulmonary effects of smoking and other problems.

Cannabis: Research Problems

Studies of the health benefits or adverse consequences of cannabis use are clouded often by confounding factors. The heavy cannabis user is likely to engage in adverse lifestyle, compounded by common types of substance abuse, such as tobacco, alcohol, and use of other illicit drugs. To separate out contributory factors that alter health status in cannabis research has proven to be difficult. As discussed earlier, studies that show correlation of cannabis use with disease often fail to establish causal links. Furthermore, there is often a concern that adverse health findings could antedate cannabis use or even operate in a causal manner to drive cannabis use.

Associations between cannabis use and adverse health effects are clear in many studies, but it is stressed repeatedly in medical literature that evidence of causality is often missing. This situation can only be cured by prospective or longitudinal studies that have been difficult to perform previously because of the many years of prohibition of cannabis use. In this book, I attempt to stress this handicap of not being able to define clear cause-and-effect relationships in many studies, especially when research has been retrospective.

Hall, W., and Degenhardt, L. ("Drug Testing and Analysis," July, 2013. doi: 101002/dta 1506) have reviewed the adverse effects of chronic cannabis use and summarized them by probability of occurrences.

Table 21. The adverse effects of cannabis use, stratified by existing evidence to invoke causal relationships (adapted with modifications from Hall, W., and Degenhardt, L. ibid. 2013)

Most probable adverse effects of chronic cannabis use	• dependence in one in nine users • cardiorespiratory problems • psychosis • low educational progress • cognitive problems
Possible adverse effects of regular cannabis use	• lung cancer • depression • mania • suicide • use of other drugs

Summary of Problems with Cannabis Research

I wish to reinforce problems that exist with cannabis research. These problems must be kept in mind when interpreting study outcome data. Studies about the health consequences of cannabis use often display disadvantages and limitations that interfere with the development of firm conclusions. As mentioned earlier and repeatedly, in most circumstances, studies are based upon associations or correlations of varying strength. This means that several factors may account for the study outcome and the demonstration of definitive cause-and-effect relationships cannot be defined. Other circumstances operate with chicken and egg arguments about what came first. For example, outcomes may be related to the presence of preexisting disorders or diseases in the study populations.

Prospective or longitudinal studies that examine potential causal relationships are much more valuable than correlative studies. Of course, these types of studies to show cause and effect are increasing but difficult to perform. The prohibition of cannabis use in the past has restricted this type of valuable research.

Chapter 4

MEDICAL CANNABIS

Cannabis for Disease Treatment

Cannabis use in the management of several diseases is rising exponentially in many locations in the United States. This has occurred most notably where state legislation exists for its recreational and more liberalized medical use. Physicians in many states in the United States (at least twenty-three states at the time of writing and increasing) are permitted to advise or prescribe cannabis for medical use, and this circumstance exists in Canada, Australia, and several European countries. Where decriminalization of the medical use of cannabis has occurred, standardized extracts of medical marijuana are in common use. Trends in the use of cannabis-related drugs or analogues (pharmaceuticals) are also growing, alongside the alarming growth of the dangerous use of synthetic pot.

General guidelines for the medicinal use of cannabis often advise the use of cannabis only after conventional treatments have been attempted and deemed ineffective. These recommendations have been stretched to include crystal-ball circumstances where conventional therapies may not be anticipated to be effective (at least in Canada). Therefore, some physicians perceive cannabis as a last-resort medication. In many circumstances a family physician (primary caregiver) can recommend or issue a prescription for cannabis use, but perceived or stated indications for use of cannabis can vary in different states of the Union and in the minds of many medical practitioners. As mentioned, medical use of cannabis tends to be more common per capita of the population in the states where recreational use of cannabis is permitted. In general, if a physician or patient elects to use cannabis where medical necessity is proven, legal outcomes (if any) are somewhat (but not always) softened.

Outcomes in several disease states permit a summary of conditions for which cannabis is prescribed or thought to be useful. The following disorders or diseases are generally agreed to be amenable to treatment with cannabis use in dosages tailored to needs, resulting in variable alleviation of symptoms or signs: nausea and appetite loss resulting from chemotherapy, radiotherapy or HIV combination therapy, palliative treatment for cancer and HIV disease, spasticity and pain associated with multiple sclerosis or spinal cord injury, chronic neuropathic (genic) pain, intractable epilepsy, and physical or verbal tics due to Tourette's syndrome.

We shall learn that the above list of conditions for which cannabis may be used is not complete, and cannabis therapy has been applied by physicians or patients in several hundred different clinical circumstances in what could be perceived as an unapproved manner. Medical professionals may be allowed to prescribe or recommend cannabis for reasons other than those listed above, with adequate purpose and documentation. For example, cannabis use has occurred in circumstances where a physician has concluded that a medical disorder is not likely to be amenable to conventional therapy, but such circumstances catalyze differences of opinion. That said, some uninformed fuddy-duddies with variable power over medical practitioners may exert little leeway on the use of cannabis. Unfortunately, laws controlling cannabis use in the United States may evolve in the future with significant variability in some states. At this stage, it is time to pause and reinforce the fact that there are many different types of cannabis in use that have different levels of efficacy and safety.

The contents of biologically active materials in cannabis (marijuana) vary by species of plant, growing conditions, ingestion of material at various times of growth, maturity of the plant, and many other influences. This means that it is almost impossible to make accurate statements about some of the effects of various mixtures of cannabis products. To attempt to match the many strains of cannabis with specific disease therapies is notoriously difficult. This situation must be understood because it has great importance in consumer conclusions about the use of different types of cannabis. Claims about certain strains and their biological effects are sometimes little more than gobble-de-gook. Medical science has a long way to go with further research to define different characteristics of whole or extracted cannabis material or synthetic analogues (drugs) or synthetic pot.

The author believes in more liberal use of cannabis than currently exists in many locations, provided that it is applied in a safe and potentially effective manner in disease states where there is good scientific agreement of potential benefits. The recreational use of cannabis is believed by the author to be appropriate providing that the user has been educated or educated themselves on the potential benefits and risks of its use. In addition, the author believes that cannabis has a clear role in integrative medicine, where it does not necessarily need to be used as a second-line drug.

Whole versus Reductionist Cannabis

Lester Grinspoon, MD, a renowned cannabis expert and the American father of cannabis research, wrote a visionary article called "On the Future of Cannabis as Medicine" (*Cannabinoids* 2007, 2, 2, 13–15). In this article Dr. Grinspoon forecasted the increasing pharmaceuticalization of cannabis, but he cautioned that drugs (analogues) based on cannabis may not be overall as effective as whole herbal marijuana. There is no doubt that he was correct.

Evidence Supporting Medical Cannabis Use

Many people are confused about the strength of the evidence that may exist for the beneficial use of cannabis in certain diseases or disorders. Attempts to rank the validity of science to support cannabis use present their own problems, because many proposed indications for cannabis use are based only on associations of the potential benefit of cannabis use with certain diseases and limited or anecdotal reports of benefit. The strength of indications for cannabis use has guided medical legislation for cannabis use, but arguments have prevailed and disagreements in research outcomes have produced variable emotional responses that may overshadow some scientific findings. The Mayo Clinic has attempted to summarize evidence that supports cannabis use in medical disorders with an attempt to rank their level of importance, based on existing medical evidence. This information has been graded without a detailed analysis of the safety and efficacy of cannabis for all medical indications. The table below provides the grades that define the rationale for cannabis use, described as grades A to F of varying scientific strength or support.

Tables 22A and 22B. Grading rationale defined in 22A and strength of data to support grade of benefit in 22B, in certain conditions, adapted and modified from www.mayoclinic.org/drugs/supplements/marijuana/evidence/ hrb,20059701

Table 22A.

 GRADING RATIONALE
GRADE A	Strong evidence
GRADE B	Good evidence
GRADE C	Unclear evidence
GRADE D	Fair evidence
GRADE F	Strong evidence against use

Table 22B.

CONDITION	GRADE	DATA SUPPORTING BENEFIT	GRADE
Chronic pain	B	Epilepsy	C
Multiple Scelerosis	C	Glaucoma	C
Amyotrophic scelerosis	C	Huntington's disease	C
Appetite stimulation	C (?B)	Neuromuscular disease	C
Atopic dermatitis	C	Quality of Life	C (?B)
Brain trauma	C	Rheumatoid arthritis	C
Adverse effects of Chemotherapy	C(B?)	Schizophrenia	C (?D)
Dementia	C	Sleep problems	C (?B)
Eating disorders	C	Tourette's Syndrome	C

Acts of Decriminalization and Legalization of Marijuana

Users of cannabis may be confused by legal terminology that is used in cannabis (marijuana) literature. The advent of increasing legal tolerance to cannabis use in many places has involved both acts of decriminalization and the development of locations of legalization for recreational use. The Indian nations of the United States have sovereign rights to grow and use cannabis on their own lands. The acts of decriminalization and legalization have important differences that exert an influence on the legal consequences of marijuana use and possession. It appears reasonable to view decriminalization trends in Europe (e.g., UK) and certain states of the Union (United States) as processes of progression toward legalization.

Several states of the Union have legislation that indicates that individuals in possession of small amounts of marijuana will not receive a criminal record for first offenses. This refers to circumstances where small amounts of marijuana (cannabis) are carried or possessed for personal consumption. For this type of offense, prison time is not usually imposed, but fines and disciplinary actions may be different, depending on the state and, of course, the judge. The quantity of drug in an individual's possession is of importance. For example, in circumstances where marijuana use has been legalized, the amount allowed for personal consumption is often no more than one ounce. However, the possession of marijuana in certain jurisdictions in greater amounts can result in significant fines or other penalties. These fines are often prorated to the amount of cannabis possessed, and felony convictions are made for large amounts, especially when intent to deal is present.

The emerging laxity in the legal systems of the control of cannabis use in areas of legalization of recreational cannabis use needs some vigilance. Vigilance is an absolute requirement in children and teenagers who are particularly susceptible to future developmental disorders in adulthood. In Colorado, Washington state, Alaska, Oregon, and Washington, DC, governments will have to continue to examine factors such as quality of product, driving under the influence of pot, and age of use, to mention a few circumstances. The author holds the point of view that regulated legalization of cannabis is a better option than decriminalization.

Several organizations have debated the benefits of legalization over decriminalization and vice versa. Table 23 gives some of the reasons that are proposed as for or against cannabis legalization and decriminalization.

Table 23. Legalization seems more advantageous than decriminalization (material modified from online NORML and Marijuana Detox Guide, 2014). A comparison of decriminalization versus legalization:

Decriminalization	Legalization
• government cost—savings	• increased tax revenue
• reduction of processing and drug enforcement activity	• elimination of much legal activity, decreased arrests
• obvious budget savings for law enforcement and cost of penalties such as incarceration	• undercut black market activity and its associated criminality, assure product quality

Toward the Clinical Use of Cannabis

While the psychoactive actions of tetrahydrocannabinol (THC) spring immediately into the minds of many individuals when cannabis is discussed, a significant expansion in knowledge exists about the biological actions of other cannabinoids and essential oils (terpenoids) found in the cannabis plant. Thus, seeing cannabis as an arch-promoter of euphoria (the high), sedation, and the munchies (appetite stimulation) are narrow but common perspectives on its use.

Starting in about 2007, there was an expansion in the number of scientific clinical studies on cannabis, but knowledge is still somewhat limited. It is apparent that cannabis and isolated cannabinoids have potential medicinal benefits for several diseases, under certain conditions of its use. These are matters of fact and the current federal government's opinion on cannabis as a "drug without currently accepted medical use" has to be reexamined. There is an acute need for the compilation of comprehensive information on the clinical outcome of the use of cannabis. Furthermore, there is need for research and development of quality cannabis products. Such research requires funding, and it is an expensive prospect that must be addressed by politicians and cannabis producers. Cannabis tax revenue may help in the development of scientific knowledge, if it is used to support the needed education and research, in an appropriate manner. That said, complaints have been made about how states with legalization have used money derived from registration fees paid for cannabis use, resulting in some legal actions.

From 1975 to 2010, at least 110 controlled clinical studies, involving more than 6,100 patients, were published on the medical potential of cannabis. These studies have assisted in understanding the endocannabinoid system and its diverse functions (Hazekamp, A., Grotenhermen, F., 2010, Cannabinoids: Special Issue: 5, 1–21).

In this book, the protean effects of cannabis on CB1 and CB2 receptors (and perhaps other receptors) are most often determined by the predominant cannabinoid content of the cannabis material in question. Beyond THC, there has been a growing interest shown in the cannabinoid known as cannabidiol (CBD). Cannabidiol has a variety of effects due to its differential actions on the endocannabinoid receptor systems. These actions of CBD include anti-inflammatory properties, anticancer effects, antispasmodic, antimicrobial, antipsychotic actions, neuroprotective effects, actions as a vascular relaxant and as a stabilizer of blood glucose, with some promise for diabetes treatment and the management of Metabolic Syndrome X. Thus, CBD (cannabidiol) appears to have a much wider range of medical uses compared with THC. For example, it has received limited orphan drug status by the FDA for specific uses such as severe seizure disorders in children (Dravet syndrome). That said, CBD is available in some dietary supplements that cannot carry specific disease prevention or treatment claims under the prevailing legislation of DSHEA (1994). CBD is not considered to be a legal dietary supplement by the FDA.

Introducing Preparations of Cannabis: The Cannabinoids

Later in this book, many aspects of the basic science, clinical effects, and potential medical use of cannabis are reviewed.

Anecdotal reports of clinical experiences with various cannabis products may fail sometimes to accurately describe or characterize the actual form or composition of cannabis that has been used in the study or observations.

> An assessment of medical cannabis literature that is presented online is difficult when uncertainty exists about the contents of the cannabis in question. Furthermore, the most common use of cannabis involves smoking, where different amounts of active ingredients are delivered into the body compared with other modes of delivery.

In a number of clinical circumstances, delta-9-tetrahydrocannabinol (THC) is often assumed to be the most important bioactive constituent found in cannabis plants. The palliative effects of THC are well recognized with the ability of this compound to inhibit chemotherapy-induced nausea and vomiting in cancer patients. However, THC is only one of approximately one hundred or more cannabinoids that are found in the cannabis plant. That said, the biological properties of only a handful of cannabinoids have been investigated in detail, and many measured cannabinoids are present as metabolites that are not known to be biologically active. The most researched natural cannabinoids, other than THC, are cannabidiol (CBD) and cannabinol.

Herbal cannabis refers to dried leaves, flowers, stems, and seeds of Cannabis sativa, but it is clear that in many types of herbal cannabis products (street varieties), different portions of the plant are used in varying amounts. As mentioned earlier in a repetitive manner, this circumstance creates problems for the health care giver or consumer to know what is being consumed with any degree of precision. Furthermore, recommendations for the use of strains of cannabis for different effects may be unreliable, even when sold in some specialty dispensaries.

It is clear that marijuana (cannabis) smoking is the common mode of ingestion of cannabis, and it delivers a number of chemical constituents that are found in the whole plant, including the products of combustion. If whole herbal products are used in clinical trials, attempts are made to standardize their cannabinoid contents. This attempt to standardize preparations of the cannabis plant has often translated into measuring THC content and expressing the amount as a percentage of dry weight of the material. More recent research has been directed to measure the effects of other bioactive constituents of the cannabis plant (e.g., cannabidiol). The main subclasses of cannabinoids are shown in table 24.

To reiterate, Cannabidiol (CBD) is one of the major cannabinoids found in the Cannabis species (sativa and indica), and it is often found in significant amounts in hemp. Versatile effects of CBD have been mentioned earlier, including antiepileptic, anti-inflammatory, antiemetic, muscle relaxing, anxiolytic, and neuroprotective actions. Cannabidiol (CBD) does not have the psychoactive effects of THC. Moreover, CBD is known to reduce or block the psychoactive effects of THC as part of an entourage effect of cannabis.

Table 24. Subclasses of cannabinoids.

This is not a complete list.

• Cannabigerols (CBG)	• Cannabichromenes (CBC)
• Cannabidiols (CBD)	• Tetrahydrocannabinols (THC)
• Cannabinol (CBN)	• Other cannabinoids, e.g. cannabicylol (CBL), cannabielsoin (CBE), cannabitriol (CBT) and others.
• Cannabinodiol (CBDL)	

Beyond herbal preparations of cannabis are a number of standardized compounds that are used in pharmaceutical prescriptions. Some of these are synthetic analogues. These drugs include Dronabinol (Marinol), Sativex (containing 1:1 mix of THC and CBD), and Dexanabinol. An attempt to use the more synergistic effects of cannabinoids (THC and CBD) has resulted in the development of the drug Cannador. This product is a whole plant extract with a THC to CBD ratio of about 2:1. It has been used with success in several European clinical trials. Oil products, derived from hemp, are sold in health food stores and large chain retail, food stores. Many of these oil products only label fatty acid contents and not levels of cannabinoids (CBD) content. Common hemp oil does not contain THC, except in traces (less than 0.3 percent THC).

Summary of the Expanding Medical Use of Cannabis

To summarize, some of the main areas of medical use and research in which cannabis and its products are used include neuropathic or chronic pain, multiple sclerosis with spasticity, HIV disease and AIDS, glaucoma, intestinal dysfunctions, nausea (vomiting and loss of appetite), and schizophrenia. Other conditions in which cannabis has shown some medical promise include cancer, relief from hepatitis C virus treatment that is not well tolerated, tics associated with Tourette's syndrome, obsessive-compulsive disorders, and several other neurological diseases (both hereditary and acquired).

Cannabis: General Observations

According to the National Institute on Drug Abuse, there has been a steady increase in the use of cannabis in young people in recent times. This trend of use has been linked to the expanding notion among drug users that cannabis is safe. Of course, these perceptions are reinforced by recent legalization and decriminalization of pot in certain states of the United States. Cannabis does not possess universal safety, and it is modestly addictive. As discussed earlier, there is an uncommon condition called cannabis use disorder, which is an accepted medical diagnosis listed in the fifth revision of the Diagnostic and Statistical Manual of Mental Disorders (DM-5).

Marijuana often has an unpleasant smell that is musty, a little sweet, and occasionally pungent. It may have a smell similar to discharge from a skunk. Dispensary technicians are often well educated on the esthetics of various types (strains) of cannabis. When smoked, marijuana releases THC, which rapidly enters the blood. In comparison, slower absorption of THC occurs when it is taken in foods or drinks. When consumed in a vaporized form, the onset of the actions of marijuana occurs in an intermediate time frame. This time frame of action occurs somewhere between the time period following the onset of effects of smoking and eating. The many factors that influence absorption, metabolism, and body distribution of cannabinoids produce variable physiological responses or symptomatic outcomes.

Marijuana has characteristic short-terms effects in users, but its longer or long-term effects are sometimes quite complex. These effects are most notable on memory. Acute effects of smoked cannabis occur rapidly, often with major effects occurring within thirty seconds or a couple of minutes. These effects can last up to three hours, approximately. As mentioned, early results vary among individuals, and tolerance may occur with both modest and heavy cannabis use. Tolerance may develop quite quickly, often within a couple of weeks following onset of intake. As noted earlier, cannabis edibles take longer to be active (greater than thirty minutes up to a couple of hours), and the duration of the psychoactive effects of edibles is longer (often hours) compared with smoking or vaporization.

The high experienced by the cannabis user is often a function of the dosage of THC, but other factors operate. The context of marijuana smoking affects initial outcomes on brain function. THC enters the brain where it acts on CB-1 receptors located on the inner and outer parts of cell membranes. As mentioned earlier, there are two types of CB (cannabinoid) receptors, CB1 and CB2, which are examples of G-protein-coupled receptors. These receptors are present in a structure that spans cell membranes several times. The other CB receptor (CB-2) is present mainly on cells of the immune system, with common presence on B cells, natural killer cells, monocytes, and polymorphonuclear white cells.

To summarize, the effects of THC (the psychoactive cannabinoid) occur by receptor binding in the brain (on CB-1 receptors). This results in changes in the amounts of neurotransmitters in the brain (chemicals that trigger nervous system functions). Notable changes occur in the concentration of dopamine and norepinephrine in the central nervous system. These transmitters are involved in causing euphoria and anxiety, but other acute effects occur. These acute effects following marijuana use include enhanced feelings of well-being, relaxation, reductions in subjective sensations of stress, happiness often due to increased sense of humor or the giggles, music appreciation, increased sensuality (mainly in women), mild hallucinations, and other psychological changes.

The early physiological effects of cannabis on body functions include accelerated heart rate, dry mouth, red eyes, muscle relaxation, reduction of pressure in the eyeballs, and change in temperature sensations in the feet and hands due to altered blood circulation. To reiterate, the short-term duration of the effects of cannabis are determined in part by its potency (content of THC), the setting in which it is used, and the route of administration (smoking, vaporization, or oral ingestion).

Sociobehavioral factors that are associated with increased risks of cannabis use are shown in table 25.

Table 25. Sociobehavioral and psychosocial issues that increase mental and perhaps physical risks for cannabis users (see reference section)

- reckless drug-seeking behavior
- selection of drug-using friends
- early onset of cannabis use (below sixteen years of age)
- underlying mental health problems
- poor social ties
- stressful life events
- social failure with hopelessness
- attraction to the cannabis lifestyle
- desires to disconnect from reality

The ability of cannabis or its analogues (drugs) to make symptoms of several diseases more bearable is often a valuable and underestimated benefit of cannabis use. This beneficial effect does not result often in the alteration of the natural history of the disease that is being treated, and it may contribute to drug dependence. Improvement of symptoms of disease is possible with many drugs, but cannabis has been perceived to go more toward managing the root cause of disease. This property of cannabis relates to its ability to exert widespread and versatile control over body functions, by modification of the endocannabinoid system.

Survey data collected between 2002 and 2013 (National Survey on Drug Use and Health, NSDUH) has been examined with a view to uncovering how young people think and behave towards cannabis use. In these studies, the national sample was broken down into three age groups: younger adolescents (age 12-14 years), older adolescents age 15-17 years and young adults (age 18-25 years).

The data show that younger adolescents (age 12-14) and older adolescents (age 15-17) have decreased their use over the past ten years and have become less permissive in their opinions about cannabis use. In contrast, young adults (18-25 years) show more acceptance of cannabis use, but increased consumption has not been noted (Christopher P. Trends in the disapproval and use of marijuana among adolescents and young adults in the United States: 2002-2013. The American Journal of Drug and Alcohol Abuse 2015, 41(5): 392 Dol10.3109/60952990, 2015).

Reducing Problems with Cannabis Use

With the cat out of the bag and the opening of Pandora's box concerning cannabis use comes the need to encourage the responsible, low-risk use of cannabis. The current increasing legalization and illicit use of cannabis has led to recommendations that individuals should understand factors that may reduce negative health and other adverse effects of cannabis use. The recognition of behavioral issues or other circumstances that aggravate the unwanted effects of cannabis permits interventions to ensure lower risks of the use of this drug. These matters that are relevant to nonmedical cannabis use have been carefully assessed by Canadian researchers (Fischer, B. et al., *Can. J. Pub. Health* 102, no. 5 [2011], 324–7).

Table 26. Reducing risks of cannabis use, based upon peer-reviewed reviews of epidemiological studies and adverse event reports of cannabis use, undertaken by Fischer ibid. 2011

This information should be viewed mainly as the work of Fischer's Group. The above cited findings by Fischer et al. (ibid. 2011) are very important, especially as the United States and other countries graduate toward a more liberal use of cannabis. Some experts argue that this type of information encourages cannabis use, but it is now time to accept planning that supports the responsible use of cannabis. The work of Fischer, B. et al. (ibid. 2011) has resulted in the development of important Lower Risk Cannabis Use Guidelines (LRCUG).

- Risks due to cannabis use are affected by patterns of use and individual factors. Risk avoidance can be achieved obviously by abstention from use.
- Early use of cannabis in adolescents increases risks of problems related to cannabis. Delaying use of cannabis until adulthood may result in less harm than adolescent use.
- Frequent or heavy use is associated with the most severe problems.
- Individuals with difficulty in controlling use should attempt to quit. Failure to quit should result in medical consultation.
- Smoking cannabis mixed with tobacco compounds health risks, as does deep breath holding during smoking (intense smoking). Vaporizers may be safer than all popular smoking methods.
- Using high-potency cannabis leads to increase levels of impairment. Titration of the dose during smoking or vaping may assist in lesser intoxication. Special care must

be exercised to avoid some cannabis preparations (notably synthetics), which are misnamed often as cannabis. Synthetic pot does not contain cannabinoids.

- Avoidance of driving, piloting, boating, or operating any machinery must be delayed after cannabis use. Delay by a period of twelve hours after use may result in greater safety, but individuals require different recovery times.
- Certain individuals should abstain from cannabis use, including pregnant women, mature males and females with cardiovascular disease, people with a history of psychosis or a first-degree relative with psychosis (e.g., schizophrenia).

Effects of Cannabis on the Nervous System

Cannabis receptors (CB-1) in the brain are found with high density in the basal ganglia, the cerebellum, the hippocampus, the cerebral cortex, and the nucleus acumbens. A summary of the site of action and some major effects of THC on CB-1 receptors are provided in table 27.

Table 27. Site of action of THC, with a list of the major effects of cannabinoids (THC) on the control of several nervous system functions

Sites of Cannabinoid CB-1 Receptors	Effects of Cannabinoids (Mainly THC)
Basal ganglia	Altered control of body movements.
Hippocampus	Changes in memory, learning to control body stress.
Cerebral cortex	Impaired cognitive functions.
Cerebellum	Coordination of body movement.
Nucleus acumbens	Known as reward center of brain with role in addictions.
Hypothalamus	Effects on body homeostasis.
Amygdala	Control emotional responses and fear

Spinal cord	Body sensation relays (e.g., pain).
Brain stem	Modulation of arousal, sleep, and motor controls with general but modest depressant actions.
Nucleus of solitary tract	Controls visceral sensations (e.g., nausea and vomiting).

The next few sections of this book provide a short review of the outcome of cannabis use on several body systems. This is a prelude to more specific disease-related information in later chapters.

Effects on Motor Tasks: Motor Vehicle and Machinery Use

Cannabis is an increasingly common cause of driving under the influence (DUI), and its disruptive effects on motor functions of the body may be sometimes compounded by simultaneous alcohol intake (dual substance abuse). There are many known associations of marijuana use with accidents. It has been made clear that motor vehicle operators who have consumed cannabis within three hours have nearly two times the risk of an accident compared with individuals who are not under the influence or drugs or alcohol (Ashbridge, M., et al., 2012, www.bmj.com press release, "Marijuana and Motor Vehicle Crashes," *Epidemiological Reviews* 34, no. 1 (2012): 65–72).

The National Highway Traffic Safety Administration has reported that about 18 percent of motor vehicle drivers may test positive for drugs other than alcohol. These data are expected to change with increases in the detection of positive drug testing as a consequence of more widespread use of cannabis. Marijuana is commonly incriminated in DUIs where alcohol consumption is involved. Recent studies show that 6.8 percent of drivers involved in accidents had positive tests for THC use. In addition, about 21 percent of these individuals, where THC was detected, had blood-alcohol levels above legal limits. These data seem to indicate that marijuana is a contributory cause of injury in drivers, and it seriously impugns the safety record of cannabis.

The safety of cannabis is questioned further with recent reports of an increased number of marijuana-positive individuals involved in fatal road traffic accidents. These reports were based on data collected after the legalization of medical cannabis in Colorado in 2009. However, it was notable that there was no significant change in alcohol-reported accidents in Colorado or states that did not have medical marijuana legalization in place. More research is required to define the causal relationship between marijuana use and fatal motor vehicle accidents, if such a relationship exists.

In brief, most people believe that the risks of road traffic injuries or fatalities are increased by cannabis use. It remains to be seen how more widespread legalization or decriminalization of marijuana will affect morbidity and mortality from road traffic accidents. However, university-based studies in US states that have legalized cannabis for medical and/or recreational use (Colorado, Montana, and Oregon) report a recent 8–11 percent decrease in deaths due to traffic accidents. These studies support the notions that drivers under the influence of marijuana have a greater recognition of their impairment, compared with those who are intoxicated from alcohol.

It is proposed that this recognition of impairment may tend to result in avoidance of driving. In addition, it is suggested that cannabis users tend to stay at home, in comparison to alcohol users. Any stay-at-home tendencies in cannabis users may change with greater availability and acceptability of cannabis use in society, even in states that permit recreational cannabis use. Smoking cannabis in public is banned in Colorado. Cannabis use has been associated with accidents involved in the occupational use of machinery and the precipitation of sports injuries. Much further study is required, but DUI with cannabis must be considered highly inadvisable.

Effects on Cardiac and Lung Function

The short-term cardiovascular effects of cannabis include increased heart rate, high or low blood pressure (with fluctuations), and alterations of peripheral blood flow, associated often with dilatation (relaxation) of blood vessels. While marijuana use in young healthy subjects is often without serious immediate consequences, its effects in older individuals with preexisting cardiovascular or cerebrovascular disease are associated with greater cardiovascular risks. These risks are compounded by short-term increases in cardiac workload, with stimulation of catecholamine amine release that occurs as a consequence of marijuana use. Thus, there is a precipitation of a stress response with cannabis smoking.

Acute cardiovascular effects of marijuana smoking may contribute to myocardial infarction and stroke. An association of marijuana use and myocardial infarction has been noted also in some young adults. Acute myocardial infarction in young otherwise healthy adults has been reported. The risk of cardiovascular events seems to be higher with heavy and prolonged intakes of cannabis. This risk is also present in heavy cigarette smokers, and, of course, tobacco and marijuana use often go hand in hand. It has been estimated that middle-aged people have a greater incidence of heart attack (about a five-fold increase) in the first hour following cannabis smoking, but these estimates have been doubted.

Many studies continue to highlight the common occurrence of mixed substance abuse, often involving cannabis use. As noted, individuals who use cannabis frequently tend to smoke tobacco and drink alcohol. In fact, lack of availability of cannabis in regular cannabis users is often associated with excessive alcohol drinking. While smoke from tobacco and marijuana is somewhat similar in composition, marijuana contains more polycyclic aromatic hydrocarbons (frank carcinogens), ammonia, hydrogen cyanide, and nitrogen oxides. Therefore, smoke from marijuana is considered potentially toxic and carcinogenic, but awareness of these potential problems is quite low in the general population.

That said, much debate has surrounded the effect of smoking cannabis on the lungs, but evidence points to inevitable precipitation of some degree of compromised respiratory function in the long term in the heavy cannabis smoker. Bronchitis and increased phlegm production are common in the cannabis smoker, and there are reports of a greater prevalence of lung infections in cannabis smokers. In some cases, lung infections occur with opportunistic pathogens, especially in individuals with impaired immune function. Furthermore, the role of adulterants or additives in pulmonary toxicity remains unclear. In addition, some studies imply, predictably, that secondhand marijuana smoke may cause health risks.

Effects on Appetite, Learning, and Memory

The munchies (encouragement to eat) following marijuana use is a consequence of the ability of marijuana to increase both interest in and appreciation of food. Stimulation of food intake by cannabis results from the direct THC activation of cannabinoid receptors (CB-1) in the hypothalamus. Contrarian effects of marijuana on appetite and food intake may occur, especially after chronic heavy use of marijuana. These circumstances can result in occurrence of the uncommon state of chronic cannabis hyperemesis (increased vomiting) syndrome. We are now entering again the realms of the paradoxical effects of cannabis.

Cannabis use compromises learning ability in a complex manner. Many studies reveal that cannabis use has negative effects on short-term and working memory (Riedel, G., Davis, SN, *2005 Handbook of Experiment Pharmacology* 168, 445–477). Some studies of the effects of cannabis on memory and thought have shown conflicting results that are not easy to explain. In such studies, the selection of the study population has material effects on outcome. This can result in a comparison of an apple with an orange. The findings of early reversible cognitive deficits after seven days of cannabis use are not consistent with findings that chronic cannabis use can affect verbal memory for up to two weeks following cessation of its intake (Pope, HG et al., 2001, *Archives of General Psychiatry* 58, 10, 909–15). However, at four weeks following cessation of cannabis use, memory problems are usually no longer detectable using standard neuropsychological testing. Other studies have confirmed that chronic marijuana use may cause selective memory deficits, but very heavy use of marijuana may cause protracted deficiencies in neurocognitive performance for about a month or more (Bolla, K. et al., 2002, *Neurology*, 59, 9, 1337–43). Some convincing research supports a greater and more longstanding effect on memory and cognition, with negative effects on brain structure.

Effects on Other Drug Use: Gateway and Closed-Gate Phenomena

There has been much discussion about cannabis as a gateway to the use of other drugs with potent effects that may have serious and greater addiction potential. There are data that support the suggestion that this gateway phenomenon operates in a significant proportion of marijuana users. How much of this tendency to progress to the use of hard drugs is a function of an individual's addictive personality or underlying psychopathology remains unclear. Again, selection of study participants can skew results in research studies in these circumstances.

There are promising recent findings that marijuana use could play a role in reducing opioid dependence and opioid drug-related overdoses. Thus, one could perceive that cannabis can be used to close the gateway to hard drug use. The Centers for Disease Control and Prevention (CDC) have characterized the alarming magnitude of the problem of death from opioid overdoses that are occurring increasingly in women. This situation is believed to constitute a serious public health issue that requires urgent attention. As mentioned, alarming statistics about this problem include the five-times increase in opioid overdose-related deaths in women with a three-fold increase in men. The CDC reports that women are more likely than men to be prescribed higher dosages of opioid drugs that are taken in the long term, but opioid-related deaths still remain more common in men.

Recent research reports indicate that there was a 24.8 percent lower occurrence of opioid-overdose deaths in states that had medical marijuana legislation in place prior to 2010, compared to states where medical marijuana had not been legalized. There is a need for more research on the relationship between the presence of medical marijuana laws and deaths from opioid analgesic use. One logical interpretation of these data is that the use of medical marijuana may form an effective adjunct for pain relief in opioid users. Of course, this may operate by resulting in a need for less opioid usage. There is some evidence to support this role of cannabis in adjunctive pain relief due to synergistic (complementary) effects between cannabis and opioids. Clearly, the safety profile of marijuana is superior to that of opioids. This is a major example of potential harm reduction due to cannabis use.

There are other links between cannabinoid effects and opioids that are quite complex. For example, CBD (cannabidiol) is an allosteric modulator of mu and delta opioid receptor sites. This is just one example of the cross reactions in the controls of body functions that are modulated by cannabinoid use, and it highlights the presence of chatter between opioid and marijuana pathways that occurs in the central nervous system. Marijuana probably chatters with other nerve pathways.

Marijuana: Focus on Health Benefits in Certain Diseases

While it may seem repetitious, I feel that it is valuable to try to focus in on the medical benefits of cannabis rather than make blanket statements about overall benefits in various diseases. For example, cannabidiol (CBD) exerts benefits in cancer management in several specific ways, but it is not a cancer cure. Of course, these matters will be addressed in later sections of this book. Table 28 summarizes some of the major health benefits in a focused manner with attempts to avoid too many generalizations about disease management. The evidence to support cannabis treatments in a variety of diseases is often quite variable and sometimes arguable.

Table 28. A focus on the specific aspects of certain diseases that may respond to cannabis

Evidence is not always cast iron, but these reports of benefits are leaning toward the demonstration of favorable outcomes of cannabis use in specific aspects of medical practice.

• analgesic actions in neuropathy	• slows progression of Alzheimer's disease
• decreases metastasis in certain cancers	• antiviral: retards the spread of HIV and hepatitis C
• management of opiate addiction	• useful in management of depression
• variable ability to treat epilepsy	• role in the management of concussions and stroke
• anxiolytic	• reduces blindness in glaucoma
• lowers insulin needs in diabetics	• ADHD and PTSD symptoms (arguable)

Is Cannabis Neurotoxic?

Cannabis may be neurotoxic, but it is a neuroprotective and neurogenic agent. This may be the ultimate paradox described with cannabis use. Studies that investigate the relationship between marijuana use and reductions in neuropsychological abilities have produced disturbing and somewhat consistent results. The Dunedin Study provided prospective information on 1,037 individuals who used cannabis. The participants in this study were born in 1972/73 and followed to the age of thirty-eight years. In this study, testing of neuropsychological function was reported at age thirteen years and thirty-eight years. This research provided valuable prospective data on cannabis use.

Moreover, heavy chronic use of cannabis was associated with irreversible declines in certain brain functions in cannabis users who started their drug use in adolescence (Meier, MH et al., *PNAS* online, Oct. 2012). These and other studies suggest that prevention strategies may be advantageous when undertaken early in the history of cannabis use in youngsters. In this book, I reiterate the absolute importance of preventing adolescent use of cannabis, which may carry a poor prognosis in some individuals.

These findings in the Dunedin Study are of major significance in the evolution of cannabis use in certain individuals, given the knowledge that about one in fifteen (or more) high school seniors use marijuana on a daily basis or near daily basis. Clearly, drug abuse and alcohol use are major risk factors that contribute to high school dropout. It is unfortunate that increasing legalization, including medical legalization, makes cannabis more available for use by teens. I cannot emphasize enough that public health measures to prevent cannabis use must be focused on these young people (echolalia).

Dosing of Cannabis

It is unfortunate to state that the dosing of cannabis for many people is often a best guess for the achievement of many desired outcomes. This is always the case if one uses illicit, nonstandardized forms of the drug. Despite general agreements that cannabis is relatively safe, there is much controversial and conflicting information about dosing regimes for medical treatments. Many users are seeking information about strains of cannabis to select the contents of different marijuana preparations, and they may inquire about some of the many factors that cause varied responses to its use. Such responses vary considerably from person to person (interindividual variation) and sometimes within the same individual from one use to the next (intraindividual variation). An important factor in determining dosage requirement over time is the development of tolerance to both the psychological and physical effects of the drug. Tolerance does occur, despite rhetoric to the contrary. As discussed earlier, tolerance may occur within a couple of weeks after the start of cannabis smoking.

Issues surrounding the definition of optimal dosages of cannabinoids for a specific effect or treatment purposes are complicated by choices of routes of administration. Routes of administration determine the amounts of the components of cannabis that get into the body (bioavailability) and their speed of absorption. High-speed absorption of THC from smoking causes the quick high. Common routes of cannabis delivery include smoking, vaporized product, edible varieties, oral sprays, sublingual forms, pills, and elixirs. Furthermore, brands can be made with different ingredients, or there may be natural variation in cannabis potency, with the result that there is sometimes inconsistency in the effects of the same brand of whole herbal cannabis products. These days, there is an increasing use of cannabis extracts where optimum dosage schedules are sometimes not clear, but they provide greater clarity of dosage applications compared with smoking cannabis.

Cannabis dosing estimates present problems for many agencies, both political and regulatory. For example, the National Institute on Drug Abuse (NIDA) has supplied prescribed dosages, in standardized amounts, for patients who are enrolled in the Compassionate Investigational New Drug (CIND) Program. The amounts involved in this study were about two ounces per week (one half a pound per month) of cannabis for smoking. The cannabis was supplied in canisters of three hundred prerolled cigarettes consumed at rates of ten or more cigarettes per day. It appears that long-term dosing with this amount of cannabis has been accepted overall as safe and effective, without much in the way of significant adverse effects.

The medical indications for cannabis treatment are used somewhat to determine duration and biological potency of which type of cannabis is selected for use. For example, patients with severe recalcitrant pain may have undertaken chronic, heavy use of cannabis, but less cannabis use can be effective in assisting in the management of transient pain disorders. Debilitated patients, with terminal illness, may have a much-reduced tolerance for cannabis. Some medical conditions require prophylactic and continuous use of cannabis (e.g., diseases such as glaucoma [raised pressure in the eye] and severe symptoms in multiple sclerosis). The variations in the clinical course of many diseases require dosage adjustments. For example, anxiety control may be possible with as little as 1–2 mg of cannabidiol (CBD) once or twice per day in some adults, but the control of epilepsy may need at least 60 mg of CBD or much more per day (even in children).

The route of delivery of cannabis and its extracts or analogues have an obvious effect on required dosages. It is clear that fast and efficient delivery of principal cannabinoids, such as THC or CBD, occurs with cannabis smoking. Smoking is the most common way of ingesting cannabis compounds, but an increasing number of users wish to avoid the uncertain risks of cannabis causing lung disease (lung structure and function alterations). When cannabis is consumed in edibles, it is estimated that eating requires higher dosages than smoking to achieve adequate psychoactive effects from THC content of the orally administered cannabis. Delivery of cannabis in food preparations requires about three to five times more than the dosage that can be derived from smoking, but this is only a rough estimate (guess). As discussed earlier, it is important to realize that cannabis taken in edible formats has actions that are spread over a much longer period of time than when the drug is taken by smoking. In addition, it should be noted again that edibles take longer than smoking to be effective.

In later chapters of this book, more details about the disposition in the body of different dosage forms of marijuana will be mentioned, especially in relationship to disease treatment. A form of cannabis delivery that is gaining increasing popularity is vaporization that uses heat without combustion. It is estimated that about twice the dose of active cannabis material taken by vaporization is required to obtain desired effects that can be obtained by smoking, but doubts exist. Many physicians believe that vaporization is safer for health than smoking, and users have found that it can be used to help to hide cannabis use in public settings.

Cannabis dosing has occurred, in a variable range, in controlled and uncontrolled observations of its effects in certain disease states. One approach to define dosage has been to attempt to study disease response (usually symptomatic improvement) in an uncontrolled or anecdotal manner. Thus, some recommended dosage schedules are relatively crude estimates that have been derived from a simple trial approach. Much more information is required from the increasing body of experience that will be acquired in formal clinical trials. One of the most complete summaries of recommended cannabis dosing is displayed in the Drugs and Supplements section of the Mayo Clinic online (www.mayoclinic.org/drugs-supplements/marijuana). Readers *must* understand that cannabis use is not allowed by federal and state law in many locations in the United States.

Table 29 is an attempt to provide a simple overview of dosing of cannabis for several common conditions, but it is incomplete in content and does not cover uses of synthetic analogues (pharmaceuticals) of cannabinoids. These analogues (pharmaceuticals, drugs) are most often used for the control of nausea and vomiting that are precipitated by chemotherapy.

Table 29. Approximate dosages of cannabis. The dosages are only rough guides, and titration against symptoms starting with small doses has been recommended (the symptom control, titration paradigm). These dosages cannot be interpreted as safe or accepted dosages for disease treatment. Users of cannabis should consult a health care practitioner for more detailed discussions. Applications for disease should be monitored by a health care professional.

Condition	Average

Anxiety	2 mg of CBD every 8–12 hours. THC may not be well tolerated in the presence of anxiety. Higher dosage may be required often for severe cases.
Sleeplessness	40–160 mg of CBD by mouth (expensive and impractical). Favorable results with lower dosages have been experienced, depending on the type of sleep disorder. THC may be combined.
Mental disease	Schizophrenia, 40–1280 mg of oral CBD for four weeks. Dosage requirement is highly variable.
Neuropathic pain	Initial dosage of 2 mg of CBD a.m. and p.m., with increase to 20 mg / 24 hours. May need THC added.
Musculoskeletal pain	Dosing variable and often individualized up to 15 mg / 24 hours of CBD, with or without the addition of THC.

Recent proposals reinforce the findings that CB-2 receptor stimulation may be a substitute for CB-1 receptor stimulation in pain control. The advantages of this include less chance of addiction and avoidance of unwanted psychoactive actions of cannabis (Deng, L. et al., *Biological Psychiatry* 77, no. 5 (2015), 475, doi: 10.1016/jbiopsych.2014.04.009).

It is important to stress that commencing with a low dosage of all cannabis (marijuana) products is a prudent approach for the initial introduction of cannabis therapy or recreational use of cannabis. This circumstance is particularly important when using cannabis edibles. Seeking the effective dosage of medical marijuana is best undertaken as a cooperative project between the patient and physician or other knowledgeable health care practitioners. There is no doubt that evidence-based guidelines must be further developed for the safe use of cannabis, especially as regulators continue to search for safe dosage limits and objective strategies for dose/response assessments in both medical and recreational uses.

If one considers the many factors that determine suitable cannabis dosing (e.g., potency of product, tolerance, and context of use, etc.), the guidelines that have been produced for cannabis use should be interpreted often as approximate at best. I emphasize again that this situation dictates a need for what has been referred to as a "self-titration dosing paradigm" (or physician-supervised titration of dosage), which is tailored to an individual's needs, ideally as a consequence of physician/patient experiences. The dosage/response relationship of the effects of components of cannabis is an important, underestimated aspect of cannabis use that should be monitored ideally in a reasonably objective manner where possible. Avoidance of highs from cannabis may reduce addiction that is precipitated, in part, by chronic use.

It is difficult or sometimes impossible to recommend dosages of cannabis for use, unless products are standardized for cannabinoid contents (as used in prescription medications). Some of the reasonable approaches to cannabis dosing of standardized or approved preparations are summarized below:

- Use the common titration paradigm applied in cannabis administration. Begin with low dosages and make gradual increases in intake as required for a desired effect or treatment outcome. Adjustments are easy in some methods of delivery of cannabis (e.g., smoking) but are quite difficult with edibles because of variable times of onset of effects.

- With prescription medications, commence with one to two doses of drabinol (2.5 mg) or one dose of nabilone (1 mg) or one spray of cannabis extract per day. When smoking cannabis, the use of one standardized joint with modest subsequent increases is recommended.
- To titrate dosages, increase by only one unit of the drug (2.5 mg of dronabinol, or 0.5 mg of nabilone, or one spray of cannabis extract containing nabiximols, which delivers 2.7 mg of THC and 2.5 mg of CBD). If side effects occur, reduce dosage by one unit.
- The maximum recommended dosage of spray cannabis extracts is twelve spray doses, and therapeutic dose ranges of drabinol are usually within the range of 5 and 30 mg per day. The daily dosage of nabilone is often 1 to 4 mg per day, and it does not usually exceed 6 mg/day.

The above recommendations refer mainly to prescription-based cannabis products (solid drugs or spray forms), and, as mentioned earlier, adjustments should be made, ideally with medical supervision and disease monitoring. Several guidelines have been proposed for the correct medical evaluation and treatment of an individual with cannabis. These guidelines are portable and have been established by the California Board for Physicians. They are summarized below:

- Take a history and conduct a good-faith examination of the patient.
- Develop a treatment plan with objectives.
- Provide informed consent, including discussion of side effects.
- Periodically review the treatment's efficacy.
- Obtain consultations as necessary.
- Keep proper records supporting the decision to recommend the use of medical marijuana.

There are a number of behavioral treatments available for cannabis dependence, which are noted below in table 30.

Table 30. Behavioral treatments available for individuals with cannabis dependence (addiction) or abuse

- motivational enhancement therapy
- group or individual therapy
- contingency management
- family-based therapies
- special programs for youngsters and teens

The results of behavioral treatments for cannabis dependence or abuse have tended in some circumstances of addiction to produce mediocre results, with an overall one-year abstinence rate of 10–30 percent. Other outcome studies have reported more favorable results.

The below information is highly relevant for people who are addicted and want to quit cannabis. This thirty-day quitting program is summarized below and is valuable for cannabis addicts and abusers. The information is adapted from McDonald Center for Student Well-Being (oede.nd.edu).

Day 1
Today is your decision to quit. For this day:
- Be proud of success to work through craving.
- Remember the advantages of quitting.
- Reward yourself at the end of the day.

Day 2
- Avoid boredom, go for a walk, buy a magazine, spend time with friends, drink water, eat an apple when cravings occur.

Day 3
Throw away all drug-use paraphernalia.
- Review reasons for quitting.
- Make a dental appointment.
- Buy a treat with the money you are saving.
- Take care of any nausea or dizziness with relaxation.

Day 4

- Find work to do.
- Drink Gatorade or soda.
- Doodle on a writing pad if antsy.
- Develop new goals.

Day 5

- Exercise day.
- Understand health benefits of not getting high.

Day 6

- Start saving for special events.
- Save money and treat yourself.
- Save for shopping or a concert or outing.

Day 7

- Consider your diet; make it healthy for good nutrition.
- Drink water, take a vitamin supplement, eat fresh fruit, and so forth.

Day 8

- Think positive and put all urges aside.
- Keep active.
- Know that relapse is possible.

Day 9

- Remember cravings will pass without cannabis use.

Day 10

- Always occupy yourself when you get a craving (e.g., play music, exercise, etc.).
- Take different routes to school or work.
- Chew gum or a toothpick.
- Explore places where you do not get high.

Day 11

- Plan all your next moves to stay drug-free and enjoy your new healthy feelings.

Day 12

- Achieve one goal from your previous promises.
- Refuse dope.
- Always say, "I quit."

Day 13

- Develop your personal motivation to quit using dope.

Day 14
- Avoid stressful circumstances where possible.
- Remember stress that causes the use of cannabis decreases achievement and work performance.

Day 15
- Do not smoke even one joint.
- Think about your efforts to date and do not spoil them.

Day 16
- Know that you changed your attitude toward dope.
- Keep saying, "I will never use it again."

Day 17
- Remember each time you have not gotten high after craving.
- Make sure you do not relapse.

Day 18
- Quitting is hard work.
- Be prepared not to relapse.

Day 19
- Think back on your compromised life when you were using and make a resolution not to go backward.

Day 20
- Say you will never touch cannabis again.
- Do not think you can try it without getting hooked again.

Day 21
- Now keep pressing all limits to quit.
- Do breathing exercises.
- Appreciate the functions of your lungs and heart.

Day 22
- Avoid rationalization for use of marijuana.
- Fight ideas of denial that you were addicted or abusing cannabis.

Day 23
- Remind yourself it takes about thirty days to really begin to feel better physically, sleep better, and see overall beneficial differences in yourself.

Day 24

- Review your progress in terms of perceived benefits (e.g., academic work, job performance, physical well-being, etc.).

Day 25

- Avoid denial now at all costs.

Day 26

- If you have used during this program or you do use again, tell yourself to stop at all safe costs.

Day 27

- Now you are on the home run.
- Never think of a high as pleasure.
- Pick nonusing friends.

Day 28

- Now get really active (e.g., play ball, go on a date, attend plays, etc.).

Day 29

- Know that all your decisions and actions were right by sticking to these plans.

Day 30

- Well done if you are sober.
- Now keep fighting relapse.
- Rejoice in your decision not to use cannabis.

I have hesitated to give any didactic guidelines for marijuana dosing because of the many factors that control outcomes other than dosage alone. These matters are the subject of great debate and some disagreement. However, the table below (table 31) provides some guidance on cannabis dosing, using CBD and THC, primarily in extract forms.

Table 31. Some directions for cannabis use (THC and CBD)

Note that many factors control or influence outcome. Start always with small doses. These statements are *not* accurate dosing guides; they are only approximations of dosage that apply to adults. In cases of doubt, please check with a knowledgeable physician.

These statements are not designed in any way to encourage the illicit use of cannabis.

- Use the titration method for acute effects of cannabis administration.
- Work with a physician or trained healthcare worker to help adjust dosages.
- Neuropathic pain. An initial 2 mg dose of CBD twice daily (a.m. and p.m.), increasing to 20 mg / 24 hours or greater, with the advice of a physician. Many individuals with neuropathic pain require concomitant THC administration for adequate relief.
- Other chronic pain. Similar to neuropathic pain management guidelines, use titration dosing. Try intermittent dosing where possible.
- Anxiety/insomnia. Start with 2 mg of CBD-rich extract taken every eight hours. May slowly add a couple of doses of CBD (about 2 mg) throughout the day. THC may provoke anxiety, and caution is required. Note similar incremental approaches, with extracts of THC and CBD, are used in the management of depression. Self-management of mental disorders is not recommended.

A typical course of progression to marijuana addiction involves steps listed below:

- experimentation (trials)
- social use
- habituation (regular use)
- abuse-use despite negative outcomes
- addiction-compulsion to use

(The above data are modified from oede.nd.edu/educateyourself.)

Synthetic Cannabis Mimics or Synthetic Pot

The Office of National Drug Control Policy has characterized the emergence of the use of synthetic cannabinoids (synthetic pot) as a rapidly emerging threat to public well-being. Some state governments have been slow to respond to this threat to public health. This is a circumstance of great social negligence. A brief overview of the emergence of this serious public health problem is present in table 32.

Table 32. Aspects of the public health problem posed by synthetic cannabinoids (adapted from information published by the administration of the Office of Drug Control policy).

Synthetic cannabinoids are not cannabinoids. They are misnamed and illegal.

- Synthetic cannabinoids are chemicals that can be mixed with plant material or added to food or snacks or candy. They may produce unpredictable psychoactive effects similar to or more pronounced than THC. They are not naturally occurring cannabinoids.
- Synthetic cannabinoids are used commonly by young people with an estimated use by one in nine youngsters in twelfth grade.
- Synthetic cathinones are chemicals related to amphetamines.
- Collaborative work among many agencies is focused toward a ban and control of availability of these potentially dangerous drugs.

As reviewed earlier, synthetic cannabinoids (misnamed) have been made available to teenagers to mimic the psychoactive effects of cannabis (marijuana) and hashish. These chemically synthesized compounds can be mixed with plant materials or tobacco, and they are sometimes described as producing a legal high in a misleading manner. There is, arguably, no legal high as a consequence of drug use, except for the use of cannabis in Colorado, Washington state, Alaska, Oregon, and Washington, DC (at the time of writing). Excellent information on synthetic cannabinoid mimics is found in material produced by the Office of National Drug Control Policy in the United States.

To review matters, a number of types of synthetic cannabinoids are labeled "not to be used for human consumption," and they are sold for a range of actual or fictitious uses including herbal incense, bath salts, or jewelry cleaner. That said, there is a common tendency for the abuse of these types of synthetic pot among youngsters. These drugs are the second most commonly used drugs among high school seniors. In fact, they are second only in use to cannabis itself. In addition, I repeat that it is alarming to see that one in nine twelfth-grade school children in America reported using synthetic pot in the year 2012. Fortunately, there are several initiatives being taken at federal, state, and local government levels to address this pernicious problem of the use of synthetic cannabinoid mimics. This topic should be approached aggressively by organizations such as DARE and the DEA.

The federal government has passed the synthetic Drug Abuse Prevention Act that is incorporated in the FDA Safety and Innovation Act of 2012. This law identifies twenty-six types of synthetic cannabinoids that are now subject to control and have been placed on schedule I of the Controlled Substances Act. Tweaking synthetic cannabinoid molecules (minor changes in chemical structure) does not afford any legal protection for the tweaker, because any molecules with chemical or pharmacological similarity to schedule I or schedule II drugs are to be classified as controlled substances under the Controlled Substance Analogue Enforcement Act of 1986. In recent times, the Drug Enforcement Agency (DEA) has moved to designate several chemicals as schedule I drugs. Nevertheless, there are some gaping holes in the law where only forty-three states have taken action to control one or more synthetic cannabinoids (at the time of writing). Such controls have been in place only for about five years.

The issuance of public health warnings appears to have done relatively little to interfere with the availability and overall use of new synthetic cannabis-mimic compounds. As mentioned earlier, there were estimated to be approximately 150 different types of synthetic pot available in the United States in 2012. Synthetic cannabinoid mimics are readily available for purchase online. While many are imported from other countries (e.g., China), they are also manufactured to a significant degree in the United States. The scary thing is that synthetic pot is quite competitive and popular when compared with natural herbal cannabis.

Some individuals have suggested that fights against marijuana legislation are best replaced by a focus on prevention of alcohol and tobacco use. These individuals argue that marijuana may be "safer than previously thought" (Ingraham, Feb. 23, online: www.washingtonpost.com/blogs/workblog.). Recent research findings in the journal *Scientific Reports* (2015)(a subsidiary of *Nature*) indicated that cannabis use was estimated to cause significantly less deaths than alcohol. This finding was based on calculations that compared lethal doses of several drugs with the amount that a typical person may use.

Symptoms of marijuana withdrawal are shown in detail below:

Physiological	Behavioral	Sleep
Nausea	Restlessness	Disruption
Perspiration	Agitation	Bad dreams
Tremors	Irritability	Insomnia
Weight loss	Depressed mood	
Appetite loss	Aggression	
High body temperature	Loss of motivation	
Anxiety		

The above data are modified from oede.nd.edu/educate yourself.

The plot thickens with recent reports in Colorado of the occurrence of severe symptoms following the consumption of what is popularly known as black mamba (*NEJ Med* 370 (2014): 389–390). The active constituent of this synthetic cannabinoid is referred to as ADB-PINACA, and it is associated with cardiac toxicity and neurotoxicity. In a group of 263 patients identified with a possible exposure to synthetic cannabinoids, there were seventy-six cases of altered mental status combined variably with tachycardia that was followed by bradycardia and occasional convulsions. While most cases were managed in the emergency room of the hospital, seven individuals required admission to an intensive care unit. It is not clear whether or not long-term disabilities have occurred in any of the afflicted individuals.

European Experiences with Synthetic Cannabinoid Mimics (Pot)

Information summarizing a body of current knowledge on synthetic cannabinoid use in Europe is reported in detail online at http://www.encdda.europa/about. Synthetic compounds that stimulate cannabinoid receptors are capable of duplicating psychoactive effects of cannabis in a highly variable manner. As mentioned earlier, these substances have been labeled incorrectly as "legal high" products, and their legality is challenged by law enforcement in a persistent manner in Europe and the United States. This large and expanding group of synthetic substances has been available since approximately 2006 in Europe, and they are an increasing public health concern. Synthetic pot is a central focus of drug compounds that are monitored by the European Early Warning System (EWS) on new psychoactive substances. I emphasize the growth of the availability of synthetic cannabinoids (cannabinoid mimics), which has gone from nine different compounds, reported to the European Monitoring Center for Drugs and Drug Addiction (EMCDDA) in 2009, to 102 compounds documented by December 2013.

Synthetic cannabinoids (misnamed) vary considerably by content and biological effects in a manner that interferes with safety assessments or predictions of adverse effects. Synthetic cannabinoids are mixed often with a number of herbs (e.g., damiana) to improve their consumer acceptance. As mentioned earlier, the most common source of synthetic cannabinoids is found in powdered compounds from China. These compounds are mixed with solvents and sold frequently on the Internet or in specialized shops. The inclusion of solvents may add to their toxicity profile. The sale and distribution of synthetic cannabinoids show several differences in Europe versus the United States, which are difficult to control. Unfortunately, the recorded prevalence of the use of synthetic cannabinoid use is potentially inaccurate, and it is based upon different methods of data acquisition. The reported data tend to show lower levels of synthetic cannabis use in Europe, compared with the United States. These differences are mainly apparent in studies of synthetic cannabinoid usage in the United Kingdom, Germany, and Spain versus the United States.

Synthetic cannabinoids are a common cause of intoxication, with anecdotal reports of the occasional occurrence of fatalities. (Who said that cannabis, or what may be thought to be cannabis, does not cause deaths?) Thus, investigators have concluded unanimously that many synthetic cannabinoid receptor agonists are more dangerous than herbal cannabis. Other serious adverse effects of synthetic cannabinoids include reports of ischemic strokes, acute renal toxicity, and psychotic reactions. Certain mixtures of synthetic cannabinoids may be particularly dangerous. These concoctions have been associated with clusters of serious toxic reactions that present to hospital emergency rooms.

Chemical substances with cannabis-mimicking properties have confusing or meaningless names. However, JWH compounds and AM compounds are named with the initials of researchers who first synthesized these compounds (these code names refer to John W. Huffman and Alexandros Makriyannis, respectively). Other labels of synthetic cannabinoids are based on chemical structures (e.g., APICA) or names derived from institutional sources (e.g., HU compounds from the Hebrew University in Jerusalem). Please note that some new cannabis analogues or drugs are synthetic compounds (synthetic cannabinoids) with reasonable safety profiles. I trust that this information solves aspects of the confusing subject of cannabis analogues or cannabimimetics.

Death from Cannabis?

News reports in recent times have described very infrequent deaths attributable to regular marijuana use (directly). I stress that these occurrences appear to be quite rare. It has been estimated that ingesting about ten times the effective dose of alcohol can be lethal, but the death risk from cannabis may be as much as one to several thousand times the effective dose of this drug (quoted as 10–40,000 but not known with precision). Are these estimates of drug dangers credible?

Three cases of death from marijuana have been a focus of media attention. Two out of fifteen cases of death linked to marijuana use were described by German physicians who were convinced of a direct causal relationship between the events in the two cases. However, some experts have claimed that there is doubt about a direct causal relationship in these cases. Moreover, these two German cases had preexisting risk factors, including a serious undiagnosed heart problem in one case, and the other victim had a history of mixed substance abuse, involving alcohol, cocaine, and amphetamines. The third highly debated case of presumed death from marijuana was reported in the United Kingdom in a female (age thirty-one years) who died from cardiac arrest associated with marijuana use. Cannabis administration or accidental ingestion of cannabis can be dangerous in pets and has caused death from the inhalation of vomit in dogs.

Synthetic pot (not regular herbal cannabis) has been reported to cause death and sickness in a significant number of individuals. Data from Russia (Oct. 2014) report more than seven hundred cases of poisoning and twenty-five deaths after smoking synthetic pot (www.sputniknews.com/russia/201411006). This problem with cannabis has gone global with recent reports of two deaths from synthetic pot in Australia (January 2015, "Synthetic cannabis deaths has sounded alarms in Australia," www.newssciencemag.org/dennis normile).

Opioid Deaths: Cannabis to the Rescue?

As a consequence of the study of death certificates from the Centers for Disease Control and Prevention (CDC), researchers at Johns Hopkins University found that death rates from prescription painkillers climbed at an alarming rate from the year 1999 to 2010. A pivotal finding in this research was that death rates from painkiller overdoses had fallen by an overall factor of 25 percent (Bachhuber, DM, et al., *JAMA* online, 2014) in states where medical marijuana use is allowed.

Many state governments have been slow to recognize the severe public health problem posed by painkiller drugs, and surveys have shown up to about a 300 percent increase in opioid painkiller prescriptions in recent times (reported also as a 425 percent increase in usage in the past decade or so). These prescriptions involve drugs such as Vicodin, Oxycontin, and

Percocet. Alternative medical approaches involve the use of topical pain-control agents purchased over the counter or prescribed in compounded pharmacy preparations. These topical agents may also assist in diminishing the excessive use of systemic opioid painkillers (Holt, S., et al., *The Topical Pain Control Revolution*, 2013).

The most recent announcements on drug-overdose deaths from the CDC, National Center for Health Statistics (NCHS) reports a doubling of painkiller drug deaths from 1999 to 2012. It is notable that deaths from heroin overdosing increased threefold in that time period. If cannabis is a gateway drug, then one may expect greater use of drugs such as heroin and opioid painkillers. However, welcome trends of reduction in opioid deaths have been noted in association with available options for the use of medical cannabis. Time will tell if cannabis can help with this serious opioid drug problem and exert a confirmed harm-reduction effect.

Cannabis Drug Interactions

There are a number of ways that cannabis use does not mix with other drug use. For example, there can be interactions among drugs based on their metabolism or amplification of the pharmacological actions of drugs. In addition, cannabis can act to decrease other drug safety and efficacy. Table 33 gives examples of commonly used drugs and their interactions with marijuana.

Table 33. Some potential drug interactions with cannabis

Drug with Interaction	Comment
Sedatives	Cannabis can often cause sleepiness and drowsiness. Excessive hypnotic effects can be experienced with cannabis and barbiturates or tranquillizers or sleeping pills (e.g., clonazepam, lorazepam, etc.).
Theophylline	Cannabis reduces efficacy of theophylline.
Disulfiram (Antabuse)	Combining disulfiram with cannabis may result in severe agitation, mood change (irritability). and insomnia. Note: alcohol abuse combined with marijuana abuse is quite common.

| Fluoxetine (SSRI) | May cause a hypomania circumstance with anxiety, nervousness, irritability, and the jitters. |
| Warfarin | Cannabis may increase effects of warfarin with occurrence of bruising and bleeding |

Characteristics of Cannabis Disposition in the Body

The pharmacological effects of cannabis are highly dependent upon the mode of administration of the drug. It is very difficult to predict the pharmacological outcome of cannabis smoking (pharmacodynamics effects). Cannabinoids are metabolized (converted in the liver by the hepatic cytochrome P450 enzyme systems to active and inactive metabolites). The oral bioavailability of cannabis components is also quite variable, with peak plasma THC concentrations occurring at any time between one and six hours, depending often on the mode of delivery. When eaten, THC is converted by liver enzymes into 11-OH-THC, a psychoactive metabolite. Cannabinoids can move into and out of adipose tissue in the body. They are lipophilic (fat-loving).

Drug Treatment of Cannabis Addiction

More widespread use of cannabis appears to cause more cases of addiction. It seems clear that about one in ten cannabis users may become dependent on or addicted to cannabis. Experts indicate that more research and development of drug treatments for marijuana dependence are required. Second only to alcohol and tobacco use, cannabis is associated with more cases of dependence than any other drug, even though its propensity to cause dependence is less than some other legal or illicit drugs. This situation occurs as a consequence of its frequency of use.

Several drugs have been proposed to assist in the management of cases of cannabis addiction (table 34).

Table 34. Drugs that may be useful in the management of cannabis dependence (addiction) (adapted from www.leafscience.com)

Note: Rimonabant is no longer in use.

Drug	Comment
Dronabinol (Marinol)	Studies have shown that dronabinol is more effective than placebo at relieving symptoms of cannabis withdrawal.
Pregnenolone	Large doses of THC produce increased pregnenolone levels in animal brains, and pregnenolone reduces the occurrence of a high.
Cannabidiol	Valid reports exist of reduction of cannabis withdrawal symptoms. Counteracts psychoactive effects of cannabis.
Sativex	Sativex has been shown to be effective at reducing withdrawal symptoms in the short term but not in the long term.
Rimonabant (withdrawn drug)	Blocks cannabinoid (THC) actions on the brain but causes severe depression and suicidal thoughts.

The approach to the treatment of drug dependence with the drug that is the cause of the dependence seems to be contrarian therapeutics. It is obvious that the administration of similar drugs to which dependence has developed is encountered with other forms of drugs of addiction (e.g., methadone substitution for narcotics). There are risks with this treatment approach, which could result in substitution of the hook of one drug to another. That said, two promising approaches requiring more research are the applications of pregnenolone and cannabidiol to treat marijuana addiction. These approaches do not involve the substitution of drugs of dependence with addictive properties.

As noted, some degree of dependence upon marijuana is common in young individuals who have had daily, heavy use over at least a period of a decade. Marijuana dependence is more common in young users with psychiatric disorders and may be associated with codependence on other drugs (e.g., alcohol and cocaine). Those with cannabis dependence may respond to treatment of underlying mental disorders by conventional means, but successful outcomes are often short-lived (www.drugabuse. gov/AvailableTreatmentsforMarijuanaUseDisorders).

While it has been stated that there are no medications available to treat cannabis abuse or dependence, promising results have been claimed with the apparent contrarian use of cannabis preparations themselves or related drugs (analogues). Most observations have been made in patients with cannabis withdrawal symptoms. One study has shown benefits in the management of cannabis dependence with the combined use of a cannabis agonist with lofexidine. The drug lofexidine is not available in the United States at present and has been used mainly for the treatment of opioid withdrawal. However, research in humans shows that this drug combination can decrease marijuana withdrawal symptoms and improve sleep. Moreover, this treatment reduces craving for cannabis and decreases relapse rate in cannabis use (reviewed at www.drugabuse.gov).

Cannabis and Work Performance

Many scientists report decreases in social functioning and educational achievement associated with cannabis use. While these associations seem clear, there is a residual debate about cause-and-effect relationships. Moreover, doubts are expressed about the role of cannabis use in causing adverse effects on sociobehavioral functions. Placing arguments aside, an analysis of forty-eight studies of cannabis use reported in medical literature has found cannabis use to be linked with poor academic performance and increased numbers of school dropouts. Adverse effects of marijuana on attentiveness, memory, and learning ability are reported to be present often in heavy cannabis users. Thus, sustained use of cannabis may diminish overall mental and physical performance to the extent that chronic heavy users can be impaired for long periods of time.

On direct questioning, cannabis users often have insight about their own poor intellectual performance, and several studies have indicated the many negative effects of marijuana use on occupational or academic performance (table 35). Again, cause-and-effect relationships are arguable.

Table 35. The negative effects of cannabis on social activity and work performance

There is considerable difference of opinion on the occurrence of these problems, and doubt exists about cause-and-effect relationships.

• reduced cognitive ability	• low levels of social interaction
• general physical health	• mental problems
• increased work absences	• tardiness
• accidents	• worker's compensation claims
• job loss	• reduced motivation

In the short term, the effect of cannabis use on general social and intellectual function appears to be almost universal, but many people compensate for their problems and remain hidden in society. One study of postal workers who tested positive on preemployment cannabis testing had more injuries, industrial accidents, and loss of work time (studies mentioned in this section were reviewed at www.drugabuse.gov/publications/research-reports).

Self-Identification of Problems with Cannabis Use

While there are classic preventive medicine approaches to cannabis abuse, it is very valuable for users to have insight and recognize problems that may result in an early identification of being hooked or dependent on cannabis. These early warning signs are summarized in table 36 and should help individuals who use cannabis to recognize problems for which interventions are required.

Table 36. Signs and symptoms that an individual is developing or has developed dependence on cannabis (modified from data provided online by Brown University, www.brown.edu/student_services/Health_Service.com)

- increasing frequency of use
- requirement for high dosages to achieve the same effect (tolerance)
- repeated thoughts about cannabis use
- economic sacrifices to purchase the drug
- poor academic compliance (e.g., missing class, late with homework, etc.)
- a preference for friends who use cannabis
- craving and discontentment without access to cannabis

Conclusion

Cannabis is poised to become a therapeutic prospect for many diseases when administered in different forms (e.g., extracts or pharmaceutical agents). Risks of adverse effects of cannabis require avoidance in certain circumstances, such as pregnancy or the presence of cardiorespiratory disease or the identification of an increased chance of precipitation of mental disorders, such as psychosis. There are no easy or clear guidelines for cannabis dosing in disease management. There must be clear advice given for cannabis use that ensures lower risks. This is a function of education. Associations of cannabis use with disease often fail to establish causal links.

Chapter 5

HEMP NUTRITION

Hemp: General Information

Hemp is derived most often from the Cannabis indica plant (species of Cannabis indica). These plants grow as many variants. Hemp is a rich source of nutrients and is gaining popularity as a source of functional foods and dietary supplements. Hemp protein applied for nutritional use is derived often from the seeds of Cannabis sativa or indica, which do not contain significant amounts of psychoactive substances (THC, the psychoactive cannabinoid). There are residual differences of opinion how to classify different forms of the genus of Cannabis, but all forms contain variable amounts and types of cannabinoids, with a predominant content of cannabidiol (CBD) in hemp versus marijuana. The most important classification systems involve the chemical characterization of the types and amounts of cannabinoid contents of the species of the plant. As described earlier, the whole family of plants is referred to as Cannabaceae, which includes the genus Cannabis and Humulus. There are considered to be three main species of Cannabis (C.), including C. sativa, C. indica, and C. ruderalis.

As mentioned repeatedly, cannabis contains two major cannabinoids, THC (delta-9-tetrahydrocannabinol) and CBD (cannabidiol). THC is the principal psychoactive component of mixed cannabinoids, and CBD is known to modulate the central nervous system reactions to THC. However, CBD is highly versatile in several positive effects on body function. There has been an important recognition of two principal types of cannabis, namely drug (psychoactive) types and preponderant fiber types (hemp). More detailed chemotypic (chemical content) classifications of cannabis include 1) the more pure drug type (high in THC, often at a concentration of 2–6 percent or greater) and lacking in CBD, 2) an intermediate type (containing mainly THC with some CBD), and 3) a fiber type (with THC levels often less than 0.25 percent and variable CBD content). Some types of modern cannabis contain up to 20 percent concentration of THC (e.g., skunk, "Made In England").

Upon review, it is clear that industrial hemp is not considered to be marijuana, which is characteristically high in THC and low in CBD. Some uninformed individuals believe that permitting hemp to have legal status is tantamount to legalizing marijuana or facilitating its availability. This opinion is nonsense. In brief, using hemp-containing CBD that is low in THC has many health benefits and will prevent the achievement of significant psychoactive reactions (the marijuana high).

In 1970, the assent of the Comprehensive Drug Abuse and Prevention and Control Act superseded the earlier Marijuana Tax Act of 1937. The 1970 Tax Act made all cannabis cultivation, including hemp, illegal in the United States. Despite this ban in the United States, there are at least twenty-nine countries that permit the legal cultivation of hemp. The sale of hemp products is permitted in the United States for nondrug uses (e.g., in garments and as dietary protein sources, using appropriate types of hemp protein). On balance, I believe that a number of concerns expressed about certain foods of hemp origin are quite arbitrary and not supported by a review of scientific studies.

Hemp has been propagated by agricultural means to contain less than 0.3 percent THC, which is generally considered as the upper level of THC in hemp that is permissible by law in the United States. It is important to note that regulations on the sale of cannabis vary from country to country and now state to state in the United States, but regulations concerning hemp use as a dietary or food supplement are quite confusing. Recent legislation in the United States is more permissive of hemp production, which is governed currently at the state level (Farm Bill of 2014, revision of 2013 Hemp Proposals).

Hemp and Nutrition: Brief Overview

Hemp seeds are a rich source of edible oils and high-quality protein. The main constituents of hemp seed are summarized in table 37.

Table 37. Main constituents of hemp-seed oil

The omega-6 to omega-3 ratio of fatty-acid content of the oil is approximately 3:1.

- Oils account for 45 percent by weight of hemp seed.
- Eighty percent of hemp-seed oils are in the form of essential fatty acids (EFA).
- EFA in hemp-seed oil are present as omega-3 and omega-6 fatty acids (linoleic, omega-6 and alpha linolenic, omega-3). Also present are gamma-linolenic acid and stearidonic acid.
- Proteins with high edestin components constitute about 30 percent by weight of hemp seed. The amino acid profile of hemp protein is considered to be complete (all essential amino acids, with some present in limited amounts).

Thus, hemp seeds present a good source of high-quality protein with a healthy content of EFA (essential fatty acids) in a desirable 3:1 omega fatty acid ratio (omega-6:omega-3).

Cannabis in the Food Chain

Cannabis sativa and indica are important and ancient sources of medicine, food, oil, and fiber. Ripe seeds of hemp and meal (made from seeds) are well-defined origins of dietary fiber and unsaturated fats (Callaway, J.C., "Hempseed as a Nutritional Resource: An Overview," *Euphytica*, 140 (2004): 65–72). Table 38 shows a representative analysis of the nutritional content of hemp seed.

Table 38: Typical nutritional content (percent) of hemp seed cv (Finola type) (reproduced from Callaway, 2004).

	Whole Seed	Seed Meal
Oil (%)	35.5	11.1
Protein	24.8	33.5
Carbohydrates	27.6	42.6
Moisture	6.5	5.6
Ash	5.6	7.2
Energy (kJ/100 g)	2,200	1,700
Total dietary fiber (%)	27.6	42.6
Digestible fiber	5.4	16.4
Nondigestible fiber	22.2	26.2

Hemp seed is a valuable source of vitamins (E and B class) and minerals. Typical nutritional values for minerals and vitamins found in hemp seed have been compiled from analysis of Finola (a Finnish variety of hemp) in studies that have been performed and reported by Callaway (ibid. 2004).

Table 39: Typical nutritional values (mg / 100 g) for vitamins and minerals in hemp seed (Finola type) (reproduced from Callaway, 2004)

Vitamin E	90.0
Thiamine (B1)	0.4
Riboflavin (B2)	0.1
Phosphorus (P)	1,160
Potassium (K)	859
Magnesium (Mg)	483
Calcium (Ca)	145
Iron (Fe)	14
Sodium (Na)	12
Manganese (Mn)	7

Zinc (Zn)	7
Copper (Cu)	2

A striking property of hemp seed is its high percentage of quality protein containing all essential amino acids. Callaway (ibid. 2004) produced a very valuable study of the amino acid content of hemp and compared this with other food sources of protein. Table 40 shows this analysis combined with information taken from reliable studies (Callaway, ibid. 2004, quotes work of Scherz et al., *Food Composition and Nutritional Tables*, 1986/1987, 3rd edition, Stuttgart).

Table 40: Typical protein content (percent) of each food is given directly alongside the name. Individual amino acid value for each food is given in grams per 100 g. Essential amino acids are indicated by an asterisk (*). Reproduced from Callaway, 2004.

Amino Acid	Potato (2%)	Wheat (14%)	Maize (11%)	Rice (9%)	Soy Bean (32%)	Hemp Seed (25%)	Rapeseed (23%)	Egg White (13%)	Whey Powder (13%)
Alanine	0.09	0.50	0.72	0.56	1.39	1.28	1.05	0.83	0.61
Arginine	0.10	0.61	0.40	0.62	2.14	3.10	1.49	0.68	0.39
Aspartic Acid	0.34	0.69	0.60	0.86	3.62	2.78	1.82	1.23	1.49
Cystine	0.02	0.28	0.15	0.10	0.54	0.41	0.39	0.29	0.17
Glutamic Acid	0.37	4.00	1.80	1.68	5.89	4.57	4.41	1.67	2.40
Glycine	0.10	0.71	0.35	0.47	1.29	1.14	1.28	0.50	0.29
Histodine*	0.03	0.27	0.26	0.19	0.76	0.71	0.72	0.28	0.29
Isoleucine*	0.08	0.53	0.35	0.35	1.62	0.98	1.00	0.74	0.85
Leucine*	0.11	0.90	1.19	0.71	2.58	1.72	1.80	1.08	1.40
Lysine*	0.10	0.37	0.33	0.31	1.73	1.03	1.49	0.74	1.15
Methionine*	0.02	0.22	0.18	0.17	0.53	0.58	0.46	0.47	0.23
Phenylalanine*	0.08	0.63	0.46	0.43	1.78	1.17	1.05	0.76	0.49
Proline	0.09	1.53	0.85	0.40	1.65	1.15	1.59	0.50	0.43
Serine	0.08	0.70	0.47	0.48	1.54	1.27	1.10	0.92	0.64
Threonine*	0.07	0.42	0.34	0.34	1.35	0.88	1.13	0.58	1.02
Tryptophan*	0.02	0.51	0.04	0.09	0.41	0.20	0.31	0.20	0.25
Tyrosine	0.06	0.40	0.36	0.33	1.14	0.86	0.69	0.46	0.47
Valine*	0.10	0.61	0.46	0.51	1.60	1.28	1.26	0.98	0.91

Hemp and Cannabinoids

Hemp is a source of cannabidiol (CBD) in preponderant amounts (usually up to about 4 percent dry weight), but hemp-seed oil can contain negligible or smaller amounts of CBD. Hemp oil may contain traces of THC, usually less than 0.3 percent, and it does not have any psychoactive properties. Less than a 0.3 percent concentration is the legal limit for hemp oil contents of THC. Many hybrids of cannabis have been produced by special selection and growing techniques where CBD contents of hemp can be increased to about 14 percent CBD per dry weight of the hemp in question.

EFA and PUFA in Hemp Seed

Hemp seed is a rich source of essential fatty acids. Approximately 56 percent of the fat in hemp seed is LA (linoleic acid, omega-6), and 19 percent is LNA (linolenic acid, omega-3), which provides LA (linoleic acid)/LNA (linolenic acid) in an optimal balance ratio of omega-6 to omega-3 fatty acids in a 3:1 ratio. Thus, hemp-seed oil contains omega-3, -6, and -9 fatty acids (linoleic acid, LA, linolenic acid LNA and gamma linolenic acid GLA, respectively). Dietary inclusion of essential fatty acids (EFA) and polyunsaturated fatty acids (PUFA) are very important in the maintenance of human health. They control eicosanoid production and cause alterations in prostaglandin activity. These compounds play an important role in normal immune function with a special role in inflammatory and allergic disease. In addition, EFA and PUFA can exert a positive influence on reducing low-density liproproteins (LDL), thereby promoting cardiovascular health. Furthermore, there is some evidence that LA and LNA reduce the time required for muscle fatigue to recover following strenuous exercise.

Hemp-Seed Protein

Hemp-seed proteins are largely composed in two main types of protein, namely albumin and edestin, which are globular and legumin-type proteins, respectively. It is apparent that amino acid profiles of hemp seed are comparable to other high-quality proteins (e.g., egg whites and soy) (table 40). Hemp protein is high in arginine, glutamic acid, and sulfur-containing amino acids (cystine and methionine). Hemp is also comparatively high in tyrosine, alanine, and aspartic acid. While hemp has been portrayed as a complete protein, especially in advertising in sports nutrition, it has some potential limitations. Although hemp seeds and hemp oil from plants contain all essential amino acids, some are present in relatively small (limiting) amounts.

The limiting amino acid in hemp protein is lysine and to a lesser extent the amino acids leucine and L-tryptophan. That said, hemp protein has a good absorption profile, and studies show that bioactive antioxidant peptides are produced from hemp protein (as studied in simulated digestive studies). In brief, hemp-seed meal has been reported to have a range of digestibility rating scores (from 50 to 86 percent approximately). Some studies have claimed a PDCAAS protein rating score of approximately 86–87 percent compared with 97 percent for casein, but hemp seeds in different forms (oil extracted or dehulled seeds) may have lower PDCAAS scores. Some studies show protein in hemp seed (whole seeds or meal) is only 50 percent digestible. This digestibility score rises to approximately 65 percent when the seed is dehulled.

Health Benefits of Hemp Seed

Studies in experimental animals (rodents) have shown that hemp seed may have positive benefits on memory and learning, perhaps by activating calcineurin. In ovariectomized experimental rats, the use of 1–10 percent of hemp seed in the diet has been shown to reduce experimental menopausal-related anxiety in a dose-dependent manner, probably as a result of its contents of specific phytonutrients.

Dietary additions of hemp seed (up to 10 percent of a total meal) raise blood levels of omega-3 and omega-6 fatty acids with modest reductions in platelet aggregation. In other experiments in healthy individuals, 30 ml of hemp-seed oil given with a regular diet for one month resulted in reductions in blood triglycerides without effects on LDL (or LDL-C). Other studies have shown similar outcomes, but not all studies have duplicated effects on the lowering of blood triglycerides with consistency.

Oral intake of hemp-seed oil (30 ml) over a period of eight weeks in patients with atopic dermatitis has resulted in a nonsignificant trend in reductions of transepidermal water loss, dryness, and itching. Furthermore, some studies suggest an effect of cannabidiolic acid (cannabidiol, CBD) within hemp oil on selective cyclo-oxygenase type 2 inhibition, but these effects are small and unlikely to be of clinical significance. Other studies show that cannabidiol (and cannabidiolic acid) have anticancer properties in one type of invasive breast cancer, and these latter effects appear to be independent of any effects on COX-2 (cyclo-oxygenase) enzymes.

Much of the alleged benefits of hemp protein focus on its potential role in the support of cardiovascular health, but detailed information on the actions of hemp protein to provide benefit in myocardial infarction, hypertension, atherosclerosis, cardiac arrhythmias, and inflammatory states are required from future studies in both animals and humans. Promising data is emerging about the arginine content of hemp protein and its potential role as a nitric oxide precursor. The bioavailability and/or biological actions of key nutritional components of hemp protein (fatty acids, amino acids, and fiber) require considerable further exploration.

Whether or not hemp-seed or hemp protein can be valuable in the prevention or management of other metabolic or cardiovascular comorbidities (e.g., diabetes mellitus, metabolic syndrome, heart failure, etc.) remains underexplored (Rodriguez-Levva, D., and Pirce, G.N., "The cardiac and hemostatic effects of dietary hempseed," *Nutr. Metab* (London) 7, 32, doi: 101186/1743-7075-7-32,

April 21, 2010). The most popular use of hemp protein in nutritional practice is found in sports nutrition.

Diet and Nutritional Status in Adult Marijuana Users

There have been several attempts to investigate changes in diet in marijuana users and their potential effects on health. Using data generated in the Third National Health and Nutrition Examination Survey (NHANES.111), dietary intakes and nutritional status have been examined in cannabis-using adults, age range twenty to fifty-nine years. In brief, differences in these measured parameters of health were not large overall. Current marijuana users, however, showed several differences in nutritional practices compared with nonusers (table 41).

Table 41. General findings of nutritional status and dietary habits in cannabis users versus nonusers (adapted from Smith, E., and Crespo, E. J., *Public Health Nutr*, 03 [June 2001], 781–6)

- A higher intake of calories and nutrients has been noted in cannabis users, but body mass index (BMI) is, on average, lower in cannabis users.
- Marijuana users consume more sodium in their diets.
- Cigarette use, alcohol use, and soda intake were higher in marijuana users.
- Nutritional status was similar in noncannabis users and cannabis users. This status was assessed in a somewhat incomplete manner by measurement of serum albumin, hemoglobin, and hematocrit.
- Serum carotenoid levels were lower in cannabis users.

The Cannabis Plant Genome

The Genomic Research Initiative is a research program at the University of Colorado that is working toward an analysis and genetic mapping of DNA in cannabis. These genomic initiatives involve a collection of DNA samples from cannabis grown in many geographic locations on a worldwide basis. These DNA samples are being investigated to provide a blueprint that can pave the way to growing specific, high-value plants. One principal research objective is to produce a greater source of cannabinoids and other cannabis components that may have special medicinal uses, but the genetic basis of the nutritional value of cannabis is also of interest.

The University of Colorado genomic research team is led by a brilliant researcher from Canada, Dr. Nolan Kane. Dr. Kane has stressed the need to identify genes (chromosomes) at an in-depth level. Earlier research (2011) has shown a sequence of the genome of Cannabis sativa in a somewhat preliminary and unrefined manner. No doubt, one may expect genetic modification to involve itself in cannabis research at some stage, but the work at the University of Colorado is not part of any genetic engineering (GMO) project. In summary, the research is restricted to working only with existing genes in the plant.

Hemp: Nutritional Summary
There are many nutritional advantages and characteristics of hemp food, which are summarized in table 42 below.

Table 42. Some nutritional advantages of hemp-containing foods

- More than 60 percent of hemp contents are essential nutrients.
- It has low allergenic potential.
- It has all essential amino acids (with limiting amino acids).
- Healthy essential fatty-acid contents—omega-3:omega-6 ratio balanced at 1:3.

- Stearidonic acid and gamma linolenic acid contents amplify benefits of other essential fatty acids.
- Hemp is a good source of cannabidiol (CBD) with versatile treatment effects.
- Hemp has valuable components (e.g., magnesium, iron, potassium, dietary fiber, antioxidants [vitamin E], and mixed phytonutrients).
- It is a useful addition to cooking, with the ability to control blood cholesterol.
- It is a sustainable, disease-resistant crop.
- It is ecofriendly, requiring less water with nondepleting properties on soil.

Eating Cannabis or Hemp

Hemp foods are rapidly gaining popularity with a perception of their superior nutritional value (table 42). The use of hemp in cooking has become particularly attractive in health-conscious young people involved in aerobic fitness. Correspondents have referred to hemp as "the new soy" (Diane Walsh, cannabisdigest. ca/hemp-foods-every-diet/). Soy has many advantages as a healthy source of protein and other nutritional factors with valuable biological actions (Holt, S., *The Soy Revolution* [New York: Random House, 1998]).

A preferred source of hemp in the diet is hemp seed, which is now popular in many health food stores and progressive supermarkets. The heart of the hemp seed is called the "hemp nut," which is the healthful source of oils and protein. Hemp seeds are eaten often in a raw form as a cereal dish or in a sprouted form. However, many other hemp-containing foods have emerged (e.g., butters, hemp tofu, milk, tea, ground forms for baking, shakes, granola-type bread, bagels, cookies, and a variety of snack foods). Hemp seeds do not need fancy preparation. They can be eaten in a raw form, packaged in foil for convenience.

Growing Cannabis

In some locations in the United States, hemp cultivation is allowed under the new Farm Bill (2013, 14). While these circumstances vary by state, they are more liberal in locations where recreational cannabis use is allowed. Differences in genetic makeup of different species of cannabis occur, and selective crossbreeding is used to change plant characteristics with a focus on the manipulation of cannabinoid contents. This process is not the same as genetic engineering (GM) product production. It is not possible to cover agricultural methods of cannabis growing in this short book, but the Internet is loaded with this information. Would-be cultivators should look for reliable guidelines for safe growing practices.

A number of other factors are responsible for good cannabis growth. These factors include sophisticated nutrient and light applications during growth cycles. Propagation of cannabis plants is usually maintained in outdoor or indoor locations in well-selected soil. However, hydroponic and aeroponic nutrient and water delivery systems combined with advanced lighting technology are now commonly applied in cannabis growing operations.

As described earlier, the main species of Cannabis include three types, notably sativa, indica, and ruderalis. The ruderalis type has the lowest concentrations of cannabinoids, and indica is usually richer, at least in CBD content. Cannabis sativa is the plant with the highest levels of THC (the principal psychoactive component), but some forms of hemp belong to the genus and species, Cannabis sativa. That said, it is clear that cannabinoid contents of various species of plant vary by geographic location, growing conditions, and many other factors. The results of their consumption can be context specific.

Modern techniques of cannabis propagation for recreational use often favor the use of sensimilla (in popular language). In this process of plant propagation, female plants are protected from pollination so that the development of seedpods can be avoided. This method of propagation results in greater yields of flowers and resin, which are the principal origins of THC. The careful selection of different strains results in desired increases in THC or CBD levels, altered plant aroma, occurrence of shortened growth periods, and different plant coloration. In brief, many selective breeding actions have produced a vast number of strains, with a vast number of meaningless names. Cannabis strains are sometimes sold with no description or an inaccurate description of their cannabinoid components, even by allegedly informed salespeople in some cannabis dispensaries in Colorado, Washington State, Alaska, Oregon and Washington DC.

Driving the Quest for Cannabis/Legalization

Federal guidelines that support marijuana prohibition have been undermined. However, many physicians and the majority of the general public do not believe that cannabis is a drug mixture without medical value and without a reasonable level of safety. As discussed earlier, favorable perceptions of cannabis safety and its medical benefits are driving its use. Recreational use of cannabis is increasing as more people become convinced about its social value and safety. It has been argued that public opinion has driven politicians to approve cannabis use without an optimal amount of research to confirm its safety and efficacy. However, there is still a cautious approach to marijuana use, especially in the presence of data that indicate that its use in youngsters may result in a generation of adults with variable degrees of social or other disabilities. Most people are starting to view hemp as legal for growing and consuming in the United States, but weakening arguments question the legality of hemp use.

Conclusion

Hemp has formed the basis of dietary supplements in many new brands and formats. So far, this circumstance remains largely unchallenged by regulators. Hemp is nutritious and has medicinal qualities as a useful functional food. The CBD content of hemp oil could present some problems because of the US Food and Drug Administration's statements that CBD is not a dietary supplement.

Chapter 6

CANNABINOIDS AND THE ENDOCANNABINOID SYSTEM

Defining Cannabinoids

The principal therapeutic components of the cannabis plant are cannabinoids (phytocannabinoids). Arguably, terpenoids within cannabis are facilitators of cannabis actions that form an entourage effect. Different cannabinoid compounds are present in high concentration in resinous glands of the cannabis plant, called trichomes. It is recognized that the effects of THC are modulated by other contents of the plant, including its various phytocannabinoids and, as mentioned, its mixed terpenoid components. As discussed earlier in this book, the phytocannabinoids in marijuana act on cannabinoid receptors, which results in a number of changes in neurotransmitter release (and function) in the central nervous system. About 480 or more natural substances are found in certain species of cannabis, and up to about one hundred of these are cannabinoids. The cannabinoid 9-delta-tetrahydrocannabinol (THC) is the main psychoactive component of the cannabis plant that has been the subject of more research than other cannabinoids, but research on cannabidiol (CBD) is rapidly advancing and catching up.

Substances produced in the human body (and in different species of animals) are able to act on cannabinoid receptors that are part of the endocannabinoid system. These endocannabinoid substances act as ligands that stimulate cannabinoid receptors. There are three distinct types of cannabinoids, which include (1) phytocannabinoids, which are found in cannabis, (2) synthetic cannabinoid analogues (drugs) (or some forms of synthetic pot), and (3) endocannabinoids, which are examples of lipid substances that are signaling molecules that activate cannabinoid receptors. In other words, this endogenous endocannabinoid system has specific receptors and ligands that permit a general understanding of the therapeutic actions of marijuana and its components.

Other cannabinoid-like effects can occur from noncannabinoid molecules, including enzyme inhibitors that prevent the degradation of endocannabinoids. In pathways of drug development, synthetic cannabinoids can be produced that are substantially similar in structure to THC and other cannabinoids. In addition, there are cannabinoid-like substances that can partially mimic the effects of various cannabinoids (e.g., eicosanoids, aminoalkylindoles, and quinolones, etc.). Finally, there are the misnamed synthetic cannabinoids that are chemicals with cannabinoid-like effects. These compounds are often toxic and should be avoided in circumstances of illicit use. They constitute a significant public health problem, especially in young people.

An Overview of Cannabinoid Actions

Endocannabinoids from within the body and phytocannabinoids from cannabis can alter many body functions. Furthermore, different species or hybrid types of cannabis can present a wide variety of different cannabinoids, some of which are metabolic products of cannabinoids themselves. However, some detected cannabinoids have been shown to be artifacts of measurement techniques in the lab. In simple terms, this means that the cannabinoid profile and content of cannabis plants are often very different. While scientific knowledge of the interactions among different cannabinoids is beginning to become clarified, the overall effects of different cannabis profiles on body functions are sometimes difficult to predict. As mentioned earlier, these circumstances form a massive jigsaw puzzle, but the components of the puzzle are dynamic or fluid.

Cannabinoids function in an entourage effect that is mainly a function of actions of several terpenes and many cannabinoids that are contained within cannabis. It is this versatile entourage effect that accounts for the many effects of cannabinoids on physiological processes (table 43). These actions are mediated by effects on CB1 and CB2 receptors (and perhaps other receptors, e.g., CB3 receptors in the brain that are not well defined).

Table 43. Endocannabinoids are able to exert control over several physiological processes in a complex manner. Their effects are protean.

• Pain modulation	• Immune Function
• Newborn suckling	• Appetite reward
• Thermoregulation	• Memory
• Inflammation	• Other effects

As mentioned earlier, the progression from soft to hard drugs is a well-known phenomenon with cannabis use (gateway phenomenon). There is a residual stubborn opinion that the gateway phenomenon does not happen with cannabis, but evidence strongly supports its occurrence. The frequency of use of marijuana is important in gateway transitions. Thus, it is recognized that the more frequent the use of cannabis, the more likely the individual will ultimately use cocaine or other hard drugs. In other words, mounting evidence exists that marijuana is a potential forerunner to the development of abuse and addiction to many other drugs, but cannabis may be of value in lowering abuse of opiate medications.

Endocannabinoids and Cannabinoids

In brief, endocannabinoids are signaling molecules produced within the body. They act as lipid ligands that stimulate cannabinoid receptors. These substances engage in the process of signaling between nerve cells (neurons, figure 6). The steps in the biosynthesis of endocannabinoids are complicated and are not fully understood. There are several endocannabinoid ligands that have been the focus of variable amounts of research (in brief, ligands are substances produced in the body that can directly activate cannabinoid receptors). Discovery of cannabinoid receptors has precipitated a search for other endogenous ligands. Examples of endogenous ligands are listed in table 44, with relevant comments about their known or suggested actions.

Table 44. Some endogenous ligands that may act on the endocannabinoid system

Actions on receptors may be direct and indirect.

Endogenous Ligand	Comment
Arachidonylethanolamine (Anandamide or AEA)	Derived from essential fatty acid (arachidonic acid). Pharmacology similar to THC with binding to CB1 receptor. Analogs of AEA possess anti-inflammatory and orexigenic effects.
Arachidonoylglycerol (AG)	Binds to CB1 and CB2 receptors and present in higher levels in brain tissue than anandamide.
Noladin-Ether (2-arachidonyl glyceryl ether)	Binds to CB1 receptor with weak binding to CB2 receptor. Argument prevails concerning classification of this compound as an endocannabinoid.
N-Arachidonoyl Dopamine (NADA)	Binds to CB1 receptor preferentially and is an agonist for vanilloid receptors.
Virodhamine (OAE)	Exerts actions as a CB1 antagonist in vivo.

To review circumstances, there are many cannabinoid receptors, often CB-1 and CB-2 types, in the brain and tissues of the body. It is believed that the cannabinoid system functions as a network of communication in the nervous system and body as a complex mechanism involved in the modulation (controls) of mood, pain, appetite, immunity, memory, the coordination and controls of movement, and so forth. These actions of cannabinoids (phytocannabinoids or analogues) make them potential therapeutic agents for a wide variety of diseases, but there is a lack of consensus on effective dosages that can be used in several potential therapeutic settings. Whether or not a consensus could exist in certain disease states is often arguable.

Endocannabinoid Signals

As discussed, the endocannabinoids are lipid compounds that are referred to as ligands that bind to cannabinoid receptors. These ligands are made as required, and they are not stored in any cellular components, but recent research has challenged this observation with the description of endocannabinoid storage vesicles. There is a continuing search for endocannabinoids (or molecules with endocannabinoid functions), but at least four main types are often discussed, including 1) arachidonoylethanolamide (ananadamide or AEA), 2) arachidonoyl glycerol or 2-arachidonyl glyceryl ether (noladin ether), 3) N-arachidonoyl-dopamine (NADA), and 4) virodhamine (OAE).

Endocannabinoids use a pathway of retrograde signaling across a synapse, whereas conventional neurotransmitter substances (e.g., acetylcholine, GABA, or dopamine) are released from presynaptic cells and move toward actions in postsynaptic cells. This form of backward transmission of signals involving endocannabinoids (retrograde signaling) is useful in regulating forward neurotransmitter traffic across a synapse. Endocannabinoids are lipophilic (fat-loving molecules) that do not diffuse for long distances in tissues. This makes their effects quite localized.

Further Insight into Endocannabinoids

Much research has clarified the interaction of cannabinoids with the CB1 and CB2 receptors. The discovery of the endocannabinoid system started with an understanding of the functions of anandamide, an endogenous (within the body) signaling molecule (receptor ligand). The sum total of the effects that cannabinoids produce is a reflection of cannabinoid receptor interactions. In general, the psychoactive components of cannabis, most notably THC, interact with the limbic system in the brain. As discussed earlier, this part of the brain is rich in CB-1 receptors that affect mood, memory, cognition, and psychomotor performance.

Other actions of cannabinoids occur within the mesolimbic pathways of the brain, and these areas of the brain are associated with feelings of reward and pain perception. In summary, the endogenous substances and receptors that affect many body functions are best described as the "endogenous cannabis receptor systems," which also include mechanisms of endocannabinoid degradation and transport. Without degradation of endocannabinoids, their actions persist.

Endocannabinoid: Overview

There is no question that a key to understanding cannabis science is possessing a working knowledge of the endocannabinoid systems of body controls. An efficient way to look at the endocannabinoid systems (ECS) is to highlight their effects in promoting body homeostasis. The ECS is a modulator of several physiological functions, and it works by altering neurotransmitter release at the synaptic level. Aside from the pivotal actions of the ECS on functions of the central nervous system, this ubiquitous controlling network exerts important regulatory actions on the autonomic nervous system, immune systems, reproductive functions, gastrointestinal functions, cardiorespiratory actions, and endocrine networks ... to name a few.

To review matters, the main conclusions of a literature search reported by Dr. J. Bostwick (Mayo Clinic) on the ECS are listed in table 45. This traces the evolution of knowledge about cannabinoid receptors and their functions.

Table 45. Conclusions on research on ECS functions (adapted from Bostwick, J.H., *Mayo Clin. Proc.* 87, no. 2 [2012], 172–86)

- Isolation and definition of the structure of THC in 1964.
- In 1990, CB-1 receptor cloned and shown to interact with THC.
- In 1992, the endocannabinoid, anandamide, was discovered.
- Thereafter, CB-2 receptor discovered with distribution mainly in tissues with immune functions.
- System is stimulated by two endocannabinoids, AEA and 2AG, and perhaps others.
- Regulation of neurotransmission by excitatory and inhibitory mechanisms.
- CB-1 receptors have psychoactive potential and are located primarily in the central nervous system.
- CB-2 receptors are generally peripheral in their actions on body defenses, cellular and humoral functions, gastrointestinal functions, and pain regulation.
- G-coupled receptors in the CNS (CB-1 receptors) are found with high density in areas of the brain that exert control over movement, pleasure, learning, memory, and pain. These areas include the basal ganglia, hippocampus, frontal cortex, and cerebellum.
- CB-1 and CB-2 receptor actions are involved in many physiological processes including coordination, motor

tone, suppression of upper motor neurone functions, tracking behavior, food intake, pain pathways, and so forth.
- Note: CB receptors are located in many areas of the body. It has been observed that activating these receptors may result in nonspecific activation effects.

Cannabinoid Receptors: Detail

There is an extensive and growing amount of literature on cannabinoid receptors. As reviewed in many areas of this book, there are two main cannabinoid receptors, labeled as CB-1 and CB-2, but others may exist. The brain contains most CB-1 receptors, which are referred to as the central cannabinoid receptors. In contrast, CB-2 receptors are sometimes called the peripheral cannabinoid receptors, due to their main location in the body, not in the brain.

There are, however, many reports of CB-2 receptors in the brain along with the presence of CB-2 receptor ligands (molecules that interact with the cannabinoid receptors). Thus, there is crossover between central and peripheral CB receptors with the presence of some CB-1 receptors in peripheral body locations. As reported earlier, it is postulated that other cannabinoid receptors may occur, such as the potential presence of a cannabidiol sensitive (CB-3) receptor.

The CB-1 receptors system has a postsynaptic location, and it assists in neurotransmitter release by retrograde signaling. The presynaptic neuron releases a neurotransmitter (e.g., dopamine), which has actions on different receptors. The outcome of the neurotransmitter release is quite variable because different types of neurotransmitter receptors exist (e.g., at least five different types of dopamine receptors).

As mentioned earlier, it is believed that endocannabinoids may be released in certain circumstances and bind with presynaptic cannabinoid receptors and inhibit the release of the neurotransmitters (e.g., dopamine). As discussed, a separate system exists for degrading or stimulating endocannabinoid synthesis, which involves regulation of enzyme actions. In summary, there is an elaborate control system affecting the endocannabinoid systems of receptors.

Clearly, there is a difference of outcomes of central and peripheral cannabinoid receptor function. CB-1 receptor stimulation tends to result in typical psychoactive effects and other mental changes (e.g., memory disruption). These changes are encountered with THC administration. Peripheral CB-2 receptor functions play a major role in immune modulation, control of liver function, and altering abnormal body metabolism, such as encountered in Metabolic Syndrome X. Thus, there are many potential pharmacological effects that can be induced by using receptor agonists or antagonists in synthetic drug form. Receptor manipulation is an obvious target for present and future drug development.

Cannabinoid Receptor: Activities

As noted, endocannabinoids (2-AG and anandamide) and phytocannabinoids (THC, CBD, etc.) bind to CB-1 and CB-2 receptors. These are G-protein coupled receptors that activate signaling cascades. There is some value in repeating information about receptor functions that are germane to the understanding of the endocannabinoid system of controls. The general effect of CB-1 activation is to alter neurotransmitter release. Neurotransmitters are suppressed at both excitatory and inhibitory synapses, resulting in short- or long-term effects. The neurotransmitters involved include glutamate, 5-hydroxytryptamine, acetylcholine, GABA, noradrenaline, dopamine, D-aspartate, and cholecystokinin (and others).

The inhibition of the release of these neurotransmitters occurs as consequence of a retrograde signaling mechanism. This involves the actions of endocannabinoids (2-AG and anandamide), which are released from postsynaptic neurons. These endocannabinoids move backward over the synapse and bind with CB-1 receptors that are present on the presynaptic neuron terminals. Activation of

CB-2 receptors plays a major role in cytokine/chemokine release and white cell migration, thereby modifying immune functions.

Cannabinoid receptors are widely distributed throughout the body, and there are more CB-1 than CB-2 receptors in the central and peripheral nervous systems. The body distribution of the two receptor types is shown in table 46.

Table 46. The body distribution of areas containing CB-1 and CB-2 receptors

Please note other areas containing CB-1 receptors include adipocytes, leucocytes, spleen, heart, lung, gastrointestinal tract, muscle, bones, joints, and skin.

CB-1 RECEPTORS	CB-2 RECEPTORS
• Cerebral cortex	• Ubiquitous in the immune tissues
• Hippocampus	• Present on leucocytes and spleen
• Amygdala	• Liver
• Basal Ganglia	• Bone
• Substantia nigra	• Astrocytes
• Globus pallidus	• Microglia
• Cerebellum	• Oligodendrocytes
• Pain pathways	• Subpopulations of neurons
• Afferent spinal cord	• Spleen
• Sparse in brain stem	• Present on other white blood cells

As discussed earlier, there are presumed to be other cannabinoid receptors, most notably the third cannabinoid receptor, GPR55. In addition, other binding sites of cannabinoids include the transient receptor potential (TRP) cation channel, nuclear receptors, such as peroxisome proliferator activated receptors (PPARs). Moreover, there appears to be close communication between pathways involving endocannabinoids and eicosanoids. Thus, there are complex intercommunicating pathways controlled by the endocannabinoids and their receptors, which, in turn, regulate body functions to create a circumstance of harmony or homeostasis. Thus, cannabis is a "chatterbox" among nervous pathways.

It is easy to see how abnormal regulation of the endocannabinoid system is linked with many different diseases. This abnormal regulation of these complex systems of control of body functions can be considered potentially protective or maladaptive, but they may be amenable to correction by exogenously administered cannabinoids that target specific receptors or alterations of metabolic pathways that affect the synthesis and degradation of endocannabinoids.

To reinforce the knowledge accumulated at this point, the characteristics of CB-1 and CB-2 receptors are summarized again in table 47.

Table 47. Main characteristics of CB-1 and CB-2 receptor activity

CB-1 Receptors

- High density of CB-1 receptors in the nerve cells of brain with lower numbers of receptors in the brain stem.
- Highest density in cerebellum, basal ganglia, hippocampus, and dorsal primary afferent areas of the spinal cord. This distribution explains effects of cannabinoids with predominant CB-1 receptor activity on pain control and modifications of motor function.
- The density of cannabinoid receptors is quite low in brain stem areas that control breathing (medulla oblongata). This is one reason why cannabinoid overdosing does not result in death by interruption of vital body functions.

CB-2 Receptors

- Immune cells express high amounts of CB-2 receptors, but there is a smaller expression of CB-1 receptors.
- CB-2 receptor activity controls immune function, such as cytokine release.
- CB-2 receptor activity may balance aspects of CB-1 receptor stimulation, e.g., inhibition of THC activity on CB-1 receptors.
- Focus of research on CB-2 receptor agonists for anti-inflammatory and antitumor properties shows promising results.

A Further Review of the Functions of Endocannabinoids: Revision

The sum of a group of lipids (eicosanoids) and their receptors constitute the functioning endocannabinoid system. This system controls many body functions including appetite, mood, pain sensation, memory, and motor learning, and it exerts psychoactive effects on the brain. To help consolidate knowledge, table 48 summarizes some of the main effects or functions of the endocannabinoid system in the body.

Table 48. Main effects of cannabinoids on the body

Function/Effect	Comment
Memory	Smoking cannabis decreases short-term memory, but higher dosages or cannabinoids can stimulate neural growth in the limbic system. That said, high-dose, long-term cannabis use most often impairs memory.
Appetite	THC acts via CB-1 receptors to increase appetite. Endocannabinoids affect taste perception and food-seeking behavior.
Energy balance	The endocannabinoid system has effects on thermoregulation, energy storage, and nutrient transport.
Stress	The endocannabinoid system can reduce stress responses by actions on the hypothalamic-pituitary-adrenal axis.
Behavior	Highly complex effects, with relaxation and passivity or antisocial behavior with aggression and anxiety.
Analgesia	Complex actions, but cannabinoids are known to suppress noxious stimuli to the CNS, e.g., injury from trauma.

Cannabinoid actions are present in natural or synthetic compounds that affect cannabinoid receptors. While phytocannabinoids were considered to be present only in

Cannabis sativa and related species, some cannabinoid-like substances called bibenzyls have been found in other plants, such as liverwort. The common types of cannabinoids found in Cannabis sativa belong to one of many classes of cannabinoids, which include most often the following types: cannabigerol, cannabidiol, delta-9-THC, cannabinol, and cannabichromene.

In review and summary, at least two cannabinoid receptors, CB-1 and CB-2, occur with different tissue distributions. These are examples of G-protein couple receptors (GPCR), which are ubiquitous in the brain, spinal cord, and peripheral nerves. The CB-1 receptors are present at the terminals of nerves, and they may inhibit or regulate the release and actions of other neurotransmitters. These actions protect extremes of activation or inhibition of the nervous system. In general, CB-1 receptor stimulation affects the psyche and circulation, but CB-2 receptor activity does not have such effects. The CB-2 receptors are present mainly on immune cells (leucocytes, spleen, and tonsils), and they control the release of cytokines.

There is evidence that the endocannabinoid system has tonic activity. Some compounds can block the effects of endocannabinoids and produce effects that oppose the results of the actions of cannabinoid receptor agonists. These changes imply that the cannabinoid system is tonically active. Tonic effects of endocannabinoids include increase in pain perception, degrees of spasticity, appetite control, and vomiting.

Revealing Terms: Tonic and Entourage Effects

The word "tonic" has several meanings, but this term was "formerly used for a class of medicinal preparations believed to have the power of restoring normal tone to tissue" (www.biology-online.org). In the context of the many components of cannabis, this is a good way of defining controls exerted by the endocannabinoid system of the body. It is crystal clear that this control system is affected by the administration of phytocannabinoids and other factors.

In this section, I raise again the concept of entourage effects. The words "entourage effects" were applied to the actions of cannabinoids in 1998 by S. Ben Shabat and Ralphael Mechoulam (Israeli physicians). Subsequently, the definition of these effects was amplified and further described by Ethan B. Russo, scientific advisor to G. W. Pharmaceuticals, UK. This use of the word "entourage" describes the ability of cannabinoids and associated compounds in marijuana to act together in a process of regulation of a number of physiological events. This cooperative biological activity involves a number of described or uncertain interactions among many compounds.

Research has revealed that terpenoids contribute to the entourage effect of cannabis. Terpenoids (essential oils) are responsible for the odor of many plants, but isolated cannabinoids have no distinctive smell. Terpenoids and cannabinoids are produced by the glandular trichomes of the cannabis plant from the precursor geranyl pyrophosphate. The therapeutic potential of terpenoids appears promising, and it would appear that they are often synergistic with cannabinoids. That said, there are estimated to be about two hundred different terpenoids in cannabis, and only a few have been studied in detail for their biological effects.

The Entourage of Cannabinoids and Other Compounds

In this chapter, a summary of the overall differences of action of many cannabinoids is discussed. This knowledge is expanding with a discovery of degrees of agonist actions of cannabinoids on cannabinoid receptors that may be tempered by antagonist actions of other cannabinoids. The principal crude classification of cannabinoids involves a differentiation between those that are psychoactive (notably THC) and those that do not possess this activity, as a dominant mode of action (e.g., CBD). In general, three principal classes of cannabinoids have been defined that do not have psychoactive properties. They include CBG, CBC, and CBD. On the other hand, THC, CBN, and certain other cannabinoids display variable psychoactive actions. Examples of the main types of cannabinoids are shown in table 49 below.

Table 49. Examples of some of the main types of phytocannabinoids

• THC	(Tetrahydrocannabinol)
• CBG	(Cannabigerol)
• CBD	(Cannabidiol)
• CBC	(Cannabichromene)
• CBL	(Cannabicyclol)
• CBV	(Cannabivarin)
• THCV	(Tetrahydrocannabivarin)
• CBDV	(Cannabidivarin)
• CBCV	(Cannabichromevarin)
• CBGV	(Cannabigerovarin)
• CBGM	(Cannabigerol Monomethyl Ether)

The most commonly occurring cannabinoid is CBD, and it has the most versatile effects on body functions (described to date). Resinous extractions of cannabis can contain up to 40 percent or more concentrations of CBD. It is important to recognize and remember that cannabinoids work in concert to alter body functions, and, as noted, other substances within cannabis operate in what has been described as an entourage effect. It is helpful to reiterate that plants with greater percentages of CBD can reduce the psychological effects of THC. In other words, high concentrations of CBD reduce the potency of the psychological impact of THC. One important property of CBD is its previously mentioned anxiolytic effect, which may be helpful in the control of anxiety precipitated by high concentrations of THC in some cannabis products.

Aged cannabis may lose significant potency by oxidation of its components. Against this background, one can see again that the variability of the outcome of cannabis use can be due to unpredictable changes in contents of the mixture of cannabinoids that are present in whole herbal cannabis. Poor storage of cannabis plant material can reduce or alter the bioactivity of a cannabis product. As noted, exposure of harvested cannabis plants to air results in oxidation of several cannabis components. Oxidation of THC produces CBN. This CBN has a minor psychoactive effect that can react with THC to reduce its psychoactive effects (c.f. CBD). Before one can delve into the treatment options that cannabis presents, it is important to know about the characteristics and general actions of various cannabinoids. These actions are summarized in the ensuing sections of this book, but this is difficult information to retain and commit to memory, especially by some heavy cannabis users.

Cannabinoids are examples of terpenoids. While all types of cannabinoids are terpenoids, the reverse is obviously not the case. The starting point ("mother of cannabinoids") of cannabinoid production is the compound Cannabigerol acid (CBG-A). Within the plant, CBG-A is converted to THC-A, CBD-A, CBC-A, and their associated metabolites.

Cannabinoid receptors (CB-1, CB-2) remain in a state of constant activity and help to set the tone of the endocannabinoid system. This circumstance occurs by constant activation of G proteins in a manner that maintains a balance of various body functions. Compounds with agonist properties activate receptors of the CB-1 and CB-2 type, and they may produce transient or prolonged effects on receptor tone. Variable activation of receptors provides some understanding about the interindividual variation in the animal or human responses to the same phytocannabinoid. In addition, receptor density in certain tissues can be altered by phytocannabinoid use. As mentioned earlier, cannabinoids are produced from precursor cannabigerol compounds, and the most studied cannabinoids are tetrahydrocannabinol THC and cannabidiol.

Tetrahydrocannabinol (THC)

Discussions that reiterate the effects of cannabinoids are considered to be highly desirable by the author, in order to reinforce learning and knowledge retention by the reader of this book. Any annoyance precipitated by this approach is a way of drawing attention to key principles in cannabis science. The recognition of the actions of THC resulted to a major degree in the discovery of the endocannabinoid system by researchers in Israel. The phytocannabinoid THC mimics the actions of anandamide, which is a principal ligand in the endocannabinoid system. The binding of THC to CB1 receptors in the brain produces psychoactive effects, and it also accounts for other actions of THC, which include relief of moderately severe pain (analgesic actions), neuroprotective effects, anti-inflammatory activity, positive stimulatory effects on neurogenesis (growth of brain tissue), and some anticancer effects.

Several isomers of THC exist, but it is 9-delta-tetrahydrocannabinol that is the principal source of psychological effects resulting from cannabis consumption. To review the main sources of THC is relevant for some degree of clarification of the effects of cannabis use. The terms cannabis and marijuana refer to the leaves and flowering tops of the plant, with the inclusion of buds that are particularly high in THC content. Hashish is composed of resinous components of the plant (Cannabis sativa) that are extracted with a solvent and subsequently consumed by smokers. Hashish contains variable amounts of THC and CBD, determined by its origin and degree of processing. It is used for dabbers or mixers with edibles. Cannabis (marijuana) and hashish are classified as schedule I controlled drugs, and the pharmaceutical version of THC is a schedule III drug called dronabinol (Marinol). Dronabinol (Marinol) is dispensed in variable dosages of 2.5, 5, or 10 mg of THC, in capsules.

As mentioned earlier, various descriptions of the effects of cannabis products have referred to properties of THC-containing cannabis as a sedative, stimulant, euphoriant, or mild hallucinogen. The problem is that varying amounts and overall composition of cannabis can produce different effects, which can occur even as a result of consumption in different contexts. The main purpose of the recreational use of cannabis is to obtain relaxation, mood-altering effects and feelings of euphoria (a high).

State laws for marijuana use specify a number of medical conditions in which marijuana may be valuable, but there are some differences among the various state acts of legislation. Most states do provide some discretion for physicians on their recommendations for cannabis use, but in all states (except Colorado, Washington state, Oregon, Alaska, and Washington, DC, at the time of writing) the recreational use of marijuana remains banned. There is a major attempt in most legislation to focus on limiting the use of THC. Thus, limitations are placed on the use of the major psychoactive component of cannabis (THC). This means that THC is recognized sometimes as a drug requiring controls of its use. Several other cannabinoids or nonpsychoactive components of cannabis such as CBD are (arguably) not considered to be drugs in the opinion of many people. While this is a simplistic overview, it is a general rule of thumb. I predict that these circumstances will change or be redefined or better defined in the future. Most people would be pleased if matters were clarified, but the FDA considers that CBD is not a dietary supplement.

The potency of marijuana for recreational use is often gauged on its THC concentration, which is often described as a percentage THC level per dry weight of material. It is worth noting that percentage dry weight can be used to refer to the content of other cannabinoids (e.g., CBD). As discussed earlier, different strains of marijuana have different compositions with varying amounts of cannabinoid content, but most attention has been placed on THC concentrations. In brief, hashish oil or resinous isolates contain about 5–40 percent (or higher) THC per dry weight, and whole herbal cannabis may have THC concentrations of 1 to about 17 percent (or higher). For example, the popular form of skunk contains often 20 percent THC per dry weight.

As mentioned, different strains at different stages of maturation are grown under different conditions, and if they are stored in an uncontrolled manner, it will affect the potency of cannabis-related products. It is now helpful to see the importance of the term "variable" when it comes to any description of cannabis composition or effects. In fact, most people who use illicit cannabis do not have any certainty about the composition of the material that they have purchased for use or grown in their own home. In brief, outcomes of cannabis use (notably for recreational use) are determined to a major degree by psychoactive potency of the product, measured as THC content. As mentioned repeatedly, the THC content is most often determined roughly by self-titration for effects when cannabis is used.

Different Modes of Delivery

The many ways of taking cannabis products (smoking, vaporization, edibles, oral sprays, etc.) result also in variable effects and timing of onset of effects. Different modes of delivery exert significant effects on the onset, duration, and potency of the actions of cannabis, at least in the short term. Rough estimates of dosage by various routes have been made, but their value in assessing dose and response information is limited. A single intake of smoke from a joint is referred to as a "hit," which can be roughly estimated to deliver about 1/20 of a gram of THC. A couple of drops of hash oil or resin are sometimes estimated to be equal in potency of a psychoactive effect to a single joint of whole herbal marijuana. I stress that these estimates are crude guesses and do not form any reliable guidelines for marijuana use. However, pharmaceutical forms of cannabis provide a way of standardizing dosage of THC, and they can be titrated over a period of time, preferably with the assistance of a health care giver, in order to define optimum dosages for disease management. Cannabis smoking materials are hard to standardize for use.

Absorption, Distribution, and Metabolism of Cannabis

There has been much research that has defined the absorption, distribution, metabolism, and excretion of cannabis components (cannabinoids) in animals and humans. Most people recognize that smoking results in rapid absorption of biologically active constituents of cannabis, notably THC. Cannabis edibles have much slower onset and more delayed actions than smoked material. The amount of active cannabis components that are absorbed and made available to the body is influenced by the body's ability to metabolize the drug mixture found in cannabis. There is extensive first-pass metabolism of cannabis components by the liver. This terminology refers to the breakdown of cannabis components as they pass through the liver, and it occurs as a consequence of the actions of enzymes in the body that break down drugs in general. Enzymes of particular note that metabolize THC and are referred to as cytochrome P450, 2C9, 2C11, and 3A (located in the liver).

These enzymes that metabolize cannabis can be induced to exert high or low levels of activity. This alteration of function is often caused by the concomitant taking of other drugs. Metabolic mechanisms alter the clearance of THC and other components of cannabis from the body. Thus, other drugs that alter these enzymes responsible for metabolism can affect drug elimination processes and the duration or magnitude of the pharmacological effects of drugs. In simple terms, this means that components of marijuana (e.g., THC) can be involved in somewhat unpredictable drug interactions. Smoking of cannabis results in rapid absorption and the psychoactive effects of THC due to the achievement of high blood concentrations. It has been reported that THC concentrations in the plasma of the blood reach levels of 100–200 ng/ml, but they usually fall to levels below 5 ng/ml in about three to four hours after cessation of smoking.

Unpredictable Effects of THC

It is recognized that THC is fat-loving (or lipophilic) and is attracted to the fatty tissues of the body where it is temporarily stored and released at varying rates. This process of redistribution of THC results in the detection of marijuana use up to several days (or longer) after its use, in many people. Many researchers have sought information about blood concentrations of THC and its relationship to psychoactive effects. It seems that it is difficult to define these dose/response relationships. For example, some psychoactive effects of THC have been noted in some individuals who do not have measurable amounts of THC in their blood that can be detected with common methods of measurement. However, there are questionable claims that a definition of the time that has elapsed from marijuana use can be used as a predictor of behavioral and cognitive changes in the individual in question. This prediction can only be considered to be of marginal accuracy. The uncertainty of the processing of cannabis by the human body is becoming a common defense in cases of an accusation of a DUI with cannabis. Enter the lawyers!

The stimulation of cannabinoid receptors in the brain by THC results in a disruption or change of the controls on body function that are exerted by the endocannabinoids. These endocannabinoids are a key part of the endocannabinoid systems of body control. The stimulation of cannabinoid receptors by THC results in the cannabis high and other changes in psychological function. It is proposed that continuing, active stimulation of cannabinoid receptors can alter brain functions such as pleasure appreciation, reward, memory, concentration, time perception, and so forth. Moreover, protracted cannabinoid receptor stimulation may result in the development of dependence and addiction. Accepting the reports of increased potency of modern cannabis due to its greater concentrations of THC, the outcome of THC exposure in greater amounts is not entirely clear. These issues illustrate the unpredictable effects THC administration.

Reviewing Effects of Cannabis on the Psyche and Body

The reader's attention has been drawn to an understanding that the pharmacological effects of cannabis use (notably THC) are altered by several circumstances. These include dosage, experience of user, context of use, tolerance, route and method of administration, and so forth. Perhaps the most protean effects of cannabis occur on psychological status. As mentioned repeatedly, feelings of euphoria, body relaxation, disorientation, lack of concentration, and difficulties in thought formation with impaired short-term memory are frequent reactions to cannabis use. In addition, occasional mood changes, panic reactions, and even paranoia may occur. These are examples of only a few psychological changes that have been documented following cannabis use, and they are a function of the presence of THC to a major degree. Please note that many of these adverse effects can be expected to be more severe with the use of hashish or synthetic pot, where THC-like effects are potent.

There are frequent changes in body functions with cannabis (THC) use. Common examples include bloodshot or reddening of the eyes, increased heart rate, dry mouth, irritated throat and airways, increased appetite, fluctuations in blood pressure, and vasodilatation (relaxing of blood vessels). Some of the most important physiological and psychological effects of smoked cannabis with significant THC content are shown in table 50.

Table 50. Signs and symptoms that may form an eclectic side-effect profile of cannabis use (short- and longer-term use)

psychosis	depersonalization
fatigue	mood alterations
paranoia	urinary retention
memory problems	constipation
motor incoordination	chronic lethargy
slurred speech	dizziness
nutritional deficiencies	lung damage
cardiovascular effects	immune problems
reproductive effects	behavioral changes

The multiple circumstances described above can be used to some degree in the detection of marijuana use or abuse, but their diagnostic ability is not always clear. There are a growing number of scientists who are interested in patterns of symptoms and signs of marijuana abuse that can be used in early detection programs of marijuana abuse (or cannabis use disorder or addiction). This approach of early detection has been suggested as a possible key to secondary preventive measures for marijuana addiction. It is proposed that early identification of marijuana abusers can result in interventions at a time when prognosis for the reversal or management of dependence with simple interventions is optimal (a form of secondary disease prevention). Moreover, these early interventions would be anticipated to be more effective in the course of the development of marijuana addiction when they are applied at a time when circumstances of dependence are easier to reverse in the emerging marijuana addict. I perceive that these ideas of secondary prevention of marijuana addiction are going to become of major significance with the inevitable legalization of marijuana use and the attendant, increasing occurrence of marijuana abuse or addiction.

Professor Wayne Hall Speaks

Professor Wayne Hall (University of Queensland, Australia) has published a review article in the journal *Addiction* that discussed the negative effects of cannabis use on mental and physical health (online: *Addiction*, 109, doi: 10.1111/add12703). This review has attracted debate, but it is a balanced view of public health warnings that sometimes accompany cannabis use. Professor Hall has reached a number of opinions from his research of modern medical literature published in the past twenty years. This information is summarized in table 51, in an adapted format.

Table 51. Summary of adverse outcomes of cannabis use (adapted from a report by Hall, W., www.addictionjournal.org)

- Acute cannabis use doubles the risk of a motor vehicle accident. This risk increases with concomitant alcohol intoxication.
- Cannabis use in pregnancy has caused reductions in birth weight of the baby.
- Persistent use of cannabis can result in the development of a dependence syndrome. Use in adolescence increases the likelihood of the development of addiction.

- An increased risk of psychosis is associated with young age of use and genetic predispositions.
- Youngsters who have used cannabis in a persistent manner tend to have lower levels of educational achievement.
- Intellectual impairment is associated with long-term, heavy cannabis use.
- Cannabis users are at risk of lung disease and myocardial infarction.

Is There a Need for Secondary Prevention of Cannabis Use?

If or when an increased number of individuals develop dependence or addiction from easier access to cannabis, then some preventive programs for marijuana addiction or frank abuse must be put in place. Certainly, there will be future modifications in political legislation that may help to prevent abuse or addiction that have started to occur in recent times (e.g., recent control of hashish production in Colorado where recreational cannabis use has been legalized). Clearly, primary prevention of cannabis use by banning this drug has not worked in a comprehensive manner. Furthermore, decriminalization of cannabis use in many locations provides a sense of comfort and relief among some users. Tertiary prevention involves the diagnosis of marijuana use at an advanced stage, where there may be established physical or mental or social problems. This stage of marijuana use is only amenable to rehabilitation at a time when the addiction is established and the prognosis for a complete recovery or abstinence is low.

I predict that there will be a further increase in secondary prevention programs for cannabis use in place. As mentioned, this form of prevention involves early diagnosis and intervention at a time when chances of recovery are more able or likely to be achieved. These strategies have been successful in the management of alcohol abuse. (Holt, S., Skinner, HA, Israel, Y., "Identification of alcohol abuse. II. Clinical and laboratory indicators," *Canadian Medical Association Journal* 124, no. 10 (1981): 1279–94. Holt, S., Skinner, HA, "Confronting Alcoholism, *Canadian Medical*

Association Journal 51 (1990): 8–9. Holt, S., "Tackling the alcohol problem: the case for secondary prevention," *Journal of the South Carolina Medical Association* 85, no. 12 (1989): 582–4.) Secondary prevention programs may be effective in the management of cannabis dependence and perhaps frank addiction.

In his valuable book titled *The Good News about Drugs and Alcohol* (New York: Villard Books, 1991), Dr. Mark S. Gold gives an interpretation of a comprehensive list of signs and symptoms of marijuana use, which are presented in a truncated form in table 52. This information is based on information compiled originally for *Psychiatric Annals* (Gold, M. S., ibid. 1991).

Table 52. Some of the main signs of marijuana use (reproduced and summarized from Gold, M.S., ibid. 1991, taken from *Psychiatric Annals*)

Many cannabis users may find some of these descriptions objectionable.

Behavioral signs	Chronic lying, memory disorders, suspicion of criminal activity (theft), abusive behavior, panic attacks, secretiveness.
Social signs	DUI, accidents, truancy or interruption of studies, underachievement, poor academic performance, laziness.
Circumstantial evidence	Smell of marijuana, disappearing for many hours, use of drug terminology, change in hygiene and attire.
Medical symptoms	Chronic fatigue, irritating cough, sore throat, headaches, persistent red eyes, impaired motor functions, general performance problems.

Cannabinoid Cascades

The biochemical pathways of the synthesis of main cannabinoids in cannabis plants are shown in table 53.

Table 53. The cascade of cannabinoid synthesis modified from D. Macpherson (www.cannabisdigest.com)

In this table, the common pathway resulting in the production of THC, CBD, and CBC starts with the presence of CBGA.

CBG-A
(Cannabigerolic acid)
↓
Synthase Enzyme
↓
CBG
(Cannabigerol)
Raw – Unheated – Undecarboxylated
↓↓↓
THC Synthase CBD synthase CBC Synthase
↓↓↓
THC-A CBD-A CBC-A
↓↓↓
(Heat/UV) (Heat/UV) (Heat/UV)
↓↓↓
THC (delta-9) CBD CBC
↓
CBN

The following sections of this book present a brief summary of the effects of various individual phytocannabinoids. In some circumstances knowledge is quite incomplete (at the time of writing).

Cannabinol (CBN)

Cannabinol has been proposed as a potentially effective antiemetic, anticonvulsant, and as a substance of value in the management of insomnia. Cannabinol (CBN) has only mild psychoactive effects and has greater affinity for the CB2 receptor than the CB1 receptor. Cannabinol (CBN) is produced by the oxidation of THC and may be an indicator of age or exposure of cannabis to heat during storage. In fact, most of the CBN (cannabinol) that is present in cannabis results from the degradation of THC by oxidation, and CBN is often found in aged cannabis that has been stored in a crude manner.

Cannabinol (CBN) is an antioxidant itself that may have similar analgesic actions as THC. This cannabinoid is almost devoid of psychoactive effects and can reduce intraocular pressure in the eye with a therapeutic effect similar to THC. The ingestion of 2.5–5 mg of CBN is quite sedative and has a similar level of sedation and relaxation equivalent to 10 mg of diazepam (a sedative benzodiazepine drug). It is recognized that a synergistic effect of CBN with THC and CBD can facilitate sleep induction.

Cannabigerol (CBG)

It is recognized that both CBD (cannabidiol) and THC (tetrahydrocannabinol) are produced in the cannabis plant from the precursor cannabigerol (CBG), in a manner that is independent of each other. Cannabigerol is nonpsychoactive, but it has several clear pharmacological effects, including alpha 2-adrenergic receptor agonist effects, properties of 5-HT 1A receptor antagonism, and an ability to bind to both CB1 and CB2 receptors. CBG appears to possess neurogenic properties (stimulating the growth of brain cells), and it can promote bone growth. Ancillary actions of CBG include anticancer effects, antibacterial actions, and sleep promotion.

Cannabichromene (CBC)

Cannabichromene (CBC) is found most often in cannabis grown in tropical climates. It is devoid of psychoactive effects, but it is described as having antiviral, anti-inflammatory, and analgesic actions. Cannabichromene (CBC) may be more effective than CBD (cannabidiol) in the potential treatment of stress and anxiety (up to ten times more effective). It is noted that THC use is not advised in individuals with major anxiety because it may exacerbate circumstances.

Tetrahydrocannabivarin (THCV) and (CBDV) Cannabidivarin

CBDV (cannabivarin) is generally found in small amounts in cannabis plants, but it has been detected in significant amounts in hashish from Nepal and India. THCV (tetrahydrocannabivarin) interacts with CB1 receptors and lessens the psychoactive effects of THC. The term "varin" refers to cannabinoids with three carbon tails, which is called tetrahydrocannabivarin (THCV). It is noted that THCV has greater psychoactive effects than THC, but its effects are of shorter duration and more energizing. For this reason, THCV has been called the "sports car" of the cannabinoids. THCV may block panic attacks without suppression of emotions. It has putative beneficial effects on tremor, bone growth, Parkinson's disease, and osteoporosis. It is a potent anorectic.

Cannabidiolic Acid (CBD-A)

Cannabidiolic acid (CBD-A) has demonstrated anti-inflammatory effects and antitumor activity. The production of hybrid cannabis plants has resulted in some modern strains that produce more CBD-A than THC.

Cannabidiol (CBD)

Cannabidiol is emerging as the therapeutic champion of the cannabinoids. Cannabidiol (CBD) has been shown to act as a 5-HT1A receptor agonist, which may account for some of its anxiolytic, antidepressant, and neuroprotective actions. In addition, CBD has been proposed to play an important role in the management of epilepsy (convulsions), inflammation, and nausea. Novel proposals for the use of CBD in medical treatment include its potentially beneficial effects on psychosis (schizophrenia), skin disease (acne), and metastatic spread of cancer (notably breast cancer).

Cannabidiol (CBD) has variable and sometimes limited affinity for CB1 and CB2 receptors, but it can antagonize some of the central nervous system effects of certain cannabinoids (e.g., THC). For example, CBD has been shown to prevent short-term memory loss induced by THC in animals. The lack of psychoactive actions of CBD is advantageous in the treatment of diseases especially in children and the elderly. This circumstance reinforces the potential value of CBD in childhood epilepsy. It has been suggested that CBD may be as effective as THC in the management of pain or the negative consequences of cancer, such as wasting syndrome, but opinions vary. There are a number of miscellaneous effects of CBD, such as calming effects, the potential of lowering blood sugar in patients with diabetes mellitus, and relieving excessive stress and/or sleep deprivation.

Cannabidiol (CBD) is the most versatile therapeutic cannabinoid that has been defined to date. The effects of CBD have been studied for its benefit in many diseases or circumstances of depressed health. These include arthritis (rheumatoid disease), post-traumatic stress disorder (PTSD), epilepsy, antibiotic-resistant infections, neurological disease, diabetes mellitus, chronic traumatic encephalopathy, insomnia, and so forth. The neuroprotective effects of CBD are becoming well defined, and much investigation is underway on its anticancer effects. It appears that CBD acts to facilitate apoptosis, and this may be due to potential actions on mutant P53 proteins that are found in cancer cells.

The list of potential applications of CBD is expanding greatly to include epilepsy, dystonia, muscle spasms (e.g., multiple sclerosis), nausea, anxiety, neurodegenerative disease, and several other disorders. It has been demonstrated that CBD may reduce symptoms of schizophrenia, perhaps as a result of its ability to stabilize the function of NMDA receptor pathways. These pathways interact with norepinephrine and GABA. These favorable effects have been found to be equivalent to those experienced with certain types of schizophrenia drug treatment (e.g., amisulpride).

Cannabidiol (CBD) reduces social and anxiety disorders, and it has a role in reducing social isolation that can be induced by THC. Some studies have suggested that CBD is effective in controlling dystonic symptoms, and it may play a role in protecting alcohol-induced neurogenic deterioration due to binge drinking. It is believed that CBD acts as an indirect antagonist of cannabinoid agonists—i.e., it works against some of the actions of some of the cannabinoids that directly stimulate CB1 and CB2 receptors and the putative receptor GPR55 (CB-3), which is expressed in the brain (caudate nucleus and putamen).

Is Cannabidiol (CBD) Legal?

This is a big question with a fuzzy answer. To remind ourselves about the current legal status of cannabidiol use is a valuable introduction to discussions about individual cannabinoid use with nonpsychoactive cannabinoids, such as CBD. The legality of CBD is highly relevant to its clinical use as a dietary supplement (nutraceutical). While the illegal status of THC is often assumed to be clear in federal guidelines, it is allowable under conditions for medical use and for recreational use in Colorado, Washington, Alaska, Oregon and Washington DC, at the time of writing. Cannabidiol (CBD) has orphan drug status in many states with cannabis medical legalization (for epilepsy in children, e.g., Dravet's syndrome, etc.). In addition, it can be used as a medicinal preparation with a doctor's endorsement or prescription in about half the states of the union, but caution is required in some legal jurisdictions. However, there is no doubt that the presence of THC in cannabis is the pivotal factor that has driven the definition of the illicit status of cannabis (marijuana), not CBD.

These days there is a further potential layer of debate concerning the legal status of cannabinoids, other than THC. Cannabidiol has formerly attracted medical use or more general use as a dietary supplement. This use has occurred in the presence of proposals by some individuals and the FDA that CBD is just another component of a schedule I drug that is illegal. However, the legality of cannabis components is far from simple, but the widespread availability of hemp-derived, CBD-containing oils in grocery and health food stores in the United States is generally interpreted as acceptance of CBD from hemp oil as legal. Recent research on CBD has defined many potential health benefits of CBD, and this has caused regulators and politicians to sharpen their pencils as they look at the complex composition of cannabis. Furthermore, CBD has emerged as a component of certain pharmaceutical preparations of cannabis (e.g., Sativex) that are approved for use in certain countries and is in clinical trials in several other countries, including the United States (at the time of writing). In recent rulings the FDA (US) stated that CBD is not a dietary supplement.

The key to the legal status of CBD may rest somewhat in its botanical origin. In general, CBD is a predominant cannabinoid in hemp, which is mainly perceived as legal providing that it contains only traces of THC (less than 0.3 percent). However, it is argued that if CBD is derived from cannabis (marijuana) with psychoactive properties (i.e., THC content), then it must be classified as a schedule I prohibited drug, even though CBD has no psychoactive actions. These circumstances have made the law a gray area when it comes to unencumbered cannabidiol (CBD) use. These arguments are superseded by the FDA's ruling that CBD is not a dietary supplement.

Although cannabidiol (CBD) of hemp origin is often considered to be legal in the United States as part of hemp oil, opinions are varied, and state legislation concerning CBD use is emerging. In brief, hemp-derived oil containing CBD is sold by some companies in the United States as a dietary supplement, which is defined as not food and not a drug. A general opinion has emerged that CBD fulfills the criteria for a dietary supplement, but clearly this opinion has been challenged as of May 2015, following FDA rulings. Clearly, regulations concerning the sale or use of CBD may vary from country to country, and importation regulations are quite variable and somewhat lacking in clarity.

As mentioned earlier, opinions exist that natural cannabinoids other than THC that are found in hemp (mainly CBD) are exempt from the Controlled Substances Act. Hemp has been distinguished as quite separate from marijuana, and this is "assumed" by some to be recognized in the 1937 Marijuana Tax Act. In fact, the Hemp Industries Association declared the exempt status of hemp in 2004 and did not receive government or DEA challenges to these declarations of exemption.

Some states have passed legislation that tends to define medical cannabis as all preparations derived from a cannabis plant. With this in mind, there has been much discussion about the increasing need for state legislation to control CBD-only products. It is argued, however, that for the treatment of certain conditions, such as uncontrolled epilepsy in children, CBD alone is not adequate without the addition of THC. At the time of writing, CBD oil (low THC with CBD) has been typically extracted from Charlotte's Web plants. It is legalized for limited medical use (orphan drug status) in thirteen states (at the time of writing). This political reform was stimulated by widespread reporting of the benefits of CBD in childhood epilepsy. It should be noted that CBD is not beneficial in all cases of epilepsy, and response rates of less than 40 percent have been reported but not completely verified. This circumstance should be hopefully clarified by newly funded research in Colorado. How these circumstances of proposed limited benefit clash with other complex arguments surrounding CBD use remains to be seen. The two main sources of cannabidiol are medical marijuana plants and hemp that is mainly grown overseas for industrial purposes. This is changing as the Farm Bill (2014) allows hemp cultivation in the United States.

As discussed earlier, CBD has been stated by some scientists and the FDA to be a schedule I drug, in common with all other cannabinoids. Cannabidiol has been assigned a code number 7372 in schedule I, even though it is considered to be safe and it has no psychoactive effects. Knowledgeable individuals conclude that the legal status of cannabidiol in the United States is not clear despite the FDA rulings, but the FDA must be obeyed. Schedule I gives a category of tetrahydrocannabinols, and despite the allocations of a statistical number for cannabidiol, it is argued that this code does not mean that it is considered illegal. These arguments are moot given recent FDA statements (May 2015).

Many companies claim that it is legal to import CBD oil to the United States that is extracted from industrial hemp grown overseas. As mentioned earlier, the limiting factor is that the hemp oil must contain less than 0.3 percent THC. These circumstances of the legality of CBD oil remain poorly defined at law. The current situation in 2014 is that CBD hemp oil with traces of THC (less than 0.3 percent) has not been subject to any major regulatory actions. If such regulatory actions occur, they should be part of a notice to cease and desist, not prosecution, because the law requires qualification and clarity, in my opinion.

Clinical Endocannabinoid Deficiency (CECD)

In 2004, Dr. Ethan B. Russo proposed the idea that there was an entity called clinical endocannabinoid deficiency (CECD). He hypothesized, in a manner that agreed with earlier comments of Israeli scientists, that there was a condition of deficiency of cannabinoids that was a causative factor in the generation of many diseases or disorders. It was suggested that these may respond to cannabis-based therapies. Russo's reasoning was based on recognition of the health benefits of an intact endocannabinoid system within the body and increasing definition of the therapeutic value of cannabinoids.

Suggestions about the number of diseases or disorders that may be alleviated or helped by cannabinoids has grown exponentially in recent years. This situation provides support for Russo's description of the entity of clinical endocannabinoid deficiency (CECD). Thus, there is an increasing acceptance of an occurrence of endocannabinoid deficiency that is amenable to replacement with exogenous cannabinoids (i.e., exogenous cannabinoids or phytocannabinoids).

Cannabinoids: Effects at a Glance

The different effects of certain cannabinoids and their analogues have been reviewed to a certain extent in other chapters of this book. This voluminous amount of material is summarized below. The data represents "cannabinoids at a glance" (modified from material online, supplied by AZ Med testing).

Cannabidiol (CBG)	Delta-9-Tetrahydrocannabinol (THC)
• Putative cancer therapy	• Analgesic
• Analgesic	• Induces relaxation
• Bone stimulation	• Anxiolytic
• Anti-bacterial	• Benefits in nerve damage
• Antiepileptic	• Antiepileptic
• Relieves muscle spasms	• Suppresses muscle spasms
• Anti-inflammatory	• Anticancer effects
• Relief of nausea	• Reverses nausea
• Vasodilator	• Anti-inflammatory
• Lowers blood sugar	• Antioxidant
• Decreases some THC side effects	• Appetite stimulation
	• Neurogenic
	• Decreases eye pressure
Cannabinol (CBN)	Cannabichromene (CBC)
• Sleep aid	• Analgesic
• Anti-inflammatory	• Anti-fungal

• Analgesic	• Anti-inflammatory
• Suppresses muscle spasms	• Bone stimulation
• Antioxidant	• Antibacterial
	• Contractile for blood vessels
Tetrahydrocannabivarin (THCV)	**Cannabigerol (CBG)**
• Appetite suppression	• Antibacterial
• Anti-obesity	• Bone stimulator
• Value in type II diabetes	• Promotes cell growth
• Some psychoactivity	
Tetrahydrocannabinol	
• Anti-inflammatory	
• Anticancer	
• Antiepileptic	
• Some psychoactivity	

Terpenoids in Cannabis

Phytocannabinoids are chemical cousins of a large group of terpenoids, which are naturally occurring compounds that are found in cannabis plants. These terpenoids include linalool, beta-caryophyllene, beta-myrcene, D-Limonene, humulene, pinene, and many others. Terpenoids (contained in essential oils) are responsible for the smell of cannabis. They have significant and versatile effects on ion channels in muscle cells and nerves, receptors involved in neurotransmission, enzymes, and second messenger systems.

The terpenoids found in cannabis are considered highly relevant to the overall effects of cannabis. Their absence in isolated compounds derived from cannabis or synthetic drug analogues is a part of a credible explanation for the limited effect of individual cannabis components (e.g., extracts), compared with the effects of whole herbal cannabis. The effects of terpenoids in cannabis are extensively reviewed by Russo, E. B. (ibid. 2011). Table 54 lists some of these terpenoids of specific interest, where their function has been identified.

Table 54. Some of the main terpenoids found in cannabis and comments about their functions. The terpenoids contribute to the entourage effect of cannabinoids (Russo, E. B., ibid. 2011).

Terpenoid	Comment
Linalool	Responsible for pleasant odor in many plants (e.g., lavender). May act as a sleep aid, anxiolytic, antiepileptic, antidepressant, and analgesic.
Beta-Caryophyllene	Has binding affinity for CB2 receptors. Found in several plants, and it has antibacterial, antifungal, anticancer, and anti-inflammatory effects.
Beta-Myrcene	Has antitumor, anti-inflammatory, and antispasmodic with analgesic effects. Increases the transfer of THC across blood-brain barrier to promote maximum effects at CB1 receptors. Found in mango, hops, bay leaves, and lemongrass. A common precursor of other terpenes.
D-Limonene	A cyclic terpene with low toxicity. Has antifungal properties. May help in management of gastro-esophageal reflux. Has antidepressant and anxiolytic effects with some antitumor properties and immune-stimulating activity.
Pinene	Alpha-pinene is a highly reactive terpenoid with uses as a bronchodilator and anti-inflammatory agent. Chemical structure readily changed into other terpenoids (e.g., D-Limonene).

In brief, it is established that the terpenoids contribute to the overall effects of cannabinoids (which are themselves terpenoid derivatives), by modulating body responses to exogenous cannabinoids and preventing some of their adverse effects. Furthermore, terpenoids have their own therapeutic actions. For example, pinene may reduce short-term memory loss caused by THC, and limonene has antidepressant effects. The terpenoid beta-caryophyllene is notable for its selective effects on CB2 receptors, with resulting analgesic and anti-inflammatory actions. The understanding of terpenes in the entourage effect requires much further research. A valuable discussion relevant to these topics is found in Dr. Russo's classic article, "Taming THC," Russo, E. B., *British Journal of Pharmacology*, 163 (2011): 1344–64.

Essential oils in cannabis, containing the terpenoid beta-carophyllene, can activate CB-2 receptors. This results in the inhibition of inflammation. This terpenoid compound (beta-carophyllene) differs in its structure to cannabinoids and has been shown to be able to reduce experimentally induced inflammation in the paws of mice. Beta-caryophyllene is also found in plants that are used as spices, notably cinnamon, black pepper, oregano, and basil, and it has demonstrated gastric cytoprotective effects (antiulcer effects).

The effects of terpenoids on the overall actions of cannabis appear to be important, but they require further investigation. The variable effects of cannabis on consciousness or psychological status may be explained to some degree by difference in terpenoid contents in certain strains of marijuana. While the cannabinoid contents of cannabis have become of prime importance in defining predominant effects of cannabis, more focus is now being placed on terpenoids as biological response modifiers. These terpenoids are believed to exert components of the entourage effect of cannabis. This knowledge has prompted growers to pay more attention to optimizing terpenoid contents with their different effects.

Table 55 below shows a terpene analysis. The appearance of terpenoids in specific stages of growth from one to eight weeks is illustrated in table 53. This table is derived from studies performed by Greenhouse Seeds and has been used in an article by Owen

Smith, entitled "How Black Pepper Relieves Cannabis Anxiety" (cannabis digest.ca/blackpepper-relieves-cannabis-anxiety).

Table 55. Concentrations of terpenoids over different growth periods (data from Greenhouse Seeds)

Terpenes Analysis Arjan's Haze #I—(Hydroponic)

Percentage	%	%	%	%	%	%	%	%
(+)-a-Pinene	1.45	7.14	15.32	29.45	35.23	47.07	58.12	75.93
(R)-(+)-Limonene	0.91	1.75	2.36	2.45	3.06	3.12	3.75	3.91
a-Humulene	0.75	1.04	1.25	2.95	3.07	3.12	3.45	3.82
(-)-Menthone	0.12	0.95	1.01	1.17	1.23	1.45	2.01	2.12
Dihydrojasmone	0.04	0.08	0.11	0.12	0.22	0.27	0.41	0.52
Nerylacetate	0.05	0.07	0.14	0.22	0.32	0.37	0.42	0.48
(-)-Guaiol	0.04	0.09	0.14	0.18	0.30	0.35	0.37	0.40
B-Caryophyllene	0.01	0.04	0.11	0.14	0.22	0.24	0.28	0.33
Weeks	1st	2nd	3rd	4th	5th	6th	7th	8th

Owen Smith (ibid. July 17, 2014) discussed the varied psychological effects of cannabis with suggestion that terpenoid/cannabinoid ratios can produce different effects. These differing effects are summarized below in table 56.

Table 56. Terpenoids (found in essential oils in the cannabis plant) have many effects on psychological reactions to THC (and other psychoactive cannabinoids). Adding essential oils can mitigate anxiety-producing effects of THC (adapted from Owen Smith, ibid. 2014).

- CBD will reduce the psychoactive effects of THC.
- Growers are tailoring plants for both cannabinoid contents and terpenoid contents. The latter may reduce unwanted effects of the psychoactive cannabinoid THC (e.g., anxiety).
- Myrcene in mangoes may increase the quality of low-potency marijuana when consumed one hour before medicating. This mango effect has been suggested by Ed Rosenthal (quoted by Owen Smith, ibid. 2014).
- Alpha pinene is altering.

- Limonene is sunshine.
- Beta myrcene is sedating.
- Pinene found in pine needles and black pepper may reduce anxiety induced by THC.
- It appears that terpenoids in cannabis may increase cerebral blood flow, enhance cortical activity in the cerebrum, kill respiratory pathogens (and some other pathogenic bacteria), and provide anti-inflammatory activity.

As compounds are discovered that amplify or diminish the effects of cannabinoids (cannabis), it may be possible to raise strains of cannabis plants with designer components. In addition, selected mixtures of essential oils containing terpenoids may be added to cannabis for other desired effects. The importance of terpenoids in entourage effects has guided the formulation of Sativex, which combines CBD and THC with some essential oils and what are referred to as ballast components. Please note that essential oils are often generally recognized as safe (GRAS) and enjoy widespread applications as food flavors.

Synthetic, Pharmaceutical-Grade Cannabinoids (Analogues)

Synthetic cannabinoids were originally created by modifying the chemical structure of naturally occurring cannabinoids, but they have been sourced more recently as modified endocannabinoids or newly synthesized molecules. A large number of synthetic cannabinoids have been tested for their activity and clinical effects. This research has major implications for the development of cannabis-related pharmaceuticals. Table 57 summarizes a list of actual and proposed medications composed of natural or synthetic cannabinoids (cannabinoid analogues). Note: illegal substances are co-mingled.

Table 57. A partial list of drugs or chemicals described as cannabinoids or cannabinoid analogues with some examples of illegal synthetic cannabinoids

Please note the use of term "synthetic" applies to drugs (pharmaceuticals of cannabis origin) and illegal substances that are used to spike cannabis. These spiking agents are toxic and dangerous (e.g., JWH-018).

Medication or Putative Treatment Agents	Characteristics
Dronabinol (Marinol)	This is delta-9-tetrahydrocannabinol (THC), used as an appetite stimulant, antiemetic, and analgesic.
Nabilone (Cesamet)	A synthetic cannabinoid and an analog of Marinol.
Sativex	A cannabinoid extract oral spray containing THC, CBD, and other cannabinoids used for neuropathic pain and spasticity, available in several countries.
Rimonabant (SR141716)	A selective cannabinoid (CB_1) receptor inverse agonist once used as an antiobesity drug under the proprietary name Acomplia. It has been used to help stop smoking but is now withdrawn from clinical use because of causation of depression and association with suicide.
JWH-018	A potent synthetic cannabinoid agonist. It is being increasingly sold in "legal" smoke blends that are illegal, collectively known as "spice." Several countries and states have moved to ban it.
CP-55,940	This synthetic cannabinoid receptor agonist is many times more potent than THC.
HU-210	About one hundred times more potent than THC.

HU-331	A potential anticancer drug derived from cannabidiol that specifically inhibits topoisomerase II enzymes.

Strains of Cannabis and Cannabinoid Content

There are many strains of cannabis, but common descriptive terms for cannabis are often based on species names (e.g., sativa, indica, or ruderalis) and other strains or hybrids. There is considerable information on the selective breeding of cannabis, and most emphasis has been placed on the development of THC-rich strains. Now researchers are becoming focused on other cannabinoids in specific disease treatments. These cannabinoids of special note include cannabidiol (CBD), tetrahydrocannabivarin (THCV), cannabigerol (CBG), and cannabidivarin (CBDV). In brief, CBDV is being investigated for epilepsy treatment, and CBG has attracted interest for the treatment of prostate cancer. While the lion's share of mixed cannabinoid research involves the use of CBD and THC, the cannabinoid tetrahydro-cannabivarin (THCV) is being investigated for its potential role in the treatment of Metabolic Syndrome X. This disorder of the variable combination of insulin resistance linked to hypertension, hypercholesterolemia, and obesity. This disorder is an important forerunner to the development of type II diabetes mellitus, and it affects an estimated seventy million American adults. (Holt, S., *Combat Syndrome X, Y, and Z* [Wellness Publishing, 2002].)

Cannabigerol (CBG) is the molecule of origin of THC and CBD. This has led to a rough and figurative comparison of cannabigerol with stem cells that are the origin of a diverse array of body tissues. The amount of CBG in most strains of cannabis is quite low because this is used as the origin of many cannabinoids. This compound (CBG) is subject to relatively rapid enzymatic conversion to CBD, THC, and some other mixed cannabinoids. Data have accumulated suggesting that CBG has antioxidant and anti-inflammatory effects, which have been researched in the treatment of inflammatory bowel disease. Moreover, CBG appears to have COX-2 inhibitor properties in high concentrations. Comparison of CBG with the therapeutic effects of nonsteroidal anti-inflammatory drugs (NSAID) is required with a promise of developing new options for arthritis treatment. The NSAID have many side effects that are not present with the use of CBG.

As a general rule, high-THC-containing strains of marijuana are used for recreation and some specific medical applications, but their obvious effects on the psyche are often perceived as their main value. On the other hand, high CBD concentrations are finding illegal applications in the development of nutraceuticals (dietary supplements), and they are becoming an increasing focus of research for pharmaceutical applications. As noted earlier, cannabidiol (CBD) is found most often in hemp oil.

Anyone searching for different varieties of cannabis or hemp by the use of the name of a strain may be overwhelmed to discover how many exist in popular language. Different strains of cannabis are often derived from the genus/species of Cannabis sativa and Cannabis indica. Such strains are often hybrids that have been bred to produce selected components within the plant. This often translates into different cannabinoid contents. The various types of cannabis strains have been classified into four major groups. These groups include wild varieties, unstable seed types, stable seed types, and clone-only varieties. However, the classification of strains by genotypic analysis is quite valuable in understanding different components of different strains. This is a highly complex and somewhat confusing subject.

As emphasized earlier, it is clear that cannabis plants with high THC contents and low CBD contents are grown for psychoactive effects, whereas those with low THC and high CBD content have found a modern and increasing role in disease management. The selection of names of strains has often been chosen by growers to involve some description relevant to the source, color, smell, or taste of the plant. This popular type of description of different strains is often quite crude, and the many applied names are of limited usefulness. Cannabis plants can, on occasion, look similar but contain different components.

Another species of cannabis is Cannabis ruderalis, which is short in height in comparison with sativa and indica. The ruderalis type of cannabis engages in auto flowering with age, and this is perceived as an advantageous property of the plant. It is understood that some indica strains are likely to have variable ratios of the contents of THC and CBD, with a low content of THC and CBD in several types of industrial hemp. Hemp can be derived from indica, sativa, and ruderalis species.

Cannabis Strains: What's in a Name?

The many popular names of different strains of cannabis may make some people's head spin. There are hundreds of names of strains including Bio-Jesus, Death Star, Sensi Kush, Vanilla Sky Cherry, Chem Dawg, and so forth, but the meaning of these names may be confused, and they seem to serve little purpose. A research scientist, Jeffrey Raber, PhD, of California, has undertaken studies of many hundreds of brands and strains of pot. Dr. Raber has not been able to demonstrate consistency of composition among the strain names.

These analytic studies performed by Dr. Raber are quite illuminating with his discovery of major differences in contents of the cannabis, which do not seem to match different species (indica or sativa) or claims about contents of materials from different cannabis plants. Dr. Raber is quoted as making a couple of highly poignant remarks about strain labels, referring to some as "flavor-of-the-week party names." He has commented on the inconsistency of "naming integrity." Thus, a buyer in a dispensary can be easily duped, especially given reports that some purveyors do not care what name is used for the pot, providing it sells (reported by Robert Meyerowitz in the *Colorado Springs Independent*, www.csindy.com, Sun., Jan. 11, 2015).

In an increasing number of locations in the United States and Europe, there is competition to produce and create strains with greater consumer appeal. In fact, there are substantially similar strains of cannabis with different popular (or common) names. These circumstances have driven illicit market sales that are hyped by both accurate and false statements about the origin of the cannabis in question. Moreover, unscrupulous suppliers may sometimes engage in fraudulent labeling of their products, even occasionally in dispensaries. The users of street cannabis should consider caveat emptor and "what's in a name?"

Cannabis Use May Be Part of an Antiaging Strategy

There is an increasing interest in the proposals that cannabis may have antiaging properties. Some of the mechanisms of these effects of cannabis include neuroprotection, antioxidation, neurogenesis, anti-inflammatory activity, and improvements in mitochondrial function. In addition, some studies have suggested that cannabis may increase amounts of brain-derived neurotropic factor (BDNF). It is recognized that BDNF exerts protective effects on brain cells and stimulates the growth of new neurons. These beneficial effects may result in retention of cognitive function and overall intellect in the aging person. This effect is most valuable in reducing the prevalence of neurodegenerative diseases, such as Alzheimer's disease. However, the short-term effects of cannabis commonly result in impairment of cognition. More evidence of the cannabis paradox emerges.

The antioxidant potentials of several components of cannabis are valuable in blocking tissue damage by free radicals. These free radicals cause inflammatory disease, and certain cannabinoids exhibit different mechanisms and degrees of anti-inflammatory effects. Cannabinoids may quench free radicals. The documented anti-inflammatory effects of cannabis presents the possibility that endocannabinoid activity may have antiaging properties that can be manifest by reduction of age-related disease, such as cancer and cardiovascular disease.

These concepts of the antiaging potential of cannabinoids have been stressed in several writings and public presentations by Dr. Robert Melamede of the University of Colorado. Dr. Melamede has championed this knowledge, along with many other scientists. It seems likely that some components of cannabis may be a useful antidote to age-related illness. Thus, cannabis may have use as a supplement to a well-controlled diet for antiaging.

Medical Conditions That May Respond to Cannabis Use

In this book I endorse the presence of significant evidence to support the medical use of cannabis in several disease states (table 54). This material is summarized at a glance in table 58 for many disease applications.

Table 58. Examples of conditions that may benefit from cannabis use, adapted from www.doc420.com

Condition	Comment on Cannabis Use
ADHD	Clinical research is limited, but anandamide levels are higher in the brain of ADHD subjects. Cannabinoid receptors are found in high concentrations in areas of the brain that are malfunctioning in ADHD (e.g., the amygdala and hippocampus).
Anorexia	Recent research implies that the body and brain create more cannabinoid receptors to compensate for persistent reduced function of the endocannabinoid system, but this circumstance is reversible. The endocannabinoid system regulates appetite, and lower levels of cannabinoids may be a positive adaptation to anorexia or starvation.
Anxiety	CBD has anxiety-relieving effects, and THC can precipitate anxiety. CBD may act on CB-1 receptors and compensate for the deficiency of natural endocannabinoids. In brief, the endocannabinoid system reduces stress and anxiety by reducing excitatory stimuli on the brain.

Arthritis	Phytocannabinoids (notably CBD) have both analgesic and anti-inflammatory actions that are valuable in the management of arthritis. About fifteen years ago CBD was shown to block progression of experimental arthritis in animals. Both THC and CBD have been shown to relieve pain and disease activity in rheumatoid arthritis. Studies show increased levels of endocannabinoids (anandamide and 2-archidonoylglycerol) in arthritic joints compared with normal joints.
Asthma	It is proposed that CB-1 receptors on nerve cells in the airways control constriction of the airways, and cannabis can reverse this effect. However, cannabis smoking may sometimes aggravate broncho-constriction (asthma), especially in the novice smoker.
Cancer	Cannabis has undoubted benefit in cancer-related problems by increasing appetite, controlling pain, reversing depression, counteracting wasting, stopping vomiting, and relief of nausea. Marijuana has several valuable antitumor properties in animals. These properties include causing cancer cell death, blocking cell replication, and antiangiogenic effects. When administered with chemotherapy, CBD can act in a synergistic manner and increase death of cancer cells.

Chronic abdominal pain	Cannabis can variably alleviate abdominal cramping pain, diarrhea or constipation, nausea, and inflammatory intestinal disease. Advancing research implies benefit in the treatment of irritable bowel syndrome, Crohn's disease, and ulcerative colitis.
Chronic back pain	Back pain is associated with advancing age, sedentary lifestyle, spinal disease, and post trauma. It affects about 25 percent of the entire US adult population. Medical use of cannabis is synergistic with many analgesic drugs and it may assist in the reduction of death from opioid overdose.
Chronic pain	Neuropathic and inflammatory pain often responded to cannabis use. Cannabinoids affect the release of endogenous opioids, and the use of opioid drugs may be lessened.
Depression	While cannabis most often lifts mood, it can sometimes cause depression. Its use in depression should be carefully monitored.
Epilepsy	Epilepsy causes fits (body convulsions) loss of coordination, depressed consciousness, and altered sensory states. Repeated seizures may respond to CBD, which is found in high concentrations in Charlotte's Web strains of cannabis. Increasing confidence in the anticonvulsant effect of cannabis has occurred recently, especially for use in children, but opinion varies on its ability to control convulsions in a reproducible manner.

Glaucoma	Marijuana tends to reduce the pressure within the eye (by a factor of 30 percent). Both central nervous system effects and actions on the production and outflow of aqueous humor may occur with cannabis use, but the value of cannabis in glaucoma therapy has been questioned.
Insomnia	Up to 50 percent of the population have episodic insomnia, with about 10 percent suffering from chronic insomnia. Both THC and CBD can promote sleep, but the effects of CBD are considered superior. That said, large dosages of CBD may be required for a hypnotic effect resulting from smoking or the consumption of edibles.
Migraine	Migraine may be present in up to 15 percent of the population. Migraine headaches are often accompanied by nausea, vomiting, and sensitivity to ocular and aural stimuli. A number of reports support migraine relief with cannabis, but more clinical trials are required.
Nausea	Cannabis can variably relieve nausea and vomiting from almost every cause. The analysis of at least thirty studies has shown cannabis to be highly effective in nausea and vomiting relief with a superior effect when compared with many other antiemetic drugs.
Muscle spasms	A significant number of animal and human studies show that THC can be effective in reducing painful muscle spasms. General surveys have shown improvement in quality of life in individuals with muscle spasms.

PTSD	Many traumatic events can trigger PTSD, not just experiences of war. PTSD has been associated with low levels of anandamide in the brain. Despite many calls for clinical trials of cannabis therapy in this disorder, politics has stood in the way.

The Widespread Use of Cannabis Therapy

It is a revelation to scan the vast number of medical disorders that have been considered to be variably responsive to whole herbal cannabis use, cannabinoids, or their synthetic analogues. One can spend much time on the Internet just putting the search terms cannabis (marijuana) and the name of the disease or disorder together. One major problem of the interpretation of the disease applications of cannabis reported on the Internet is sometimes the lack of disclosure that the observations have been made in animal, preclinical studies, or in cell preparations. Sometimes the effects described in some human diseases are mere anecdotes or are part of hyperbolic or false claims.

These issues have led to a call to accept only controlled studies as a reasonable basis to predict a positive benefit of cannabis in a certain disease state. The list of medical disorders displayed below shows links to cannabis use (sourced at www.unitedpatientgroup.com/resources/illnesses-treatable) and should not be interpreted as final proof or adequate proof of benefit of cannabis-derived compounds for the listed disease (table 54). Most of the disease links shown in table 59 are not supported by significant degrees or amounts of scientific evidence.

Table 59. Highly variable positive benefits described or merely mentioned with the use of cannabis or cannabis analogues. Not to be used as any form of recommendation for cannabis use. Reviewing a list of potential treatment targets for cannabis is a daunting task (adapted from www.encod.org). Readers are referred to the website www.encod.org, which provides several hundred potential medicinal uses of cannabis, with links to information on many other websites. Examples include:

Agoraphobia	Hepatitis C
AIDS-related illness	HIV/AIDS
Alcohol abuse	Hospice patients
Alzheimer's disease	Huntington's disease
Amphetamine dependency	Hypoglycemia
Amyotrophic lateral sclerosis (ALS)	
Anorexia	Inflammatory bowel disease (IBD)
Anxiety disorders	Insomnia
Arthritis	Lyme disease
Asthma	Lymphoma
Attention deficit hyperactivity disorder	Major depression
Autism	Malignant melanoma
Autoimmune disease	Mania
Autoimmune-mediated arthritis	Multiple sclerosis (MS)
Back pain (acute and chronic)	Muscle spasms
Bipolar disorder	Muscle dystrophy
Brain tumor, malignant	Myeloid leukemia
Cachexia	Nightmares
Cancer	Obesity
Cancer, prostate	Obsessive-compulsive disorder
Chronic fatigue syndrome	Osteoarthritis
Chronic pain	Parkinson's disease
Colitis	Peripheral neuropathy
Constipation	Persistent insomnia
Crohn's disease	Post-traumatic stress disorder (PTSD)
Cystic fibrosis	Post-traumatic stress disorder (PTSD)
Damage to spinal cord nervous tissue	Psoriasis

Degenerative arthritis	Pulmonary fibrosis
Diabetes, adult onset	Radiation therapy
Diabetes, insulin-dependent	Restless legs syndrome (RLS)
Diabetic neuropathy	Rheumatoid arthritis
Diarrhea	Rosacea
Diverticulitis	Schizophrenia
Eczema	Sedative dependence
Emphysema	Seizures
Epilepsy	Severe nausea
Fibromyalgia	Sinusitis
Gastritis	Skeletal muscular spasticity
Genital herpes	Sleep apnea
Glaucoma	Sleep disorders
Glioblastoma multiforme	Spasticity
Headaches, migraine	Tourette's syndrome
	Viral hepatitis
	Wasting syndrome

Further Defining Medical Uses of Cannabis

It was not my intention to confuse or overwhelm some readers of this book by producing an adaptation of a gargantuan list of potentially treatable diseases with marijuana. It is becoming clear that mounting evidence exists for the use of cannabis compounds or their synthetic analogues in many clinical circumstances. How do we approach the development of a process that will form a logical plan for further research on cannabis as an empiric treatment of different diseases?

Among the vast amount of information that has accrued about cannabis use, there is a significant amount of conflicting information on clinical outcomes in various diseases. I have stated, with intentional repetition, that crude, illicit plant preparations of cannabis may result in different benefits, no benefits, or untoward effects, in comparison with single pharmaceutical-type cannabinoids or limited cannabis extracts. Add to this, paradoxical actions of cannabis that can be at the basis of what I have termed the double-edged sword. Moreover, it must be acknowledged that evidence derived from preclinical studies to support the potential use of cannabis in human-disease management does not always predict the therapeutic outcome.

Very important information that is relevant for matching diseases with cannabis treatments has resulted from two review studies of a number of clinical trials with cannabis and cannabinoids. These reviews were made in the time periods 1975–2005 and 2005–2009. The first study period was published by Dr. Amar M. ("Cannabinoids in Medicine: A Review of Their Therapeutic Potential," *J. Ethnopharm* 105 [2006]: 1–25), and the second clinical study period was published by Drs. Hazekamp, A., and Grotenheimen, F. ("Review on Clinical Studies with Cannabis and Cannabinoids 2005–2009," *Cannabinoids* 5 [2010]: 1-21). The latter study (by Hazekamp and Grotenhermen 2010) identified several disorders or diseases in which controlled studies on cannabis and cannabinoids have been published. This study (2005–2009) was mentioned earlier in this book, and it reported on outcome of thirty-seven well-constructed studies that had the objective of documenting the therapeutic effects of cannabis and cannabinoids. The eight different disorders covered by the studies included 1) neuropathic or chronic pain, 2) experimental pain, 3) multiple sclerosis and spasticity, 4) HIV/AIDS, 5) glaucoma, 6) intestinal dysfunction, 7) nausea/vomiting, and 8) schizophrenia (with other mental diseases). Overall, results were often favorable. Of course, it is relevant in this book to expand on evaluation of the treatment applications of cannabis and cannabis-based preparations (cannabinoids).

A Note on Cannabis Tea, Soda, and Edibles

Absorption studies of THC often show uptake with unreliable or unpredictable outcomes. There are many factors that control the speed of absorption of drugs, including gastrointestinal motility or disease, drug characteristics, drug solubility, and so forth. It has been reported that an oral dose of 20 mg of delta-9-THC results in a systemic bioavailability of only 4–12 percent of this cannabinoid.

In this circumstance, peak plasma concentrations of delta-9-THC of around 6 ng/mL were noted between one and two hours, with multiple peaks for several hours (up to about six hours).

These erratic absorption kinetics of delta-9-THC carry several implications. For example, the impatient user may prematurely take extra amounts of edibles or smoke in a concomitant manner. Moreover, oral liquids containing THC (tea or soda) also have variable timing of onset of effects, which may be anticipated to work faster in onset of action but exert weaker effects due to rapid first-pass metabolism in the liver. In addition, there is poor solubility of delta-9-THC in water (tea or soda).

The Range of Cannabis-Derived Products

As described earlier, for use as a medicine or in clinical trials, whole herbal cannabis is most often standardized for its content of THC and measured in percent of dry weights. Some trials focus on other cannabinoids (e.g., CBD) for treatment outcomes, but the content of THC is necessary for optimal recreational and selected medicinal uses. A well-accepted use of THC is in the palliative care of cancer and HIV disease, where it can be used to inhibit chemotherapy-induced nausea and vomiting.

Cannabidiol has versatile effects on body functions in a manner that is not completely understood. Cannabidiol (CBD) is perched to be a blockbuster dietary supplement (or drug) as a consequence of its potent and versatile therapeutic actions. Several mechanisms to explain the effects of CBD have been proposed. These mechanisms of effect are listed below (source Hazekamp, A., and Grotenhermen, ibid. 2010).

- CBD antagonizes (works against) central CB1 receptor effects and sometimes inhibits effects of THC.
- CBD stimulates the vanilloid receptor type 1 (VRI) with a maximum effect similar to capsaicin (peppers).
- CBD inhibits the uptake and metabolism of anandamide, thereby increasing its concentration.
- CBD may increase blood levels of THC as a consequence of inhibition of the cytochrome P-450 oxidative system.

Drugs Related to Cannabis

Dronabinol is the isomer of THC that is present in the cannabis plant. Oral capsules are marketed under the brand name Marinol (Solvay Pharmaceuticals, Belgium) which is a synthetic version of THC. Marinol is indicated for the treatment of anorexia with weight loss caused by AIDS (HIV disease). It is also used for nausea and vomiting caused by cancer and chemotherapy, most often in patients who have failed to respond to antiemetic drugs.

Nabilone (Valeant Pharmaceuticals, United States) is a synthetic analogue of THC. This drug is marketed under the trade name Cesamet, and it is indicated for antiemetic purposes, but off-label use sometimes occurs.

Sativex (G W Pharmaceuticals, UK) is a combination product containing THC and CBD in a 1:1 ratio. This drug is delivered in an oro-mucosal spray (mouth spray). It contains other nonstandardized components (ballast components), such as other cannabinoids and terpenes in small amounts. Sativex has been used for cancer pain and neuropathic pain in adults with multiple sclerosis.

Cannador (Society for Clinical Research, Germany) is a capsule for oral use that contains THC and CBD in standardized dosages with a ratio of 2:1, THC to CBD. This mixture of CBD and THC has been used in conditions of cachexia resulting from cancer, postoperative pain, and spasms in patients with multiple sclerosis.

While most interest has been shown in CB-receptor agonists, there are several antagonist compounds that have been developed. One example of a cannabinoid antagonist is Acomplia (rimonabant) (Sanofi Aventis). This drug was used for the treatment of obesity, but it was withdrawn because of serious adverse effects (depression and suicide). Several drugs (cannabis analogues) are shown below in table 60.

The pharmaceutical industry has accelerated cannabis-based, drug development programs as medical cannabis legislation spreads in the United States. There is an array of current cannabis-based medications that involve different modes of delivery and the demonstration of benefits in specific disease states. The main examples of these drugs are summarized in table 60 and include Sativex, Marinol, and Cesamet.

Table 60. Drugs based on cannabis in use or in development

Several are pending FDA approval in the United States.

Drug	Comments
Sativex	A mouth spray produced with natural cannabis extracts focused on delta-9-THC and CBD (cannabidiol). Used in neuropathic pain, spasticity in patients with multiple sclerosis, and for analgesia in cases of advanced cancer. Approved in several countries and is in advanced phase III new-drug application studies in the United States (at the time of writing).
Dronabinol/Marinol	Synthetic delta-9-THC used in nausea and vomiting in cancer patients as an appetite stimulant in patients with AIDS and for neuropathic pain in multiple sclerosis. Classified as schedule III drug.
Nabilone/Cesamet	Synthetic cannabinoid with chemical structure similar to THC, used in the management of nausea and vomiting in patients receiving cancer therapies. Off-label use in some countries to treat chemotherapy-related neuropathic pain.
Dexabinol	Synthetic cannabinoid without psychoactive effects that blocks NMDA receptors and inhibits cytokine and chemokine production with prominent neuroprotective actions. Assists in preventing brain damage after cardiac surgery. Assists in memory functions and improvement in manifestations of traumatic brain injury.

CT3/Ajulemic Acid	A synthetic potent analogue of the THC metabolite THC-11-oic acid. Anti-inflammatory properties, useful in arthritis and management of spasticity and pain in multiple sclerosis.
Cannabinor/PRS-211, 375	Synthetic compound that binds to CB-2 receptors with anti-inflammatory effects, analgesic (neuropathic pain) actions, and assists with bladder control.
HU 308	Synthetic compound that binds to CB-2 receptor with potential value in treatment of hypertension and inflammation.
HU 331	Synthetic compound with broad actions on CB-1, CB-2, and other non-CB receptors. Research for weight control, loss of memory, appetite stimulation, anticarcinogenic effects, analgesia, and inflammation.
Rimonabant/Acomplia	An effective synthetic compound that blocks endocannabinoid entry into the brain and suppresses appetite. Drug not safe due to depression and suicide risk. Withdrawn from use because of adverse effects.
Taranabant/MK-0364	Effect on appetite suppression by action as a CB-1 receptor inverse agonist. Promise as an antiobesity drug.

Denbinobin: Another Cannabis Gem

Denbinobin is a member of the family of anthraquinones, which have demonstrable antiviral activity. It has been isolated from Cannabis sativa, and it exerts its antiviral effects on HIV by inhibiting virus replication through a pathway of cellular activity involving NF-KB. (Sanchez-Duffhues, G., et al., *Biochem Pharma.* 76, 10 (2008): 1240–50). Denbinobin has other potential treatment effects (e.g., in cancer). It is found in other botanical sources (e.g., Ephemerantha lonchophylla, which is a herb used in traditional Chinese medicine).

Allergy to Cannabis

Acute allergic reactions to cannabis are usually examples of type 1 hypersensitivity reactions. Allergy in this type of hypersensitivity reaction is quite acute and is caused by IgE antibodies. Symptoms usually occur within approximately one hour of exposure, causing effects that are summarized in table 61. The prevalence of cannabis allergy is not known, but it seems quite uncommon.

Table 61. Allergic reactions to cannabis can cause many symptoms and signs

• Sneezing	• Asthmatic attacks
• Watery eyes	• Urticaria
• Dry cough	• Eczema
• Nasal congestion	• Pruritus
• Runny nose	• Headaches

Homeopathic Cannabis

In the mid-1800s to date, cannabis was proposed to be an ideal source of homeopathic remedies. This perception grew from the observations of the protean effects of cannabis on body functions. Historical studies on cannabis, performed in the late Victorian era, led to recommendations of cannabis homeopathy in the treatment of a number of medical conditions (table 62).

Table 62. A list of some medical conditions that were or are believed to be amenable to cannabis homeopathy. Please note that homeopathic medicines involve serial dilutions of active compounds, often to levels of undetectable amounts.

• **Treatment of delusions**	• **Muscle cramps**
• **Urinary tract infections**	• **Backache**
• **Tremors**	• **Pneumonia**
• **Heart palpitations**	• **Tinnitus**

Two Decades of Cannabis Use

As discussed earlier, a recent review article in the Journal Addiction presents an excellent summary of the physical and psychological effects of cannabis use (Wayne Hall, *Addiction*, 2014, doi: 10.1111/add 12703, summarized at www.sciencedaily. com/releases/2014/10/14/007092449.htm7). The main findings of this review are summarized below in table 63 (adapted from www. sciencedaily.com).

Table 63. A pivotal recent study (adapted from Hall, W., 2014 and published at www.sciencedaily.com)

Acute Cannabis Use	Adverse Effects
• Problems with driving or operating machinery	• Substance increase in accident risk with operating vehicles
• Increased road traffic accidents	• Increases in fatal road traffic accidents
• Reduces birth weight of infants	• Other risks in pregnancy— increasing definition of problems
• **Chronic Cannabis Use**	• **Adverse Effects**
• Development of cannabis abuse and dependence (addiction)	• One in six to nine adolescents may develop addiction
• Precipitation of psychosis	• More common with teen onset of use and family history of the disorder
• Lower IQ and lower educational achievement	• Arguable in terms of a causal relationship, unclear if reversible
• Causes gateway phenomenon	• Arguments prevail, but data show increased use of illicit drugs in addition to marijuana

• Adolescent use doubles the risk of schizophrenia or psychosis in adults	• Particular susceptibility with family history of psychosis
• Lung disease	• Debatable, but airways damage (chronic bronchitis) occurs
• Cardiovascular risks	• Definite risk with existing coronary artery disease

A Brief Review of the Medical Use of Cannabis

In anticipation of the need to provide some in-depth discussion of cannabis in specific disease states, this section of the book attempts to provide a macroscopic view of treatment options with cannabis or cannabinoids. There is value in estimating the level of evidence to support the use of cannabis in certain diseases or disorders. As mentioned earlier, much evidence supports the use of cannabis and its specific cannabinoid contents in the following circumstances:

- nausea and vomiting as a consequence of cancer chemotherapy
- anorexia caused by AIDS (HIV disease) and appetite stimulation
- chronic pain, especially of neuropathic origin
- spasticity in multiple sclerosis and spinal cord injury

Less evidence of benefit but promising use of marijuana are noted in epilepsy, pruritus, depression, Alzheimer's disease, brain injury, and glaucoma. In addition, anecdotal reports are assessed as promising in several other medical problems. These matters are summarized in the next few pages as a prelude to more in-depth information provided later in this book. Knowledge building on the effects of THC and CBD is provided in figure 1.

Figure 1. Knowledge building on the general effects of CBD and THC on body functions

Effect	CBD	THC
ANALGESIC — Relieves Pain	✓	✓
ANTIBACTERIAL — Kills or slows bacteria growth	✓	
ANTI-DIABETIC — Reduces blood sugar levels	✓	
ANTI-EMETIC — Reduces vomiting and nausea	✓	✓
ANTI-EPILEPSY — Reduces seizures and convulsions	✓	
ANTI-INFLAMMATORY — Reduces inflammation	✓	
ANTI-INSOMNIA — Aids sleep	✓	✓
ANTI-ISCHEMIC — Reduces risk of artery blockage	✓	
ANTI-PROLIFERATIVE — Inhibits cell growth in tumors/cancer cells	✓	

Effect	CBD	THC
ANTI-PSORIATIC — Treats psoriasis	✓	
ANTIPSYCHOTIC — Tranquilizing, used to manage psychosis	✓	
ANTISPASMODIC — Suppresses muscle spasms	✓	✓
ANXIOLYTIC — Relieves anxiety	✓	
APPETITE STIMULANT — Stimulates appetite		✓
BONE STIMULANT — Promotes bone growth	✓	
IMMUNOSUPPRESSIVE — Reduces function in the immune system	✓	
INTESTINAL ANTI-PROKINETIC — Reduces contractions in the small intestines	✓	
NEUROPROTECTIVE — Protects nervous system degeneration	✓	

At present, about 350,000 Americans are using medical marijuana (cannabis) under state laws. As noted, the therapeutic or adverse effects of cannabis are sometimes highly variable, and it has paradoxical effects in some circumstances. Much of the ensuing information is referenced at the end of the book.

Nausea and vomiting as a consequence of chemotherapy has been defined as responsive to cannabis and its synthetic analogues in more than four-dozen studies. Cannabis or synthetic analogues may amplify the effects of certain antiemetic drugs, and it has been used in other clinical circumstances of protracted nausea and vomiting, which may occur in patients with AIDS and hepatitis, in a manner that is aggravated by treatment. Clearly, the appetite-stimulating effect of THC can assist in maintaining body weight, and this has been documented in several circumstances, including patients with Alzheimer's disease who refuse adequate food intake. The positive effect on appetite can be present for several months, but enhancement of body weight in responsive individuals is often due to fat deposition rather than increases in lean body mass. It has been suggested that appetite stimulation should be used with an exercise program for more healthy weight gain. Nevertheless, this weight gain from cannabis often imparts a sense of well-being.

Movement disorders (altered motor function) and spasticity may be quite responsive to THC, nabilone, and cannabis. Many benefits have been observed in patients with disorders of the central nervous system that result in spasticity and associated symptoms of pain, tingling sensations (paresthesia), and tremor. Movement disorders show a variable response to cannabis or synthetic analogues (drugs) with reported benefit in circumstances of tardive dyskinesia and dystonia. A very promising effect of cannabis is described in Tourette's syndrome, especially in relationship to the control of tics. There are conflicting observations in the management of tremor and rigidity with the use of cannabis in Parkinson's disease, but the symptom of dyskinesia due to L-Dopa therapy may respond favorably.

The effects of cannabis or its analogues on pain control are accepted by many health care givers, but this medical indication has been questioned surprisingly by some state legislation governing the use of medical marijuana. Marijuana may act synergistically with opioid medication and even help to reduce death rates from opioid overuse. Reports of pain control due to neuropathic causes are sometimes impressive (e.g., pain caused by multiple sclerosis, HIV infection, or brachial plexus damage). There are many anecdotal reports of the benefit of cannabis in pain caused by cancer, inflammatory arthropathy (rheumatoid disease), migraine, general causes of headache, menstrual pain, different types of neuralgia, and digestive disease (irritable bowel syndrome and Crohn's disease).

Epilepsy is variably responsive to cannabis, and synergistic activity is apparent with several other anticonvulsant medications. There is orphan drug status for CBD-containing preparations in the management of epilepsy in children. The value of cannabis in the management of psychiatric disorders is debated extensively, but improvements are quite well defined in reactive depression and some mood disorders. It is clear that cannabis use should be supervised in the presence of all psychiatric disorders, especially those that are serious (e.g., schizophrenia or psychosis).

Therapeutic benefits of cannabis have been variably confirmed in dysthymia, sleep disorders, bipolar disease, and anxiety disorders. I emphasize that much difference of opinion exists as a consequence of contrarian findings in some studies (e.g., observations of the precipitation of convulsions and occasional exacerbations of psychiatric disorders, such as schizophrenia or depression, by herbal cannabis and its analogues). There have been some reports that modifications of dosage of cannabis could actually be used to reverse its own undesirable gateway tendency that causes a switch from soft to hard drugs. In particular, favorable observations have been made in the management of drug dependency on opiates, alcohol, and tranquillizer drugs (e.g., Valium and other benzodiazepines).

One highly promising application of cannabis is a combat against the common problem of inflammation. Inflammation is involved in the pathogenesis (causation) of much disease and has an accepted role in aging. There are many reports of an ability to reduce dosages of anti-inflammatory drugs (e.g., steroids and nonsteroidal anti-inflammatory drugs, NSAID) when cannabis is used, especially in cases of arthritis. Recent studies in Israel confirm the ability of cannabis to reduce drug use in many other disorders. It has been noted that cannabis could play a role in managing certain allergies, and its role in the treatment of autoimmune disease appears somewhat promising.

I have made it clear that the possible treatment applications of cannabis are legion. To do complete justice to all of the literature on the medicinal use of cannabis is unfortunately not possible in this short book. Conflicting findings in clinical trials and statements made on evidence derived from preclinical studies in animals act to both clarify and cloud the picture on the study of cannabis use.

We have learned that the important controls that cannabinoids exert on many body functions form a treasure chest of chemicals to fight disease, which have been viewed to be a consequence of "cannabinoid deficiencies" in humans and animals (E. B. Russo).

Long-Term Consequences of Cannabis Use

Opinions that support the safety of cannabis seem to clash with a significant amount of data that warns of its potential adverse effects, especially in the long term. While liberalization of the use of cannabis is advancing on a global basis, it is not possible to ignore any social changes and risks to physical or mental health that may occur as a consequence of its use.

The behavioral consequences of marijuana use are described in a number of surveys. There is a notable trend for young cannabis users to have poorer academic performance and higher educational dropout rates than nonusers. Much survey data has been accumulated, often in an anonymous manner of self-reporting. Such data is suspect, especially when collected from specific groups who have been arrested or have interacted with law enforcement agencies. Arrests for dealing cannabis are quite common. However, it is clear that many of the behavioral characteristics of cannabis users may often be very different from those present in dealers.

Some opinions smolder on the lack of addictive potential of marijuana, but a general consensus identifies the relatively common development of drug dependence. It is estimated that approximately 10–20 percent of cannabis users who smoke cannabis on a daily basis will develop varying degrees of dependence. Higher rates of marijuana dependence occur in young-onset cannabis users. To get an idea of dependence risks with other illicit substances helps place cannabis use into a general perspective. It is known that the addiction potential for cannabis is lower than that experienced with the hard drugs such as cocaine and heroin, but it is higher than LSD or mescaline. Of special interest is the greater addiction potential of legal drugs, such as alcohol, tobacco, and caffeine, compared with cannabis. However, use of these legal substances of potential abuse is common in cannabis users. While this book is not a comprehensive account on the management of drug dependence, it is clear that there is no single cure for drug dependency. Dependence on drugs may have to be managed by psychotherapy, motivational guidance, and lifestyle therapies, sometimes in a residential rehabilitation facility (e.g., Dream Recovery, Boca Raton, Florida). However, some health care practitioners and facilities wish to avoid the special challenges posed by drug dependence.

While negative changes in learning, attention, psychomotor abilities, and short-term memory are the hallmark of the early effects of marijuana use, long-term effects continue to be debated.

It has been suggested that long-term exposure to cannabis may result in permanent cognitive impairment when used in some children or adolescents, but this risk is not clear in adult-onset users. It would appear that the lifetime use of cannabis from a young age exerts significant influences on the development of long-term adverse consequences. This is especially the case in children and early adolescence, where risks of future problems are increased by cannabis use. These circumstances are confounded sometimes by the presence of several factors, including underlying psychiatric disease in cannabis users, interindividual responses to cannabis use, social factors, and so forth.

As mentioned earlier, the entity of cannabis use disorder is a well-accepted diagnosis that is described in the Diagnostic and Statistical Manual of Mental Disorders (DSM-5). The presence of this disorder is a clear indication for treatment. In brief, I continue to emphasize that high dosage and frequency of cannabis use from an early age forms a high risk for the future development or aggravation of mental and developmental disorders.

It appears that cannabis plays a role in the occurrence of acute and chronic psychosis. There are many reports of increased hospital emergency room attendances and admission for acute cannabis-related mental problems, particularly in young individuals. Moreover, there are individuals in the general population who have a greater tendency to psychotic reactions. Such individuals are often not readily identifiable. Psychotic disorders or diseases appear to be more common in the presence of established psychiatric disease (e.g., schizophrenia) and in individuals with a genetic tendency to the disorder. Childhood trauma and the presence of vulnerabilities determined by the environment (e.g., urban versus country upbringing) are important variables in the cause of psychosis. An emerging nefarious influence on health and well-being is the emergence of the common use of synthetic pot.

Whether or not cannabis exerts negative or positive effects on schizophrenia remains debatable. The factors that determine psychological or behavioral responses to cannabis use in the presence of schizophrenia are far from clear, but there are reports of better cognitive performance in some schizophrenic users of cannabis. Cannabis with a high THC to CBD ratio appears to be best avoided in schizophrenics, but CBD has been shown to possess antipsychotic effects, presumed to result from its antagonistic effects on THC. Several reports seem to suggest that CBD may be effective in both the prevention and management of schizophrenia, but more evidence is required. Unsupervised self-medication with cannabis for major psychiatric illnesses is quite common, but it should be avoided.

Suicidal activity and depression go hand in hand. Suicide risk with cannabis use seems to be present more often in individuals who started its use in childhood and persisted into adulthood. While cannabis has emerged as a risk factor in suicidal tendencies, many other circumstances operate to promote such tendencies. These include presence of depression or mood disorders, stress, social isolation, personal problems, and so forth.

It is reported that cannabis users exhibit no difference in the occurrence of major depressive disorders than nonusers. That said, risks of depression and negative moods with impulsive behavior in cannabis users may contribute to the evolution of psychological disorders later in life. Again, long-term heavy users of cannabis appear to be vulnerable to the development of depression, but much contention surrounds opinions that marijuana has major physical and negative health consequences. However, many physicians agree that further research is required before several firm conclusions can be made.

Differences of opinion exist about whether or not marijuana is carcinogenic (increases cancer risk). Various mentions have been made of an increased occurrence of cancer of the testicles, head, neck, lungs, and bladder with long-term cannabis use over the past two decades. Perhaps most evidence of cancer risk exists in the potential association between cannabis smoking and lung cancer, but this association has been refuted by some studies, where this risk has not been identified in pooled patient data. That said, the association of lung cancer and cannabis use is likely at high levels of smoking cannabis due to exposure to carcinogens. There is a relationship between head and neck cancer and cannabis smoking.

Cannabis smoking has been reported to be associated

with adverse respiratory symptoms such as cough, bronchial irritations, increased phlegm production, bullous lung disease, and bronchitis. A recent literature review from the British Lung Foundation has highlighted the difficulty in separating the effect of cannabis smoking alone from tobacco use. This situation is present because of the widespread use of cannabis and tobacco by the same person (common dual substance use).

Cannabis use has been stated to have significant negative effects in pregnancy, including fetal growth retardation, miscarriage, and cognitive problems in the neonate. The characterizations of these effects on the newborn are reminiscent of but somewhat different from adverse outcomes in the fetal alcohol syndrome. I believe that there may be a cannabis equivalent of the fetal alcohol syndrome, which may deserve the label "fetal cannabis syndrome." The effects and outcome of maternal cannabis use on human offspring may include attention disorders, language problems, and poor cognitive performance. There has been a suggestion that these effects could be persistent in children, and an association between maternal cannabis use in pregnancy has been made with adolescent delinquency. Unfortunately, the circumstances are clouded by correlation only without demonstrated causal links.

Many people continue to stress the lack of toxicity of marijuana because of its ability to be used in large dosages without recorded fatalities. However, this does not mean that cannabis has little or no effect on death rates. This association is becoming clearer as cannabis use is associated with a number of road traffic fatalities. The indirect contribution of cannabis to mortality is underestimated and may be expected to grow as the liberalization of cannabis use evolves. There seems to be little doubt that synthetic pot can cause deaths.

Cannabis and Motor Vehicle Accidents

The consumption of cannabis interferes with motor skills and impairs the operation of machinery and driving. It is estimated that individuals who drive within three hours of cannabis use are approximately twice as likely to cause a motor vehicle collision. These estimates came from comparisons with controls, consisting of drivers who were not under the influence of alcohol or psychoactive drugs.

Measurement of impairment by cannabis can be undertaken by laboratory testing. The negative effects of cannabis that cause impairment include poor reaction times, attention deficits, slow hand-eye coordination, and overall lack of vigilance. There is research that implies the presence of cannabis dose-related interference with driving capability. Added to these risks of cannabis use are poor or slow decision-making capabilities. It is argued that cannabis users are often able to compensate for the impairment caused by cannabis use, but such compensations are unpredictable. Some studies have concluded that cannabis use presents only modest risks of motor vehicle accidents in comparison with the use of several other drugs, including alcohol, some sleep drugs, medication used for the control of anxiety, and the use of hard drugs, such as cocaine and opiates.

There have been several recent news captions implying that "driving stoned" is safer than driving drunk, but this is not a reason to conclude that road traffic accident risks are low or lower with cannabis in all circumstances. It does appear that increasing perception of the safety of cannabis in the past ten years or so has led to greater use of illicit cannabis and an increasing prevalence of DUI associated with cannabis use. However, combined information on crash risk in states where medical use of cannabis is permitted has shown decreases of traffic related deaths by a range of 8–11 percent. Several hypotheses have been formed to explain this lowering of mortality, which could be a chance occurrence. It has been suggested that drunken drivers (alcohol excess) exhibit more reckless behavior than cannabis users, but cannabis is associated with risk-taking.

Testing for Cannabis Use

There are increasing needs for efficient cannabis testing to define driving "under the influence" or workplace use. The metabolism of cannabis and its storage in body fat produce circumstances of potential long-lasting detection in urine and blood samples. Most laboratories consider a level of 50 nanograms of THC metabolites per millimeter (ng/ml) to be a positive test. New Breathalyzer tests for the detection of cannabis use are being developed.

Earlier positive testing for cannabis was set at a lower level of 20 ng/ml in blood samples, but many false tests resulted in raising a positive test level to 100 ng/ml. However, the positive test is now 50 ng/ml, since its redefinition in 1995. It has been reported that the inhalation of secondhand cannabis smoke can result in a positive test level under circumstances of heavy exposure, but doubt exists.

Teen Cannabis Use Is Clearly Associated with Adult Disorders

Researchers have examined relationships between cannabis use in teen years and developmental outcomes up to the age of thirty to forty years or so in young adults. These measured outcomes included events such as suicide or attempts at suicide, occurrence of depression, suboptimal academic performance, failure to achieve educational milestones, subsequent use of other illicit drugs, and needs for social welfare in adulthood. In some of these studies, there were no clear links to depressive illness and dependence on welfare, but adolescents who used cannabis were eight times more likely to use other illegal drugs. In addition, there was a seven times greater likelihood of cannabis users to attempt suicide.

Many of these valuable observations were made in Australia at the National Drug and Alcohol Research Center at the University of New South Wales. In Australia, there is a growing interest in cannabis legalization. This future legalization will tend to make marijuana more available for unapproved use by adolescents (as may be now occurring increasingly in Colorado, Washington state, Alaska, Oregon, and Washington, DC, United States). Use of cannabis in youngsters in an illegal manner is well recognized but still poorly defined. It has been argued that this situation presents real concerns because of the predictable relationship between an increased risk of developmental problems in youngsters and daily use of cannabis. It has been argued that these aforementioned studies illustrate clear links between cannabis use and many problems, but they are not regarded as proof of direct causal associations. An important conclusion of these studies was the potential social and health benefits of efforts to delay the use of cannabis until adulthood.

Studies on cannabis use in teenagers, performed by the National Institute of Drug Abuse in the United States, indicate that approximately 7 percent of high school students are daily or frequent cannabis consumers. In summary, combining the results of these studies point to use of cannabis in adolescent or early teenage years as a cause of several negative developmental outcomes in adults. If this is the case, youngsters impaired by cannabis use are likely to become disadvantaged adults. I cannot apologize for my repeated attack on the dangers of cannabis use in youngsters.

The Cannabis Literature

As mentioned earlier, inaccurate reporting about cannabis use tends to continue to plague the development of clear understandings among the public, politicians, and physicians. Expressed opinions about cannabis are not always backed by scientific evidence (or social studies) and biased opinions can be detected in many types of cannabis literature. The ensuing sections of this book focus on cannabis use in various diseases or disorders, with attempts to convey accurate information from peer-review medical literature. The bias of opinion that has crept into cannabis literature requires a consideration of opinions that come from both sides of the fence. This fence separates protagonistic from antagonistic points of view about cannabis (marijuana). However, the dice have been loaded against complete knowledge on cannabis use in medical reporting. This has occurred because of many years of research that has focused on the negative outcome of cannabis use.

Many reviews of the scientific literature on cannabis use follow a predictable pathway of in vitro research, followed by preclinical animal studies, where some degree of premature truncation of research pursuits often exist. This is part of the legacy created by prohibition where human studies have been blocked or not encouraged to occur. Of course, the most valuable information about cannabis use comes from controlled human research, but this area of research is starting to be dominated by studies on drug analogues of cannabis or proprietary extracts. Of course, this research direction is encouraged because proprietary products, not whole herbal cannabis, present the dominant economic opportunity for the cannabis and pharmaceutical industries.

Many individuals have been anxious to see data that has been derived from recent recreational legalization of cannabis. This information is now recorded in a 188-page report released by the State of Colorado (Monitoring Health Concerns Related to Marijuana in Colorado: 2014, Colorado Department of Public Health and Environment htts://www.colorado. gov/pacific/sites/default/files/DC_MJ-Monitoring-Health-Concerns-Related-to-Marijuana-in-Co-2014.pdf). I find the report disappointing because it does not provide much new data on marijuana research. However, it provides a review of "limited existing studies." (Kristen Wyatt, Marijuana Research: Colorado issues 188-page report on health studies, www. thecannabist.co/2015/02/02 marijuana-research-colorado-health-effects-asthma-cancer-stored-driving/28946/.)

Kristen Wyatt of the associated press (K. Wyatt, ibid. 2015) summarized several highlights from the Colorado Government Report (State of Colorado, ibid. 2015). This summary is extracted and repeated below in table 64 from the work of K. Wyatt (Associated Press, ibid. Feb. 2015).

Table 64. This information is taken directly from Kristen Wyatt (ibid. Feb. 2, 2015). Much of the comments are verbatim quotes from Kristen Wyatt's highly accomplished synopsis of the Report from the Colorado Department of Public Health and Environment (2014) (www.colorado.gov).

- The risk of a motor vehicle accident doubles among drivers with recent marijuana use.
- Heavy marijuana use is associated with memory impairment persisting a week or more after quitting.
- Maternal use of marijuana is associated with negative effects on offspring (e.g., decreased academic ability, cognitive function, and attention).
- Regular marijuana use by adolescents and young adults is associated with psychotic symptoms and disorders such as schizophrenia in adulthood.

- The Colorado Department of Public Health and Environment review has been ordered by state lawmakers. A panel of doctors met for several months to compile the survey, which was delivered to lawmakers at the end of January 2015.
- The report laid out areas where there is limited evidence or where research is lacking.
- Doctors noted little available research on the health effects of edible or concentrated marijuana.
- Marijuana smoke contains many of "the same cancer-causing chemicals as tobacco smoke."
- There is limited or mixed evidence to suggest pot smoking is associated with greater risks of lung cancer or other respiratory health effects.
- Physicians suggested additional education about the health effects of marijuana and requested more public health surveys about how people use pot.

It is early days in the collection of data from the monitoring of the health effects of marijuana since its legalization for recreational use in Colorado on January 1, 2014. In brief, Section 25-1-5-110 on Monitoring Health Effects of Marijuana from The Colorado Department of Public Health and Environment states:

> The Department shall monitor changes in drug use patterns, broken down by county and race and ethnicity, and the emerging science and medical information relevant to the health effects associated with marijuana use. The Department shall appoint a panel ... To monitor the relevant information ... the panel shall establish criteria for studies to be reviewed ... making recommendations, as appropriate ... The Department may collect Colorado specific data that reports adverse health events involving marijuana use ...

The above truncated version of the monitoring of the health effects of marijuana will be delayed to some degree depending on funding by recommendations of the general assembly. Only time will tell on changes experienced with more widespread cannabis use.

Cannabis Treatment of Developmental and Behavioral Disorders

The wide range of potential clinical benefits of cannabis use in adults contrasts with the lack of evidence of its value in childhood developmental disorders and behavioral problems (Scott, E., et al., "Medical Marijuana," *Journal of Developmental and Behavioral Pediatrics* 36, no. 2 (2015): 115, doi: 10.1097/DBP.00000000000001 29). The lack of information on the outcome of cannabis use in children with developmental or behavioral disorders should result in caution concerning cannabis use in youngsters. Whether or not negative effects of cannabis are a cause of disease exacerbation in these young patients is not always clear.

Specific problems with cannabis use in adolescents may occur, including declines in intelligence, increased risks of addiction, major depression, anxiety disorders, and psychosis. The senior author of the study of medical marijuana for children with development and behavioral disorders (Scott, E. et al., ibid. 2015) stated that "as marijuana policy evolves and the drug becomes more readily available, it is important that practicing clinicians recognize the long term health and neuropsychiatric consequences of regular (cannabis) use."

This recent review of the literature questions the use of cannabis as treatment of developmental disorders in adolescents such as autism spectrum disorders (ASD) and attention-deficit hyperactivity disorders (ADHD).

In Jump the Lawyers

In a responsible manner, the Colorado Department of Public Health has released $7.6 million to fund a variety of valuable research projects on marijuana. The money to fund this research emanates from registration fees paid by patients to be placed on the state's medical cannabis register. A surprising response from the Patient Caregiver Rights Litigation Project was to file a lawsuit in 2014 to block the funding of research on marijuana. Allegations in the lawsuit include overcharging of patients by the Colorado Department of Health and Environment and inappropriate use of these funds, which are argued to be best used for administrative costs.

Revising Cannabinoids: Simple Perspectives

Medical reviews state that there are between sixty and more than one hundred types of cannabinoids in the cannabis plant, which constitute ten groups of related cannabinoids. Many of these different cannabinoids differ in minor ways in their structure, and not all of them have well defined or specific functions. In fact, many of the measured cannabinoids in cannabis are metabolites or intermediary compounds or end-products metabolism. Thus, the bioactivity of these cannabinoids is highly variable, and their effects are being increasingly defined in modern research.

A valuable classification of the ten groups of cannabinoids is shown in table 65. This information may not be accurate as more compounds are defined.

Table 65. Cannabinoids in cannabis, based on data presented in the Institute of Medicine Report, March 1999: "Marijuana and Medicine: Assessing the Science Base"

Please note that these data will change as more cannabinoids are characterized (displayed on www.procon.org/cannabis).

Cannabinoids in Cannabis

Cannabinoid Group	Abbreviations	Number of Known Variants (Changing)
Delta-9-tetrahydrocannabinol	9-THC	9
Delta-8-tetrahydrocannabinol	8-THC	2
Cannabichromene	CBC	5
Cannabicyclol	CBL	3

Cannabidiol	CBD	7
Cannabielsoin	CBE	5
Cannabigerol	CBG	6
Cannabinidiol	CBND	2
Cannabinol	CBN	7
Cannabitriol	CBT	9
Miscellaneous types		11

Conclusion

Cannabis has created many horizons for the potential treatment of a variety of diseases, especially as an adjunctive medicinal agent. It is clear that whole cannabis herbal preparations may not have the same effects as cannabis-related drugs. Comparisons of dosage/responses of different types of cannabis or cannabinoids have not been studied often, and many factors operate to affect interindividual and intraindividual responses to cannabis administration.

In the next few sections of this book, I have relied on information for health care professionals presented by Health Canada. This excellent review of the effects of cannabis and the cannabinoids has been compiled by many distinguished authors. It may be viewed on the Internet at www.hc-sc.gc.ca/dhp-mps/ marihuana/med/infoprof-eng.php, editor H. Abramovici, June 12, 2013, and August 24, 2014. This work is highly recommended and is referred to often in this book as a primary source of information.

Chapter 7

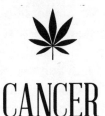

CANCER

Major Effects of Cannabis in Cancer

Certain cannabinoids (e.g., THC and CBD) have dual roles in cancer management. First, they can variably relieve nonspecific symptoms or consequences of cancer (e.g., nausea, pain, loss of appetite, fatigue, wasting syndrome, and sleeplessness); and second, they possess specific anticarcinogenic (antitumoral) effects. The most researched cannabinoids in cancer therapy are delta-9 tetrahydro-cannibol (THC) and cannabidiol (CBD). The notion that cannabinoids are a cure for cancer is a gross overstatement that may create false hope for patients and may encourage them to adopt some wrong ways of cancer treatment. However, many studies in animals and in vitro (in the lab) have shown the promise of cannabinoids for the adjunctive treatment of different types of cancer. This situation is a promising stimulus to oncological research.

In summary, there are several explanations for the putative actions of cannabinoids in cancer management. Moreover, the effects of cannabis or related substances analogues can be different in different types of cancer. For example, in laboratory experiments (in vitro), cannabidiol (CBD) seems to have pronounced effects on the inhibition of the growth and spread of breast cancer cells, whereas some other types of cancer (e.g., central nervous system tumors and prostate cancer cells) seem to be quite responsive to THC. However, these observations are mainly part of preclinical studies that may not be predictive of the effects of specific cannabinoids in human cancer treatment.

The role of cannabis and related compounds is a highly complex subject. The organization, Cancer Research UK, has produced a list of commonly asked questions to illustrate the role of cannabis in cancer management. This information is a good starting point for understanding cannabis research in cancer (scienceblog.cancerresearchuk.org/ 01/07/25/ cannabiscannabinoids-and-cancer-the-evidence-so-far).

This chapter reports that cannabinoids can be considered to be a novel class of anticancer drugs that interfere with cancer cell proliferation, reduce cancer spread, and inhibit blood supply to tumors (antiangiogenesis).

Applying Medical Cannabis

Cancer treatments such as chemotherapy, surgery, and radiation ("cut and burn" treatments) are perceived often as unattractive management options. These approaches seriously impair quality of life and sometimes result in only modest improvements in cancer treatment outcomes. Federal guidelines, set forth by the United States attorney general in 2009, seem to discourage the prosecution of medical users of cannabis with serious diseases, but problems with the law may occur in states where there is no formal legalization of the medical use of cannabis, even if the individual has cancer or other types of disabling disease. This situation is absurd and preposterous. That said, law courts have tended to act toward the decriminalization of cannabis use, especially if medical necessity for cannabis is present. Medical necessity is a powerful defense used against any penalty or prosecution imposed on cannabis use by the government.

Medicinal use of cannabis may provide options for the amelioration of some of the general adverse effects of cancer chemotherapy with improvements in nausea, anorexia (loss of appetite), and variable alleviation of reactive depression and pain. One advantage of cannabis use is its potential for immediate or early symptomatic benefits when smoked or vaped (administration by vaporization). In summary, there is a general opinion that marijuana can ease adverse effects of cancer therapies, with added benefits of specific anticarcinogenic actions. Disease symptoms appear to be often better tolerated with cannabis use.

There are versatile delivery systems for whole herbal cannabis, which include smoking, vaporization, additions to edibles, or infusion in teas or sodas. In some cases, physicians or caregivers may advise the use of synthetic analogues such as Marinol (THC analogue) in cancer management. Many physicians have discussed perceptions that whole herbal cannabis may be more effective than pharmaceutical analogues, but further research is required to define these circumstances in detail. Marinol is a drug that contains synthetic THC, and it is very expensive, with an estimated need for payment of several hundred dollars per month. In general, insurance companies do not pay for cannabis prescriptions. This situation drives the illicit use of cannabis. Furthermore, while THC analogues are expensive, some CBD-rich products may cost up to several thousand dollars a month (e.g., Charlotte's Web in high dosage). This is consumer gouging.

Table 66 is an intentional reiteration of some of the side effects of medicinal cannabis that have been discussed in earlier sections of this book. Some of these effects can limit cannabis use as a cancer therapy.

Table 66. Examples of side effects of cannabis preparations

Other risks or negative outcomes of cannabis use are present when illicit cannabis use occurs as a consequence of the presence of adulterants (other chemicals) or microbial contamination.

behavioral change	anxiety
drowsiness	thirst, dry mouth
memory loss	insomnia
euphoria	appetite increase
gastrointestinal intolerance	avoidance of driving
accidents at work	sensitivity to surroundings

Stephen Holt, MD, DSc

As mentioned earlier, the side effects or psychoactive consequences of cannabis use can sometimes result in noncompliance with treatment. It is arguable whether or not psychoactive effects of cannabis should be viewed as a side effect or a desired effect. Illicit cannabis use results in unpredictable outcomes in cancer treatment because cancer presents multifactorial challenges that may be amenable to the versatile and favorable effects of cannabinoids in specific dose ranges.

The relevance of cannabinoids in cancer management includes their effects on immunity, pain control, inflammation, cell proliferation, programmed cell death (apoptosis), and other effects. In fact, cancer manifests itself by lack of control of cell division combined with ultimate cell death. The ability of cancer cells to proliferate and spread is caused by loss of control or damage to many different genes, and these effects can be inhibited to varying degrees by cannabinoids (THC and CBD). Reductions in cell proliferation by cannabis compounds were first well documented in the mid-1970s. A lot of research with laboratory studies of cancer has shed light on how cannabinoids and their receptors alter uncontrolled cell division, metastatic events (spread), and cell death.

Knowledge is advancing rapidly, but the underlying mechanisms of the effects of cannabinoids in cancer development and progression are not fully understood. The dual effects of some cannabinoids on programmed cell death (proapoptosis and antiapoptosis) imply a pivotal role of the endocannabinoid receptor system in the development or natural history of cancer. In medical reviews of the therapeutic implications of the endocannabinoid system and cancer, scientists have described dysfunction of the endocannabinoid system. In addition, paradoxical effects may enter the picture of cannabis use in cancer.

Cancer promotion and immunosuppression are described in some recent research that has indicated that cannabinoids can trigger the development of large numbers of myeloid-derived suppressor cells (MDSCs). These cells function to suppress the immune system. Other studies have shown that MDSCs may promote cancer growth and reduce the ability of immune cells to kill cancer cells. Furthermore, cancer cells can produce interleukin-1-beta, which also stimulates the growth of MSDCs with their immunosuppressive and cancer-promoting actions.

While a large body of opinion supports the value of cannabinoids in cancer-associated vomiting and pain, evidence for these effects accrued from several studies performed in the 1970s and modern results of similar studies have been sometimes equivocal. Recent studies of Sativex (THC:CBD in a 1:1 ratio) in cancer pain in comparison to placebo have been undertaken. However, the administration of THC alone in some studies did not result in significant reductions in pain scores. While some recent studies have implied that cannabis may not always induce significant levels of analgesia, it seems to be able to induce tolerance to pain. These qualities of cannabis may be due to alterations in the emotional status of individuals with pain. Support for these opinions that involve emotional status comes from correlated changes in functional magnetic resonance imaging (FMRI) studies of the brain. These studies were performed in Oxford, England.

In these FMRI studies, twelve healthy volunteers received an oral dose of 15 mg of THC or a placebo. The test materials were then crossed over. After applying a pain-inducing cream of capsaicin (1 percent) to their skin, repeated MRI scans were undertaken. In other words, these scans were performed with and without pain-provoking cream and with and without THC-containing tablets or placebo. It was observed that pain induced by capsaicin did not bother the study participants to a major degree, but the burning sensation experienced by the volunteers persisted unchanged. The FMRI scans showed reductions in brain activity in areas of the brain where the emotional aspects of pain are registered (the anterior midcingulate cortex). Also, changes were observed on scans in the right amygdala, an area of the brain that is primed by pain. Thus, complex highways of communication in the brain that control pain sensations are altered by THC. Many other studies using different methodologies have confirmed the value of THC in pain control.

Carcinogenicity of Cannabis Smoke

An excellent review of the carcinogenicity of cannabis has been produced by the California Environmental Protection Agency (August, 2009) (www.oehha.gov/prop65/hazard_ident/pdf). Cannabis smoke has been placed on the Proposition 65 list of chemicals recognized by the state of California to cause cancer. The evidence for the association of cancer risk and cannabis use is apparent in both human and animal studies. Animal studies involving both the inhalational and skin exposure of rodents to cannabis smoke have shown the development of malignant and benign neoplasia, respectively. Cannabis smoke is genotoxic and toxic to the immune system. Moreover, cannabis-induced disruption of endocrine function and altered cell signaling pathways are proposed as support for a potential carcinogenic effect of cannabis.

The chemical composition and toxicological profile of cannabis smoke are similar in many respects to those of tobacco smoke. This causes a problem in separating carcinogenic effects between cannabis and tobacco, which both contain numerous carcinogens. While there is argument over the carcinogenic effects of cannabis, most evidence points to its possession of a carcinogenic potential.

Laboratory and Clinical Research in Cancer

It is important to note that the majority of evidence that supports cannabis use in cancer treatment comes from laboratory experiments on cancer cells (in vitro) and research in animal models of cancer (in vivo). The effects of cannabis in lab or animal models cannot be assumed to be accurate predictors of similar effects occurring in humans. One potential problem that has not been addressed in detail is potential gender differences in responses to cannabis. Do males respond differently than females to cannabis? Perhaps they do because of the known presence of close hormonal/cannabis links (e.g., estrogenic influences).

A number of valuable review articles have presented discussions on the various effects of natural cannabis or its pharmaceutical analogues on pathways of cancer initiation, growth, and spread. These pathways are highlighted in table 67.

Table 67. Effects of various cannabinoids on cancer

Please note specific cannabinoids have different affects depending on their cannabinoid receptor interactions (CB1 and CB2), and effects of cannabis on cancer tissue have been observed sometimes in a manner independent of CB receptor interactions.

Cause apoptosis (cell death)	Inhibition of cell division (antiproliferative)
Antiangiogenic (interference with blood vessel growth in tumors)	Antimetastatic (stopping cells from moving and invading local tissues)

Cause autophagy (speeding up cells waste disposal)	Synergistic effects with anticancer drugs (stronger cancer kill may occur by combining treatments)

Guzman's Classic Cancer Studies

There have been few controlled clinical trials in humans with cancer. One notable study was performed by Dr. Manuel Guzman and his team of researchers in Spain. In this study, nine patients with a severe form of brain malignancy (glioblastoma multiforme) were treated with THC, which was directly instilled into the brain. Certain degrees of favorable responses were noted in eight out of nine individuals, but all patients died within a year. Survival in individuals with glioblastoma multiforme is very limited, and the early deaths in this study were consistent with the aggressive nature and natural history of this tumor.

In addition to the experiences of Dr. Guzman and his colleagues, there have been isolated cases of cancer treatment with variable degrees of success, but many of these reports are anecdotal. While the observations of cancer therapy with cannabinoids is promising, at the time of writing, there is a lack of evidence that comprehensive cancer treatment can be effective with cannabis or its analogues alone. However, some evidence of potential adjunctive treatment benefit with other cancer treatments has emerged.

A Brief Overview of Cancer and Its Responses to Cannabinoids

It is difficult to do justice to a large amount of basic laboratory research that points to the potential efficacy of cannabis therapy in treating certain types of malignancy. Table 68 represents a brief summary of different forms of cancer and their potential response to cannabinoids. These findings have been derived often from preclinical studies, and much further research is required.

Table 68. Responses of different types of cancer cell lines to cannabinoids, in the lab and in animal models. Data may not be portable to humans.

Cancer	Comment
Breast cancer	CBD administration decreases 1d-1 expression in metastatic breast cancer cells, resulting in a reduction in tumor aggression.
Lung cancer	THC administration reduces tumor growth and number and severity of lung metastases in mice. Cannabidiol inhibits lung cancer cell invasion and metastases via effects on intercellular adhesion molecule-1.
Pancreatic cancer	Cannabinoids cause apoptosis of pancreatic cancer cells by action on CB2 receptors, with ceramide upregulation of P8 and endoplasmic reticulum stress-related genes (ATF4 and TRB3).
Prostate cancer	Prostate cancer cells express CB-1 and CB-2 receptors, which when stimulated cause increased apoptosis, decreased androgen receptor expression, and reduced cancer cell viability.
Colorectal cancer	Cannabidiol has chemo-preventive actions and reduces cell proliferation by multiple mechanisms.
Ovarian cancer	Cannabinoid receptors have been defined as a target for ovarian cancer therapy.

Hematological malignancy	CB2 receptors on human leukemia and lymphoma cell lines may be a target to induce apoptosis.
Skin cancer	Cannabinoids induce apoptosis and inhibit blood vessels supply to tumors (antiangiogenesis). Value in melanoma.
Hepatocellular cancer	Certain cannabinoids (THC) and JWH-015, a CB2 receptor agonist, reduce the viability of hepatocellular cancer cell lines. THC has shown potential in retarding cell growth and metastases in cholangiocarcinoma in lab experiments.
Other cancers	Cannabis smoking may decrease the risk of bladder cancer. Cannabidiol impairs invasion of human cervical cancer and human lung cancer cells.

While the majority of the effects of cannabis or selected cannabinoids on experimental cancer appear favorable (table 53), there may be certain potentially negative effects. The laboratory observations that THC in high dosage can kill cancer cells under some circumstances are confounded by observations that cannabis may sometimes encourage cancer cell growth (a paradoxical effect). Different responses of cancer may result from several variables, including the density of cannabinoid receptors on some cancer cell types and the dosage of consumed cannabinoids.

There has been a suggestion that activating CB2 receptors may reduce the immune system's ability to target and destroy cancer cells. Again, many of these conclusions rely on observations in preclinical studies and cannot be projected reliably to circumstances in humans. On the other hand, certain synthetic analogues of cannabinoids appear to enhance specific immune functions in cancer studies in animals. The development of resistance to the anticancer effects of cannabinoids in cancer cells has been proposed as a potential problem.

Cannabinoids and Malignancy of Immune Origin

Malignant cells of immune origin present in lymphoma and leukemias are quite susceptible to the apoptotic (all death) effects of cannabinoids. More than a decade ago studies demonstrated that human leukemia and lymphoma cell lines (e.g., Jurkat cells and Molt-4) expressed mainly CB-2 receptors. Apoptosis was facilitated in these cell lines by a variety of cannabinoids or analogues, including THC, HU-210, Anandamide, and JWH-015. Apoptosis induction occurs by several mechanisms, and these effects hold promise for the development of drugs to treat malignant immune cells (Amcaoglu, S. et al., *Immunobiology* 215, no. 8 (Aug. 2010): 598–605).

Cancer Pain and Cannabinoids

Pain reduction by cannabinoids occurs primarily as a consequence of interactions with cannabinoid receptors (CB-1), but it can result from specific anti-inflammatory effects or effects of phytocannabinoids and related substances. One interesting discovery is the ability of CB-2 receptor stimulation to reduce the release of inflammatory substances from many cell types, including mast cells. This reduction of histamine and serotonin release may be associated with a release of natural opioids in the body. Opioid release would act to reinforce pain relief, because opioids and certain cannabinoids have synergistic actions on pain control. In fact, cannabis has demonstrated opioid-sparing effects in the presence of pain.

It has been shown in animal models that synthetic agonists of CB-1 and CB-2 receptors may produce potent relief of pain with an equivalence to the effects of morphine. As stated earlier, the most important cannabinoid receptor in pain control is the CB-1 receptor, which is present in both peripheral nerve junctions and areas of the brain that are involved in the processing of nociception. It is recognized that endocannabinoid production in the spinal cord can actually enhance pain by dampening the activity of inhibitory neuronal networks in some circumstances (Grotenhermen, F., *Cannabinoids* 5, no. 1 (2010): 1–3). In brief, this is a key mechanism whereby cancer and other types of pain may be promoted. This potential role of endocannabinoids may change over various time periods as a consequence of the development of a reduction of the dampening effects on inhibitory pathways that cause pain.

Most research has focused on THC use in the relief of pain, but there have been observations of the favorable analgesic effects of CBD, notably in hashish users. Hashish may contain more CBD than THC in some circumstances. Comparisons of THC plant extracts and Sativex (THC and CBD, cannabidiol), involving a placebo arm of study, showed significant reductions of pain scores (Numerical Rating Score) with Sativex but not with THC. In one study, THC extract was noted to reduce pain using different measures of pain improvement (Brief Pain Inventory-Short Form, BP1-SF) (www.cannabis-med.org). An interesting inference from this study was that the study medications influenced different aspects of pain perception. Some studies, however, have failed to define a clear role of CBD in pain control studies.

Cannabis is gaining increasing popularity in the management of chronic pain, but few studies have examined its safety profile in this important therapeutic application. Canadian researchers have undertaken a national multicenter study that examines the safety of cannabis use in groups of patients suffering from chronic pain (Ware M A et al. Cannabis for the Management of Pain: Assessment of Safety Study (COMPASS), The Journal of Pain, 2015; DOI: 10.1016/j.pain. 2015.07.014). In brief, this study showed that daily cannabis users had no greater risk of serious adverse events compared with controls. In these studies the average intake of cannabis was 2.5 grams per day (smoked, vaporized or consumed as edibles). The researchers described mild to moderate side effects in cannabis smokers, but there were no major effects on cognitive function. However, levels of pain, mood and quality of life were improved in comparison to controls.

Advocacy for Cannabis Use in Cancer?

The Internet is endowed with many anecdotal reports of success with the use of cannabis to treat cancer. At present, one cannot conclude that cannabis cures cancer. The value of cannabis in cancer treatment is debated, but it is somewhat reinforced by many animal studies that show varying degrees of treatment success, at least at a cellular level of study. Many factors coalesce to support the use of cannabis in cancer treatments. Discussions about these factors are reinforced by contents of some Internet blogs and a plethora of favorable reports of cannabis use in cancer that are displayed on YouTube. However, this information cannot be interpreted currently as evidence to confirm the efficacy of cannabis as a cancer cure.

Does Marijuana Cause Cancer?

The jury remains out on whether or not cannabis smoking can cause lung cancer. Early studies of lung cancer risk in males who smoked tobacco and marijuana showed that lung cancer risk was doubled for men who used marijuana and tobacco. Other studies have suggested that lung cancer risk is increased in heavy, long-term users of cannabis. There is clear evidence that cannabis smoking causes inflammation and cellular damage with the occurrence of precancerous changes in lung tissue. Furthermore, many of the carcinogens found in tobacco are present in cannabis, often in larger amounts. It has also been proposed that immune system changes (immunosuppression) occur with cannabis use in a manner that may favor cancer formation.

Cannabis use has been associated with the risk of testicular cancer. In a study of 455 men in California, it was found that those who had used cannabis were two times as likely to have developed aggressive testicular germ cell tumors. The actions of cannabis in the cause of testicular cancer are not known, but animal studies show that cannabis smoking and THC administration reduce levels of circulating testosterone. The risk of testicular cancer seems to increase with young age at the time of the first use of pot and high amounts of cannabis use.

The association of marijuana use with cancer occurrence remains unclear. A recent epidemiologic review of marijuana and cancer reinforces uncertainty about causal links (Huang, Y. J. et al., "Epidemiologic Review of Cannabis and Cancer: An Update, Cancer Epidemiol," *Biomarkers Prev* 24, 11 (2015): 15–31). Studies on head and neck or lung cancer reveal evidence of increased or decreased cancer occurrences, perhaps because no association exists or other factors operate and cloud the picture. While a relationship between cannabis use and testicular cancer may exist, the development of other types of cancer with cannabis use is not clarified due to lack of sufficient information.

More Anticancer Observations

An excellent source of information on the antitumor effects of cannabis is present at www.cancer.gov.com/cancertopics/pdg. I reiterate that a number of animal studies have shown that certain cannabinoids can inhibit the growth of different tumors. A study of two years' duration was undertaken in rats and mice that received THC by gavage (forced feeding). These studies showed a reduction in the development of a variety of tumors, including a decrease in hepatic adenomas and hepatocellular cancer in mice. In rats, there was a decreased occurrence of polyps and adenomas (benign tumors) in different locations in the body. In separate investigations, delta-9-THC, delta-8-THC, and cannabinol administration resulted in inhibition of Lewis lung cancer growth. It seems that selected cannabinoids can kill cancer cells without affecting healthy cells. In addition, there may be some protective effects of cannabinoids from cell death in healthy tissues. For example, certain cannabinoids are noted to protect normal glial cells (brain cells) from apoptosis (cell death).

Studies in 2014 at the University of East Anglia in the UK (in association with Universidad Complutense in Spain) have shown that targeting of human cancer cells in mice with THC resulted in interactions with two cannabinoid receptors (CB2 and GPR55). These two receptors appear to interact jointly to cause anticancer effects.

A popular model for animal cancer studies is the subcutaneous placement of xenografts (cancer cell transplants) in a special species of rodents, referred to as nude mice. This animal model is believed to be a predictor of the anticancer effects of various test substances on humans, but there are many differences in body functions between humans and nude mice. That said, impressive anticancer effects of delta-9-THC or a synthetic agonist of the CB2 receptor have been noted in xenografts of hepatocellular carcinoma and other tumors in nude mice.

Studies in mice have produced somewhat conflicting results concerning the study of the development of cancer. On the one hand, THC-treated mice may show significant inhibition of cancer growth by its ability to exert antiproliferative effects, but on the other hand, some studies have shown enhanced tumor growth in some nude mice with certain types of xenografts. Cannabinoids may play a favorable role in modifying the circumstance of inflammation that promotes certain types of cancer (e.g., colon cancer sequences in inflammatory bowel disease). These findings and other studies have formed the basis of suggestions that cannabinoids may be valuable in reducing the risk of cancer formation that can be promoted by inflammation (e.g., colon cancer occurrence in ulcerative colitis).

More detailed studies of antitumor mechanism show both promotion of apoptosis and cell death as a consequence of activation of stress pathways in the endoplasmic reticulum (inner cell contents) of cancer cells. These cellular stress pathways stimulate the occurrence of autophagy (a form of cell degeneration). Loss of viability of cancer can occur as a consequence of programmed cell death, which can be induced by cannabidiol CBD (noted specifically in breast cancer cells). Laboratory studies show that CBD inhibits the growth and survival of breast cancer cells in a manner that does not rely on the function of CB-1, CB-2, or vanilloid receptors. In this circumstance, cell death from apoptosis has been shown to increase with increasing dosages of CBD. There are data that show that the administration of CBD may increase the entry of cytotoxic drugs into cancer cells. This property of CBD contributes to a synergistic effect between chemotherapy and CBD. This observation is worthy of much further investigation.

Other mechanisms may operate in the ability of CBD to exert antitumor effects. Studies of the role of intercellular adhesion molecule-1 (ICAM-1) indicate that occurrence of this substance seems to be associated with a decreased metastatic risk of cancer. Research shows that ICAM-1 can be increased by CBD administration, with a consequential decrease in cancer invasiveness. Of particular note are the demonstrated cancer-prevention properties of CBD in colon cancer that can be experimentally induced by a carcinogen. In detailed investigations, it has been shown that CBD directly reduces cancer cell proliferation, increases endocannabinoid concentrations, and acts as an antioxidant.

Anticancer Effects of Cannabinoids: Revision

Cannabinoids emerged in the medical literature in the early 1970s as a palliative way of managing cancer patients. To review matters, the ability of cannabis and its analogues to exert positive benefits in cancer management include (1) the well-established reduction of chemotherapy induced vomiting and nausea, (2) appetite stimulation, and (3) pain management. While these effects are highly valuable adjuncts in treatment, cannabis has some well-defined antitumoral (anticarcinogenic) properties in laboratory experiments and some promising observations in humans.

There are many studies that link the endocannabinoid system and the emergence of different types of cancer. As described earlier, there is a concept that the tone of the endocannabinoid systems in the body influence disease occurrence and progression. This tone is believed to be a significant factor in controlling the malignant potential of several types of tumors. As one may expect, the expression or occurrence of cannabinoid receptors is different in malignant cells compared with normal cells. There appears to be a situation where differences in receptor expression on cancer cells are likely to exert significant influences of selected cannabinoid therapies. One reasonably consistent factor has emerged in the study of endocannabinoids and cancer. This relates to the observation that levels of endocannabinoids are often elevated in cancer tissues, notably glioblastoma, prostate cancer, colon cancer, pituitary adenoma, and others (Abramovici, H. et al., www.hc-sc.gc.ca).

As discussed earlier, there are an increasing number of experimental studies in animals that can pave the pathway to further potential use of cannabinoids in cancer treatment. As noted earlier, cannabis receptors can work in diverse ways, which include metastasis prevention, cell apoptosis, cell cycle arrest with direct growth inhibition, antiangiogenic actions, and inhibition of cell migration. To confuse the circumstances, the anticancer effects of THC may differ at different dosages. It is suggested that low or high dosages of THC may result in different degrees of cell proliferation. However, these findings are not consistent.

The wide-ranging biological effects of cannabinoids in malignancy are modified by many circumstances. Alterations in experimental conditions in animals with cancer may influence effects of cannabinoids in a rather profound and unpredictable manner. These influences include differences in the cancer cell type under study, differences in cannabinoid receptor expression, prevailing hormone levels (notably estrogen), and the occurrence of regulatory mechanisms that are separate from any actions on cannabinoid receptors. Promising findings have emerged with the use of cannabinoids as a potential combination therapy with cytotoxic chemotherapy, but these research data involving combination therapy are restricted currently to animal experiments of tumor transplants. Human data are needed in this area of research.

As noted earlier, the most significant human experiences with cannabinoids and cancer in human clinical trials revolve around the work of Dr. Guzman and his colleagues in Spain. These important studies involved observations of THC effects in nine patients with highly malignant brain tumors (glioblastoma multiforme) that had failed standard therapies for their disease. Beneficial outcomes were noted with THC administration by anticancer effects, which were most likely due to direct inhibition of cell proliferation and decreased viability of the tumor cells. It has been noted, in separate experiments, that the addition of CBD to THC amplified antitumor effects. It is clear that CBD and THC may form a dynamic duo in the fight against certain types of cancer.

Conclusion

The value of cannabis in cancer management has emerged with significant strength (Abramovici, H. et al., www.hc-sc.gc.ca). Nonspecific effects of cannabis on symptoms of cancer and benefits in the palliation of malignant disease are apparent. The specific anticarcinogenic effects of cannabis appear potent and versatile in many circumstances. While it is premature to characterize cannabis as a cancer cure, its potential adjunctive benefits in cancer therapy are increasingly clear. Human studies in cancer research are required, with a degree of urgency.

Chapter 8

MENTAL DISORDERS

Links between Mental Illness and Cannabis

Cannabis can cause or contribute to a variety of psychiatric disorders. In contrast, a significant amount of emerging literature supports the use of cannabis in the treatment of certain types of mental illness. In some circumstances, concerns about provoking mental disease have inhibited the use of psychoactive preparations of cannabis by practicing clinicians. That said, self-treatment of psychiatric disease with marijuana has become quite attractive to some patients, but this unsupervised practice should not be encouraged. Unwanted psychoactive effects of cannabis are a common reason for lack of compliance with conventional treatments for psychiatric disease, and they can lead to the cessation of prescribed cannabis use, due to side effects. In other words, the potential beneficial effects of cannabis are confounded by variable levels of patient acceptance or tolerance of the psychoactive effects of cannabis. One man's meat does appear to be another man's poison.

Psychiatric disorders are associated with cannabis use, but they are not necessarily all linked in a causal relationship. These disorders are shown in table 69.

Table 69. A number of psychiatric disorders or behavioral problems associated with cannabis use but not necessarily causally linked.

• Psychotic episodes	• Anxiety
• Panic attacks	• Depression
• Mood swings	• Anhedonia
• Antimotivational syndrome	• Self harm/suicide
• Impulsivity	• Other substance abuse or addiction

It is clear that the use of cannabis in the management of psychiatric disorders and behavioral abnormalities remains controversial. Conflicting opinions about its value, or dangers, have emerged from observations in both controlled research and uncontrolled clinical circumstances. As mentioned earlier, many individuals with psychiatric disorders self-medicate with illicit cannabis. There is good reason for patients not to have confidence in the use of illicit sources of marijuana, and there is a loud call among the medical profession for the greater availability of standardized cannabis materials. Such materials would be expected to be safer and more efficacious for their selected purpose of use. In addition, they may be more predictable in their effects. The pharmaceutical demand for double-blind controlled clinical trials of cannabis treatments is shared by many scientists, but a large unknown proportion of the general public does not subscribe to this notion. However, this situation is perhaps moot for some people, given increasing legalization of cannabis. Cannabis use has been encouraged in recent times by an unjustified common reputation of being universally safe.

Clearly, support for the illicit use of cannabis comes from perceptions of the safety of cannabis. This perception has been reinforced by decriminalization and variable legalization of cannabis in many locations in the United States. Many people have noted that there is well-established dual status of cannabis, defined by its illicit versus legal use. While herbal cannabis is a substance with highly variable composition, consumers may not recognize the advantages of standardized marijuana produced by good growing and manufacturing practices, or they may be swayed in their choice by economic issues. Illicit cannabis is often cheaper than medical prescription cannabis, and it often feels the same or even better when used, as judged by its psychoactive effects. This is a major dilemma!

The Association of Substance Abuse with Mental Disease

The simultaneous occurrence of mental disease with substance abuse is an important component of modern clinical practice (Rach Beisel, J. et al., "Co-occurring Severe Mental Illness and Substance Abuse: A Review of Recent Research," accessed 2/17/15, ps.psychiatryonine.org/doi/abs/10.11176/ps.50.11.1427). Recent research has confirmed a significantly higher occurrence of substance abuse by individuals with severe forms of mental illness. It has been concluded that the natural history of mental illness is affected in a negative manner by concomitant use of drugs of abuse, of which cannabis is a common example. Strategies to manage this co-occurrence of severe mental illness with substance abuse include (table 70).

Table 70. Treatment strategies using an integrative medicine approach for co-occurrence of severe mental illness and substance use disorders (Rach Beisel, J., ibid.)

- harm reduction
- staged treatments
- motivational interviewing
- cognitive behavioral interventions
- modified twelve-step self-help groups
- well-selected pharmacological interventions and drug substitution
- a variety of alternate medical treatment strategies

The end results of substance abuse in patients with mental disease include aggravation of symptoms, increased hospital visits and admissions, lack of treatment compliance, disruptive behavior, and poor social interactions (Mueser, K. T. et al., "Comorbidity of Schizophrenia and Substance Abuse: Implications for Treatment," *Journal of Consulting and Clinical Psychology* 60 (1992): 845–56). An excellent source of information on what has been termed the "double jeopardy" of substance abuse and mental illness is the book *Double Jeopardy: Chronic Mental Illness and Substance Abuse* (Drake, R. E., Mercer McFadden, C., edited by Lehman, A. F., and Dixon, L. B., New York, Harwood Academic, 1995).

With an estimated frequency of use of cannabis in one out of every ten adults in the United States, it shines as the most commonly used illicit drug. Some scientists have been suspicious about the accuracy of public reporting of cannabis use for many reasons, not the least of which is the continuing stigma applied to its use. This book attempts to examine some of the varying attitudes to marijuana legalization in many locations in the United States, but it seems that there is an overall opinion among mental-health workers that cannabis may result in common adverse effects in people with mental disorders. This opinion is reinforced by many factors including the occurrence of the trouble with law enforcement. This trouble includes criminal behavior, developmental difficulties in young adults, or the potential gateway phenomenon. The sociobehavioral and psychological or psychiatric consequences of marijuana use precipitate a variety of problems in society, and such problems may be somewhat hidden or occult.

Individuals with mental illness have a greater tendency toward negative emotions (e.g., depressed mood and anxiety). These tendencies may also be present in the cannabis user who does not have overt signs of psychiatric illness. Tolerance to the effects of cannabis serves to make many users increase their cannabis intake, and sociobehavioral disturbances are principal hallmarks of cannabis withdrawal.

Table 71. Withdrawal symptoms, usually seen in heavy users of cannabis

loss of appetite	irritability
insomnia	dreaming
weight loss	restlessness
cannabis seeking	craving

The relationship between marijuana use and mental illness is most apparent in individuals with psychotic illness, such as schizophrenia. It is estimated that about one-third of all individuals with schizophrenia use marijuana on a somewhat regular basis. Most of this cannabis use involves illicit sources of the drug. Evidence suggests that individuals who are more susceptible to developing schizophrenia are at the greatest risk of the development of psychotic reactions to cannabis. This situation implies that genetic or hereditary tendencies operate in mental reactions to cannabis. Individuals with a high risk of schizophrenia who use cannabis tend to develop this serious disease at a younger age, respond less to appropriate treatment, and tend to have more hospital admissions for their illness.

Cannabis Benefits in Psychiatric Disorders

Cannabis has been perceived to exert beneficial effects in the treatment of a variety of psychiatric disorders (table 72). However, patients with psychiatric disorders have to be carefully selected and monitored.

Table 72. Claims of potential benefits of cannabis in several neuropsychiatric disorders

Note: much information on the Internet is anecdotal and sometimes represents opinion alone, without any substantiation.

anxiety	depression
post-traumatic stress disorder (PTSD)	attention deficit disorder
sleep disorders neurodegenerative disease	withdrawal from drugs of addiction obsessive-compulsive disorders

Many physicians agree that the treatment of most psychiatric disorders with existing medications is more effective in the absence of marijuana use, but patients may not agree. There are many individuals with mental disorders that continue to use marijuana, but these people tend to be noncompliant with standard psychiatric drug therapy, and they may be generally unreliable in comparison to abstainers. It is important to stress the twist on the interpretation of data on cannabis and mental illness. On the one hand, cannabis may be used by individuals to self-medicate their illness, but, on the other hand, cannabis may be a cause of certain types of mental disorders, especially transient mental disorders. Individuals who causally link cannabis use and mental disease have been accused of furthering antidrug agendas. However, the link between serious mental illness and cannabis use is still not entirely clear. Moreover, it appears that a significant number of individuals with serious forms of depression and schizophrenia are more likely to have used cannabis over long periods of time. Scientific or reliable data on these issues remains limited, but it forms an area of intense research interest (Abramovici, H. et al., ibid. 2014).

While marijuana has been used in the treatment of depression with some beneficial outcome, other studies imply that cannabis is a cause of depression. One important Australian study in school children (age range fourteen to fifteen years) found a higher risk of depression in children who used cannabis, but children with a past history of depression did not appear to be more likely to use cannabis. As discussed earlier, studies have shown that young cannabis users are at a greater risk of the development of psychotic disorders, such as bipolar disease or schizophrenia. Furthermore, individuals who appear to be genetically at risk of psychotic disease or those that exhibit schizoid personalities appear to be quite vulnerable to the adverse mental effects of cannabis. Cannabis use has been reported to precipitate relapses in patients with schizophrenia.

More on the Association of Cannabis with Mental Illness: Genetics

There have been a number of recent scientific studies that have focused on the potential ability of cannabis to cause mental illness. The association of cannabis with mental disorders is most apparent in the relationship of the use of the drug and the development of psychosis, anxiety, and depression. As noted earlier, scientific studies have indicated that there is a relationship between cannabis use and the development of psychosis, especially later in life, after cannabis onset of use in adolescence.

To review matters, marijuana use has a tendency to exacerbate symptoms in patients with psychosis due to schizophrenia or individuals with a family history of psychosis or schizophrenia. As mentioned earlier, the development of psychosis or psychotic reactions to cannabis are dependent on several factors, including precipitation of these disorders by long-term heavy use of cannabis that started at an early age and genetic predispositions. Therefore, a family history of psychosis is an important predictor of potential psychotic-producing effects of cannabis.

As noted in many mental disorders, a relationship often exists between genetic vulnerability and the development of psychiatric disease. This circumstance is illustrated by studies of individuals who used marijuana as teenagers and had a specific variant of the gene for an enzyme that is involved in the metabolism of certain neurotransmitters (dopamine and norepinephrine). This gene controls the expression of the enzyme catechol-o-methyltransferase.

There are several other documented associations of cannabis use with mental illness that are listed in table 73.

Table 73. Some of the main mental disorders associated with cannabis use

• Antimotivational syndrome	• Gateway disorders
• Depression	• Anxiety
• Suicidal thoughts	• Personality disorders
• Psychosis	• Cognitive disorders

There has been debate about the relationship of antimotivational syndrome and gateway disorders with cannabis use. Gateway disorders are included in the list because the psychological factors or vulnerabilities that lead to a switch from marijuana to hard drugs are somewhat unclear. The major concern is that the operation of the gateway phenomenon with marijuana will result in an overall increase in the use of hard drugs, such as cocaine and heroin.

More on Cannabis Use in Schizophrenia

As mentioned repeatedly, many informed scientists believe that cannabis use (THC) is contraindicated in the presence of schizophrenia because of its potential to provoke psychotic reactions and other mental problems. Definite alterations in the endocannabinoid systems of control are present in disorders associated with psychosis or schizophrenia. Such alterations include the presence of elevated anandamide levels in the cerebrospinal fluid of schizophrenic individuals and an upregulation of CB-1 receptors in the cingulate gyrus and frontal regions of the brain.

Changes in the type and pattern of use have emerged as exerting a major effect on the occurrence of psychosis in cannabis users. Researchers in the UK at King's College Hospital, London, have undertaken a case control study of patients with a first episode of psychosis attributable to the use of high-tetrahydrocannabinol-potency marijuana (DiForti, M. et al., "Proportion of Patients in South London with First-Episode Psychosis Attributable to Use of High Potency Cannabis: A Case Control Study," www.thelancet.

com/psychiatry. Published online February 18, 2015, http//dx.doi. org/10.1016/s2215-0366 (14) 00117-5).

In this latter study, DiForti et al., ibid. 2015) tested the hypothesis that the ready availability of high-potency cannabis in South London (UK) may have generated in a greater number of cases of first onset psychosis. This situation was believed to be attributable to high-potency cannabis use in a sustained manner. This research concluded that the risk of psychosis was three times higher for users of potent skunk-like cannabis compared with nonusers. Overall, the risk was estimated to be five times higher in individuals who used skunk-type cannabis on a daily basis. The skunk-types of cannabis contain higher levels of the psychoactive cannabinoid, delta-9-tetrahydrocannabinol, and they contain little cannabidiol.

In public interviews, the lead researcher, Dr. DiForti, quoted sources from the UK police that UK has become a leading producer of skunk-like products that are exported to the United States and other European countries. Psychotic reactions can precipitate major degrees of destructive paranoia and suspicion among certain cannabis users. The Home Office of the UK made strong statements that indicated, "this report serves to emphasize how they can destroy lives and communities." However, the researchers have been cautious to warn that the studies (DiForti et al., ibid. 2015) do not prove causal links, but it is difficult to place noncausal arguments in this important case control study. Of course, ironclad-controlled longitudinal (prospective) studies are preferred to be confident about clear causal links.

The present studies identify a basis for public interventions that may reduce the occurrence of psychosis in cannabis users who elect to engage in continuing dosing with skunk-like cannabis, because study results imply that there could be a prevention of 25 percent of all cases of psychosis if individuals stopped smoking high-THC-potent cannabis.

> Marjorie Wallace (CEO of the mental health charity SANE) summarized the negative outcome of skunk use in statements to the BBC News, February 16, 2015: "While scientists and politicians debate (in the UK), we face the daily heartbreak of young people whose minds and thoughts have been altered through continued use (of cannabis) and whose families feel helpless. What we need is a strong uncompromising message so that parents, teachers, the police and young people themselves know that a significant percentage who take skunk risk acute, and in some cases lasting, mental illness."

As patterns of use and types of cannabis used change, risks and outcomes of cannabis use are likely to change. This section shows a very important consequence of changing habits with marijuana use that have major public health implications. These changes in outcome appear to be of special impact in youngsters. This book recommends shielding of youth from cannabis use in an intentionally monotonous manner.

> The common link between illicit drug use and the presence of psychotic disorders or schizophrenia can be explained in a couple of ways. One argument suggests that self-medication of schizophrenia with cannabis provides relief of symptoms, and other arguments postulate that a tendency to drug addiction is present in many schizophrenic patients. It has even been suggested that schizophrenia or a tendency to psychosis share a common causality with drug addiction. Certainly, evidence points to a role of genetic tendencies in the development of schizophrenia, but the role of certain genetic polymorphisms remains unclear

The actions of THC seem to be a principal precipitator of psychosis. Added to the inextricable linkage of cannabis use and psychotic reactions are direct observations that the intravenous administration of THC can sometimes precipitate psychotic reactions. This THC administration can result in both transient symptoms of schizophrenia in individuals without a prior history of psychosis, and it can unmask schizophrenic symptoms in schizophrenic patients. These circumstances have favored an overall conclusion that cannabis or THC use in schizophrenia or persons susceptible to psychosis is most likely harmful, and any benefits are outweighed by risks.

The potential dangers of THC use in schizophrenia may be avoided by using cannabidiol (CBD) without any THC content. It is heartening that CBD can be shown to reduce psychosis in rat and mice experimental models. This favorable outcome has been observed in human clinical experiences where the intravenous administration of 5 mg of CBD was found to inhibit the onset of psychotic reactions. An important observation of the benefit of CBD in schizophrenia has resulted from the comparative study of CBD and amilsupride (a dopamine D2/D3 antagonist not available in the United States, at the time of writing). These matters are summarized below.

Treating Schizophrenia with CBD

While the use of THC may worsen symptoms of schizophrenia, the cannabinoid CBD (cannabidiol) has anxiety-controlling effects and works against the psychoactive effects of cannabis. In a research study performed in Germany at the University of Cologne, scientists treated thirty-nine patients with schizophrenia who were admitted to hospital with psychosis. About one half of the patients received treatment with an antipsychotic drug (amisulpride), and the others received cannabidiol (CBD). The results of this four-week trial showed that there was no difference between the outcome of CBD use versus drug (amisulpride) treatment. These groundbreaking studies are particularly important because they suggest that CBD is a potential viable alternative to some antipsychotic drugs. Antipsychotic pharmaceuticals are fraught with adverse effects such as movement disorders (sometimes permanent), increased risk of diabetes, weight gain, and general reductions in motivation with occasional pronounced feelings of sadness.

Stephen Holt, MD, DSc

Light has been cast on mechanisms whereby cannabis can act to precipitate or suppress psychosis in certain circumstances. It has been proposed that when tolerance occurs to THC, there may be a circumstance that reduces the positive effects of the endocannabinoid anandamide on mental function. Furthermore, it appears that CBD could facilitate the actions of anandamide by preventing its breakdown.

Cannabis and Bipolar Disorder

Cannabis use is quite common in individuals with bipolar disorders, and a number of human studies have explored this circumstance (Agrawal, A. et al., *Psychiatry Research* 185 (2011): 459–461) (Stinson, F. S. et al., *Psychol. Med.* 36 (2006): 1147–60). In a valuable prospective survey, it was found that cannabis use increased the risk of developing manic symptoms in a dose-dependent manner. Moreover, in a five-year prospective study, it was found that cannabis use was associated with greater periods of time in affective episodes (mixed or manic) and it promoted rapid cycling of bipolar disease.

Perhaps the most important study on cannabis use in bipolar disorder was the European Mania in Bipolar Longitudinal Evaluation of Medication (EBLEM Study). This study was designed to assess the effects of cannabis use and cannabis exposure on clinical and therapeutic outcome measures. The results indicated that over a one-year period treatment, cannabis users showed less treatment compliance and increased levels of mania, psychosis, and general illness severity compared with controls who did not use cannabis. The use of cannabis in the management of bipolar disorder requires much more research.

Attention-Deficit Hyperactivity Disorder

Attention deficit hyperactivity disorder (ADHD) is present in up to 10 percent of school children and about 5 percent of adults in the United States. The presence of ADHD is sometimes accompanied by other diseases of the central nervous system, including bipolar disorders, obsessive-compulsive states, depression, anxiety, and altered sleep patterns. Patients with ADHD show a significant

256

tendency to self-medicate with a large variety of substances of potential abuse, some of which are addictive or toxic.

One major factor in the cause of ADHD is related to low levels of dopamine in the central nervous system. These changes in dopamine levels are often treated by stimulant drugs such as Ritalin and Vyvanse. Many drugs used in a recreational manner can increase dopamine levels (e.g., cocaine, tobacco, and alcohol) in the brain, and the ability of a drug to raise dopamine may be linked to likelihood of the development of drug addiction.

Evidence for the benefits of cannabis in ADHD is based largely on preclinical research. There appears to be a close link between endocannabinoids and dopamine handling in the brain. Moreover, cannabinoid receptors are found in greater numbers in regions of the brain that are linked to the generation of the symptoms of ADHD (amygdala and hippocampal regions). These areas of the brain play a role in emotion, memory, and common mental disorders, such as anxiety and depression (Abramovici, H. et al., ibid. 2014).

While ADHD treatment with cannabis holds promise, drawbacks to its use are present, especially in children. Youngsters are at risk of several developmental disorders with cannabis use, and about one in ten or more may develop a cannabis addiction. However, contemporary research implies that the brain can adapt itself to the chronic use of stimulants, which, in turn, increases the rate of dopamine elimination. It remains to be seen if this kind of tolerance can develop with cannabis use in ADHD.

As mentioned earlier, attention-deficit hyperactivity disorder (ADHD) is a complex disorder that causes distractibility, impulsivity, and hyperactivity. While ADHD is most commonly diagnosed in children, there is an adult equivalent of this disorder that often occurs without overt signs of hyperactivity. The prevalence of ADHD has grown fast in last fifty years, and it is estimated that more than one in ten children receive this diagnosis. This prevalence can be as high as one in six in some locations in the United States.

The conventional treatment of ADHD involves the use of drugs that stimulate the central nervous system, most notably Adderall, Ritalin, and Concerta. These medications have a chemical structure that is similar to methamphetamine and cocaine, and, as mentioned earlier, they work mainly by increasing dopamine concentrations in the brain. Dopamine is a neurotransmitter that exerts major effects on cognition, memory, and attention. Cannabis exerts a beneficial action in ADHD by increasing dopamine's availability. Cannabis may cause a slowing down of mental activity, which can promote an individual's ability to focus thoughts and actions. It is hypothesized that the brain of the person with ADHD receives too much information that cannot be readily handled, and cannabis ameliorates these circumstances.

Recent survey studies (2012) of certain subtypes of ADHD show that the hyperactive-impulsive type of ADHD may be more responsive to cannabis use than inattentive types of this disorder. Research findings imply that specific forms of ADHD (subtypes) may show greater benefit from cannabis therapy. Researchers have found alcohol abuse and marijuana use to be more common in ADHD, with a 14 percent prevalence of alcohol use in youngsters with ADHD (age range fifteen to seventeen years). There may be several reasons for these observed links between ADHD and alcohol and cannabis use. These reasons may involve underlying mental instability or perhaps the presence of shared genetic tendencies (Abramovici, H. et al., ibid. 2014).

While cannabis or related compounds are commonly used by individuals with ADHD, its use in a form containing THC is limited overall. This is because most cases of ADHD occur in children, where THC use is not advisable. As mentioned earlier, the disease ADHD is associated with low levels of dopamine in the brain, and this situation is linked with a tendency for drug addiction. One mechanism proposed to explain the occurrence of ADHD involves the presence of disorderly controls that are exerted by the endocannabinoid system, which have significant effects on neurotransmitter function.

One cannot discount the risk of developing a substance abuse problem when THC containing cannabis is given to adolescents to manage ADHD. It is quite clear that there are problems with standard medications for ADHD that are essentially stimulants (e.g., Ritalin, Adderall, and Dexedrine). These drugs have some tendency to provoke dependence themselves with a number of physical side effects.

To review matters, certain regions of the brain (hippocampus and amygdala) play a role in emotion, memory, anxiety, depression, or bipolar disorders. Cannabinoid receptors are found in high density in regions of the brain that control these mental activities. There is an increased occurrence of certain mental disorders in ADHD that may be amenable to the effects of both THC and CBD, but human research in this area is still limited.

Withdrawal from Cannabis

An area of great interest is the management of the consequences of drug withdrawal in individuals who have abused drugs or been addicted. Individuals who withdraw from heavy cannabis use, defined as consumption greater than one hundred cigarettes per week, will inevitably exhibit symptoms or signs of withdrawal. Most notable among withdrawal effects are sleep disorders, which result in less sleep time, difficulty falling asleep, and reduced slow-wave sleep. Thus, many aspects of sleep disturbance emerge in circumstances of withdrawal. In some circumstances, it is not clear if the individual has a preexisting sleep disorder that was being self-medicated with cannabis or the drug withdrawal caused the adverse effects (or both of these factors).

The Clinical Spectrum of Cannabis Abuse

There are many accounts of the cannabis high, but cannabis abuse and toxicity result in a wide range of unwanted effects. To summarize key points, the acute effects of cannabis use during periods of marijuana intoxication include poor memory, acute cardiovascular effects, impaired cognitive functions, and psychotic episodes in susceptible individuals.

Intermediate and long-term effects seen in chronic cannabis abuse are variable but not often permanent. Persistent or intermediate duration of cannabis use causes sleep problems and impairment of educational performance or work performance. In the long term, cannabis use may lead to the following problems listed below.

Table 74. The consequence of marijuana abuse in the short, intermediary, and long term (adapted from www.drugabuse. gov). These data are relevant to understanding how cannabis exacerbates or complicates mental disease.

- addiction, which affects one in nine users or more
- risk of mental problems, most notably exacerbation of schizophrenia or psychotic episodes
- lung disease—a highly debated area, but general agreement exists on the development of increased bronchitis, inflammatory changes, and small alterations in lung function (breathing)
- risk of antimotivational syndrome
- mood change with increase in depression and anxiety

Marijuana Dependence and Addiction

There is a potential major public health concern with the possibility of cannabis legalization causing future increases in cannabis abuse, dependence, or addiction. This situation is based on the logic that the greater the number of cannabis users, the greater the public's risks of dependence or addiction. This concern is reinforced by the findings of several recent studies.

As mentioned earlier, approximately 9 percent of individuals who use cannabis develop drug dependence of variable severity. This risk may increase to one in six people in individuals that commenced cannabis use at a young age (adolescents). Perhaps one of the most alarming statistics is the proposed increase in risks of dependence to 25 to 50 percent in daily heavy smokers of cannabis. Moreover, a study of identical twins showed that a twin who had used cannabis before the age of seventeen had a greater tendency to use other drugs and develop problems related to drug taking in their adult years, compared with a nonusing twin. The inevitable increase in marijuana use that accompanies legislation to permit recreational and perhaps medical use may result in greater cannabis use by children and teenagers.

Withdrawal from heavy, prolonged cannabis use may often result in relapse because cannabis use (e.g., especially smoking cannabis) often gives rapid relief from withdrawal reactions. That said, it should be noted that heavy cannabis use may sometimes interfere with sleep in an unpredictable manner. This is another example of the double-edged sword that is wielded by cannabis. Further components of sleep disturbance such as bad dreams, night sweats, and perceptions of nonrestful sleep can be experienced in circumstances of cannabis withdrawal. Cannabis suppresses REM sleep and dreaming. The withdrawal symptoms in cannabis users are often present for a couple of weeks or more following cessation of cannabis intake.

Marijuana and IQ

Considerable argument persists on whether or not cannabis use can result in decline in IQ among young people. An eye-catching study from Duke University has linked IQ decline with cannabis use in teenagers (Meier, M. H. et al. *PNAS* 109, no. 40 (2012): E2657-64). In this study, the persistent use of cannabis resulted in measurable declines in neuropsychological testing from childhood to midlife. This study examined participants in the Dunedin Study, which analyzed a cohort of 1037 individuals from birth (1972–73) to age thirty-eight years. These individuals underwent sequential tests of neuropsychological function that showed variable decline in IQ scores (at ages eighteen, twenty-one, twenty-six, and thirty-eight years). These findings underscored the perceived dangers of neurotoxic effects of cannabis with recommendations for the preventive efforts focused on adolescents and young teenagers. It was not long before these conclusions were questioned when Dr. Ole Rogeberg presented data that implied that IQ changes observed in the Dunedin Study were "confounded" by differing socioeconomic status among the individuals in the study. Claiming flawed methods in the study, Ole Rogeberg described the claim of causal relationships between marijuana use and the compromise of IQ as "premature" (Rogeberg, O., *PNAS*, 110, 11 (2012): 4251–54).

UK studies of IQ and cannabis were based on a larger number of participants than were examined in the Dunedin Study (Meier, M. H. et al., ibid. 2012). In this UK study of 2,612 children born in Bristol, England, in 1991–92, confounding factors on any conclusions were considered and eliminated where possible. There seemed to be no clear relationship between heavy cannabis use and lower IQ scores in this study, but there was a trend in heavy users to have small reductions (3 percent) in examination scores, measured at age sixteen years. It has been argued that other lifestyle factors exert significant effects on IQ development and academic performance, in a manner independent of cannabis use.

Why is it important to solve the issues of causality in these circumstances? This circumstance has major implications for assessing the risk of cannabis use in youngsters and for the development of sociobehavioral problems in cannabis users in later life. Furthermore, it may help to predict the positive or negative outcomes of decriminalization or legalization of marijuana on a wider scale than currently exists.

Recent analytic studies by the Center on Juvenile and Criminal Justice show that legalization or decriminalization of cannabis do not lead to universal negative outcomes that are predicted to occur by the antagonists of more liberal marijuana policies. Circumstances that support this point of view are emerging. For example, in California where decriminalization of cannabis occurred on January 11, 2011, the report from the Center on Juvenile and Criminal Justice does not describe negative consequences of this policy. In fact, there was no increase in young people involved in crime, drug overdosing, driving under the influence, or increases in high school dropouts. Most revealing in these studies was that teenage behaviors actually improved in general after cannabis legalization in California!

These findings place a further burden on antagonists of cannabis legalization to show that associations between adverse events or outcomes associated with cannabis use are directly causal associations and not just correlated findings. Moreover, links between cannabis legislation to permit more widespread drug use and negative outcomes require careful definition and not just assumptions. (Ingraham, C., www.washingtonpost.com/blogs/workblog/wp2014/10/15). The debate concerning the long-term effects of cannabis on the brain continues to gain momentum as scholarly articles associate long-term marijuana use with a number of neuroadaptive changes (brain changes) that require prospective studies for clarification (Filbey, F. M. et al., *PNAS* 111, no. 47 (2014): 16913–18, doi: 10.1073).

Memory and Marijuana

Animal studies have shown that prolonged exposure (for eight months) to THC results in premature loss of hippocampal nerve cells, compared with controls that were not exposed to marijuana. This situation seems to be somewhat contrarian to the observations of neuroprotection and neurogenic properties of cannabinoids.

Memory is attenuated by THC, which changes information processing in the hippocampus. Cognitive activity in young rats is also impaired by THC administration. Moreover, rats exposed to THC in utero (the fetus), in both infancy after birth and during adolescence, tend to show impairment of memory and learning tasks when they mature. Cognitive problems later in the life of marijuana-dosed rats are often correlated with neurone loss in the brain and abnormal function of the hippocampus (Abramovici, H. et al., ibid. 2014).

These animal studies mirror effects that have been noted in human adolescents who use cannabis. It seems clear that the early onset of heavy marijuana use creates more problems in memory and cognition in young adults. This legacy of neurological problems from cannabis use has been documented in several studies. What is the ability of cannabis abusers to reverse cognitive problems that have been created by cannabis? The answer to this question is debated by scientists in a fierce manner.

It is believed that the compromise of memory and learning caused by cannabis may be partially reversed by taking nonsteroidal anti-inflammatory drugs (e.g., ibuprofen). This treatment approach to memory and learning impairments is reinforced by the finding that delta-9-THC administration causes increases in cyclooxygenase-2 (COX-2) enzymes levels in the brain regions of rats that control learning and memory. Thus, COX-2 inhibitor drugs may be valuable in the mitigation of learning and memory problems that tend to occur in cannabis users. In addition, researchers have found that neuronal dysfunction caused by Alzheimer's disease in rodents can be reduced by THC administration. Furthermore, these beneficial effects are present with the coadministration of COX-2 inhibitor compounds.

An important animal study has indicated that long-term effects of cannabis on the brain are persistent to a variable degree. In contrast, other animal studies have shown reasonable evidence of restoration of cognitive functions and memory at about four weeks following the cessation of marijuana intake.

Regional Brain Shrinkage and Expansion?

Animal studies have suggested that the structure and function of various portions of the brain can be altered by cannabis administration. There is a clear recognition that chronic alcohol use can result in brain shrinkage, and recent data suggest that cannabis smoking can also reduce gray matter in the human brain (Filbey, F. M. et al., *PNAS* 111, no. 47 (2014): 16913–16918, doi: 10.1073.PNAS). However, there has been ongoing debate about the ability of chronic marijuana use to affect brain structure.

In recent research, medical resonance imaging (MRI) has shown that marijuana users have significantly less bilateral orbitofrontal gyri and higher functional connectivity in the orbitofrontal cortex, compared with controls (nonmarijuana group). These findings have been questioned in terms of their validity because the studies were not longitudinal and preexisting factors could have operated.

The finding of less gray matter in the orbital frontal cortex in marijuana users is intriguing. This area of the brain is intimately involved in reward systems, motivation, decision making, and addictive behaviors. The "chicken and egg" argument applies to these findings because it is possible that the smaller orbital frontal cortex of marijuana users could be either a cause or result of cannabis use.

Earlier studies have shown that individuals with a reduced size of their orbital frontal cortex at age twelve years were more likely to start cannabis use by the age of sixteen years. It has been suggested that deficiencies in this brain region make substance abuse more likely. A further observation in this study was lower IQ scores in the marijuana group. This is another area of dispute in cannabis science when it comes to cause and effect.

Cannabis Altering Brain Structure and Function

Clearly, circuitous arguments exist about the ability of cannabis to alter brain structure (morphology) and function. It would appear that despite limitations of study designs, changes in brain morphology do occur with cannabis use. A valuable review of these issues is presented in an article published in 2014 (Lorenzatti, V. et al., *Curr. Pharm. Des.* 20, no. 13 (2014): 2138–67). These researchers examined medical literature with a view to answering several questions about brain structure and function, altered by cannabis use. One pivotal question answered by this work (Lorenzetti, V. et al., ibid. 2014) was the convincing evidence of altered brain structure in regular cannabis users.

A consensus opinion derived from medical literature reviews indicates that regular cannabis use is associated with structural changes in the medial, temporal, frontal, and cerebellar regions of the brain. These changes were more pronounced in individuals that had engaged in chronic heavy marijuana consumption, but the association between changes in brain structures and measures of cannabis use were not always clear. While there are limitations in many studies in terms of sample size and types and extent of utilized imaging methods, this valuable review linked alterations of brain morphology with cannabis use in a convincing manner (Lorenzetti, V. et al., ibid. 2014).

Studies published in April 2014 by Boston researchers show clear changes in brain morphology associated with cannabis use (Gilman, J. M. et al., *Journal of Neuroscience* 34, no. 16 [April 16, 2014]: 5529–38). This Boston study has been widely quoted in recent literature, but it has been described as possessing limitations that do not support a causal relationship of altered brain structure due to cannabis use. Again, it has been argued that other factors could have caused the changes in brain morphology in this study. The main conclusion of the study by Gilman, J. M. et al. (ibid. 2014) was that marijuana exposure caused changes in brain morphology in the nucleus accumbens and amygdala. These areas of the brain control reward/aversion centers that control drug addiction. These reported changes in the human brain seem to mirror changes noted in several animal studies.

Cannabis and PTSD

Post-traumatic stress disorder (PTSD) follows major stress and is manifest by the development of a number of behavioral and psychiatric symptoms. Such symptoms involve difficulties with adjustment to new environments, intrusive thoughts about painful or stressful experiences, and inaccurate or aberrant memory. Other symptoms of PTSD are displayed in table 75.

Table 75. Common manifestations of PTSD

persistent thoughts of stress	skewed memory
intrusive recollections	numbing
reliving of traumatic events	avoidance behavior
increased arousal	dreams and flashback to trauma

When one considers the role of the endocannabinoid system in the control of emotion, cognition, thought, and understanding, it is not surprising that endocannabinoid function and the spectrum of disorders in PTSD are linked. There are a number of animal models that have been developed to study the treatment and characteristics of PTSD, but their relevance to human cases of PTSD has been questioned.

One prominent clinical trial of nabilone in forty-nine individuals, in dosages less than 6 mg per day for the treatment of PTSD, produced favorable results. In this non-placebo-controlled trial, benefits of nabilone were observed, including reduction in bad dreams, a lessening of unpleasant flashbacks, and some control of night sweats. There were no serious side effects in this study, and tolerance to the effects of nabilone was not observed.

Although preclinical studies offer support for cannabis in the treatment of PTSD, there is only a small amount of research to date on the human clinical outcome of cannabis use in this disorder. Inhibition of CB1 receptor stimulation, using pharmacological antagonists in animals seems to promote the preservation of memories that are traumatic or aversive. On the other hand, in some circumstances stimulation of the CB-1 receptor seems to enhance the extinction of such memories. This latter effect is desirable in the management of PTSD.

At the time of writing, there are no convincing clinical studies on the ability of THC to extinguish bad memories in people with PTSD, but many anecdotal reports of this phenomenon seem convincing. It has been noted that phobias present a number of problems that are similar to aspects of PTSD. This situation has prompted some researchers to examine the potential benefits of cannabis for the management of phobias, but outcomes are inconclusive. The conundrum of PTSD has major political implications. In 2014, there was considerable controversy about the firing of a researcher at the University of Arizona who intended to do in-depth research on cannabis and PTSD.

Autism and Cannabis

Autism can be a devastating disease, resulting in an individual living in social isolation in his or her own world. The condition is of varying severity, and it affects about 2 percent of all children in the United States. The hallmark characteristics of autism include impaired and reduced communication, compromised social relationships, and repetitive behavioral activity.

The cause of autism remains unknown, but it has been associated with the genetic disease of fragile X chromosome. Symptoms of autism usually become apparent within the first three years of life, resulting in a wide spectrum of social and mental disabilities. It is reasonable to state that autism is often poorly responsive to medication, which includes stimulant drugs and antipsychotic medications that have onerous side effects, such as the precipitation of heart disease and weight gain.

The use of cannabis in autism management is supported by anecdotal human experiences and animal studies. In animal models of fragile X syndrome, levels of the endocannabinoid 2-AG,

(2-archidonoylglycerol) were found to be low, and interventions to increase 2-AG levels were found to reduce some of the manifestations of fragile X syndrome. Subsequent research has shown that cannabinoid receptor type 2 (CB-2), but not CB-1, has increased dominance in blood mononuclear cells in children affected by autism, but the significance of this finding remains unclear (Abramovici, H. et al., ibid. 2014).

Other studies have indicated that children with autism have borderline regulation of their immune system, presumed to be related to alteration of CB-2 receptor functions. The role of altering CB-2 receptor activity as a focus for drug development in autism treatment is quite promising, especially in the midst of concerns about the toxicity of standard drug treatment for this condition (e.g., Risperdal).

Value of Cannabis in Alcohol and Opioid Withdrawal

A body of evidence, derived largely from animal studies, suggests that cannabis could play a positive role in alcohol or opioid withdrawal. Not only are there many complex changes in endocannabinoid function caused by alcohol, there is suggestion that the endocannabinoid system may play an important role in symptoms of alcohol withdrawal. In the absence of many convincing clinical studies of the benefit of cannabis in opioid withdrawal, there are research studies that show similarities in the effects of cannabis and opioids on the brain. These similarities support the notion that cannabis may be used as a partial substitute for opioids, with a view to diminishing opioid withdrawal symptoms and dangerous opioid toxicity.

Antimotivational Syndrome

Antimotivational syndrome due to cannabis use has variable symptomatology. It occurs most often in adolescents and young adults and is characterized by several sociobehavioral changes that are summarized in table 76. In essence, the antimotivational syndrome has been likened to a minor vegetative status.

Table 76. Behavior encountered in the cannabis-induced antimotivational syndrome

• apathy	• fatigue
• poor motivation	• loss of interest
• impaired judgment	• difficulty with communication
• poor academic performance	• loneliness
• social isolation	• poor life planning

The antimotivational syndrome is aggravated by loss of short-term memory that disrupts learning. There is a failure for an individual to apply him- or herself to daily tasks and routines. Antimotivational cannabis users cannot easily integrate themselves into social groups. These individuals tend to attract each other, sometimes to form idle groups of nonachievers. There is a spectrum of severity of antimotivational syndrome. Descriptions of this disorder have created offense among cannabis users, but it is a condition of fact and reality. This syndrome is usually found in the chronic, heavy cannabis user.

Cannabis and Violence

There appears to be a reasonably consistent association of marijuana use with aggressive behavior and interpersonal violence, but the prevalence of these problems is not clear. Cross-sectional and longitudinal studies confirm these findings with a specific association between marijuana withdrawal and violent behavior (Moore, T. M., Stuart, G. L., Agression and Violent Behavior 10, no. 2 (2005): 171–972). That said, arguments prevail.

Other studies have doubted a clear relationship between violent behavior and marijuana use in otherwise healthy individuals. It has been suggested that preexisting mental disorders (e.g., temporal lobe dysthymia), the context of use of cannabis, and other factors operate in the precipitation of violent behavior in cannabis users. Is this a paradoxical effect? After all, many cannabis users are often mellow.

Cannabis and Brain Injury

Research in Israel has uncovered the benefit of very low dosages of THC in protecting the brain from damage following injury, seizures, lack of oxygen supply (hypoxia), and exposure to certain toxic drugs. The most important aspect of this research is the discovery that extremely small amounts of THC given over a period of one to seven days before, or up to three days after brain injury, can protect brain structure and function to a variable degree. The use of small dosages of THC appears to be acceptable therapy in these circumstances, with a low prevalence of side effects.

The reported results of low dose THC have included a significant impact in the brain on prevention of cell death, the promotion of the production of growth factors, and positive effects on cell signaling. Experiments in mice demonstrated the neuroprotective effect of small doses of THC, where prevention of long-term cognitive damage caused by brain injury has been noted.

It has been proposed that minor damage induced by THC results in neuroprotection against more severe injury. This research illustrates the potential ability of very low dose THC to be used in prophylaxis against certain forms of tissue injury in the brain and perhaps injury to other tissues, such as the heart. There is some evidence that low-dose THC may be cardioprotective. Is this a modified homeopathic effect, akin to the alleged actions of cell salt therapy?

Chronic Traumatic Encephalopathy

Cannabis has shown promise in the management of chronic traumatic encephalopathy (CTE). This degenerative disease affects individuals who have suffered repeated head trauma (e.g., boxers and football players). Commercial companies (KannaLife Sciences) are attempting to produce cannabis-based treatments for CTE in cooperation with the NIH. These new treatments are designed to have preventive and therapeutic properties for CTE management. These targets are based upon preclinical studies that demonstrate a clear neuroprotective effect of cannabis, with added properties of their ability to induce neurogenesis.

Public interest increased in this situation as a consequence of the filing of a class-action lawsuit against the National Football League (NFL), which alleged that the NFL had covered up the effects of concussions on players.

Conclusion

Cannabis use shows promise for amelioration of several mental disorders. Cannabis has become an attractive self-medication for individuals with a variety of psychiatric disturbances, but this trend may be dangerous in some individuals where exacerbation of psychiatric disorders may occur. Identification of cannabis use with a view to supervision or monitoring of cannabis use in mental disease is required. This situation constitutes an important public health issue that may become more prevalent in society with uncertain outcomes.

Chapter 9

THE GASTROINTESTINAL TRACT

The Brain-Gut Axis

In common with much of cannabis research, studies of the effects of cannabis on gastrointestinal function have been most often restricted to animal experimentation, but this circumstance is rapidly changing. Cannabis can be anticipated to play a major role in modifying digestive function, given the pivotal position of the endocannabinoid receptor system as a controlling link between the gut and the central nervous-system function. The brain plays a significant role in modulating digestive processes. These concepts underlie the presence of a brain-gut axis, which is a well-accepted entity. This axis operates in a reciprocal manner in the overall control of digestive function, with major effects of cannabinoids on eating behavior and other gastrointestinal activities.

Areas of the brain that control stress or emotion are rich in CB-1 receptors, and certain gastrointestinal hormones can exert direct effects on emotion (e.g., ghrelin- and gastrin-releasing peptide). Moreover, these hormones can work in concert with other body controls to regulate satiety (a feeling of being full) and produce appetite control. These events exert an important function of initiating reward processes in the brain.

There are four major components of endocannabinoid receptor system, which is best viewed as a synchronized unit. These receptor systems (CB-1 and CB-2) can be viewed in functional terms as (1) receptor interactions with the endocannabinoids (anandamide and 2-arachidonoyl glycerol), (2) alteration in function of the enzymes that synthesize and metabolize these and other endocannabinoids, (3) the role of reuptake transporters, and (4) effects of administered phytocannabinoids and analogues. Of course, such controls occur in three major locations, including (1) the nervous system, (2) adipose tissue, and (3) the gut. This is the expanded concept of the brain-adipose-gut axis of coordinated events that contribute to body homeostasis (Frider E).

The Brain-Adipose-Gut Axis and Its Regulation

In review of the role of the endogenous cannabinoid system in the function of the brain-adipose-gut axis, Dr. Ester Frider, a prominent cannabis researcher, reached several conclusions. She proposed that the endocannabinoid receptor system closely links the brain and digestive functions, and regulation of eating is a remnant of initiation of feeding in the newborn. Moreover, there is an obvious role of the actions of endocannabinoid receptors in controls of digestive functions. These circumstances indicate that cannabinoids may form a basis for the development of useful treatment compounds for gastrointestinal disorders (modified from Frider, E., *Cannabinoids* 2, no. 2 (2007): 5–12). Table 77 lists medical conditions in the gastrointestinal system that may form a focus for cannabinoid-based treatments.

Table 77. Disorders that may be amenable to treatment with cannabinoids. Data are considered from animal studies and limited human clinical observations.

loss of appetite (anorexia)	failure to thrive
peptic ulcer	obesity
nausea	irritable bowel syndrome
inflammatory bowel disease	vomiting
secretory diarrhea	gastroesophageal reflux disease

Cannabinoid Receptor Effects and the Gut

The interplay of the local nervous tissue networks in the gut (enteric nervous system) with the brain is the focus of much research, which is now expanding with knowledge about the important regulatory roles of the endocannabinoid system on body functions. Added to the complexity of feeding and digestive controls are the roles played by a large number of hormones that act on the brain and local tissues in the digestive tract. These hormones also play a role in the communications between the brain and adipose tissue (e.g., cholecystokin, leptin, and oxrexins A and B).

The effects of exogenously administered cannabinoids on the gut-brain-adipose tissue axis require much further elucidation. Research over the past decade has indicated that stimulation of the CB-1 receptor is a major factor in the control of alimentary function and food intake (eating). In the application of exogenous cannabinoids (phytocannabinoids and analogues) for digestive function, several types of cannabinoids have been noted to have CB-1 receptor stimulatory properties in the absence of psychoactive properties. These compounds include cannabidiol (CBD) and some of its chemical analogues.

A brief overview of the known alimentary effects of the endocannabinoid receptor systems is shown in a summarized form in table 78. It is modified in its presentation and content from the excellent review by Frider, E. (ibid. 2007).

Table 78. Alimentary controls and effects on adipose tissue exerted by the endocannabinoid receptor system (adapted from Frider, E. ibid. 2007)

Location of Receptors in Brain, Gastrointestinal Tract, and Adipose Tissue	Main Effects of Endocannabinoid Receptor System
CNS—forebrain including hypothalamus	Rewarding food intake and digestion and an orexigenic effect.
CNS—hindbrain	Reduction of gastric and intestinal secretions, antiemetic effects with reduced gastric and intestinal motility.
Mouth	Reduction in saliva production.
Lower esophageal sphincter	Both relaxation and failure of relaxation described.
Adipose tissue	Enhanced lipogenesis.

Much data supports the importance of the endocannabinoid receptor system in the regulation of digestive function. While CB-1 receptors are found throughout the gastrointestinal tract, their occurrence is more common in the stomach and the upper parts of the large intestine. Research in animals with limited observations in humans has highlighted the effect of endocannabinoid receptor activity on secretory and motility functions of the gut. It appears that endocannabinoids alter gastrointestinal transit (movement) of food with an overall delaying effect.

Several studies indicate that smoking marijuana or taking certain synthetic cannabinoid analogues is an effective approach to the control of vomiting caused by chemotherapy. The synthetic cannabinoids nabilone and dronabinol have been used effectively as antiemetics, alongside cancer chemotherapy. These drugs have shown promise in treating nausea and vomiting caused by radiation therapy and anesthesia. In addition, these drugs may be of value in helping patients to tolerate chemotherapy for HIV disease and treatments that are used in the management of hepatitis C virus infection. Cannabinoid therapy in several of these circumstances appears to be a popular patient choice, despite the variable occurrence of significant psychoactive effects, such as euphoria, sedation, depression, and hallucinations.

Cannabis: Gastrointestinal Controls

In summary, the endocannabinoid system is ubiquitous in the digestive tract and serves several basic aspects of regulatory control over the following functions (table 79).

Table 79. Regulatory actions of the endocannabinoid system in the gastrointestinal tract. Recent studies indicate that there may be genetic mutations affecting the controls of the endocannabinoid system in gastrointestinal disease.

• food intake	• ion transport
• nausea and vomiting	• visceral sensation
• gastric secretion	• inflammation
• gastric cytoprotection	• cell proliferation
• gastrointestinal motility	• bowel habit

Cannabis (cannabinoids) exerts control over gastrointestinal function by actions on the enteric nervous system, cells lining the digestive system, organ-specific receptors in the liver and pancreas, and immune-competent cells (e.g., spleen, tonsil, and Peyer's patches). The molecular basis of these controls involves several receptor systems.

Table 80. Molecular actions of cannabinoids. These effects have been investigated extensively in animals with a view to developing new drugs. Effects on endocannabinoid degradation and synthesis, with resulting changes in endocannabinoid levels, can participate in the altered functions of the digestive system.

- cannabinoid receptor actions
- transient receptor potential Vanilloid-1-receptors
- alpha receptors
- peroxisome proliferator activated receptors (PPAR)
- orphan G-protein coupled receptors (GPR55 and GPR119)

Explaining the Munchies

Marijuana use is often a cause of increased appetite that is referred to in popular language as "the munchies." Recent studies in animals indicate that THC may act on the olfactory bulb (smell and taste center) to promote enhanced smell and taste of food. The exposure of mice to aromatic oils (banana and almond oil) creates interest for the animal, but this interest is quelled by a process of "olfactory habituation." It appears that THC can prevent olfactory habituation, thereby promoting appetite.

Other mechanisms operate to produce the munchies. The effects of THC on the nucleus acumbens of the brain promote dopamine release and the sensation of pleasure. It has been hypothesized that THC reproduces sensations of food deprivation that trigger eating behavior. This animal research work was produced in a collaborative effort among several European scientists, and whether or not these mechanisms operate in humans requires clear demonstration (Soria-Gomez et al., *Nature Neuroscience* 17 (2014): 407–15).

Cannabis and Cotton Mouth

Cannabis smoking inhibits secretion by the salivary glands. This results in the development of a dry mouth or "cotton mouth," in popular language. It appears that smoking is apt to produce this problem, which results, in part, from inhibition of secretory stimuli from the parasympathetic nervous system to the submandibular glands. There may be both central and peripheral actions of cannabis in blocking salivary secretion (www.ncbi.nlm.nih.gov/gov/pubmed/16946411, Prestifullippo, J. P. et al., 2006).

Cannabis and Bowel Function

The effects of cannabis on bowel function are not completely clarified. Cannabis is reported to both relieve and cause constipation. Dr. Lester Grinspoon was among the first US scientists to report a patient with multiple sclerosis and irregularity of bowel actions that were improved by cannabis (Grinspoon L. Marihuana, *The Forbidden Medicine*, [New Haven, CT: Yale University Press, 1997], 91). There are reports that cannabis has been used to manage constipation in the practice of traditional Chinese medicine for many years (Emperor, Shen Nung). Cannabis has similar described uses in Ayurvedic medicine.

Cannabis has been reported to have a long history of use for the treatment of diarrhea, especially in cases of Crohn's disease (inflammatory bowel disease, IBD). Benefits in IBD would be expected to be present because of anti-inflammatory effects of cannabis and its ability to reduce intestinal motility. In brief, paradoxical reactions are reported in the effect of cannabis on bowel function. That said, bowel function is most often unaffected with cannabis use. Clearly, further research is required, and effects of cannabis on bowel actions may be related to other factors, including the cause of diarrhea or constipation and the dosage of administered cannabis.

Anti-inflammatory and Hormonal Effect of Cannabinoids in the Gut

There are indications that abdominal obesity in humans is associated with disturbances of the overall effects of CB-1 receptors. Moreover, there seems to be a specific association between the hormone leptin and the endocannabinoid receptor system. Leptin is secreted by fatty tissue (adipose tissue). It enters the central nervous system and alters food intake. Injections of leptin into rats have been shown to lower levels of certain endocannabinoids, resulting in changes in appetite and food intake. In addition, the regulation of the activity of endocannabinoid-degrading enzymes, such as fatty acid amide hydroxylase (FAAH), can also affect endocannabinoid functions. The endocannabinoid receptor system in humans is responsive to the significant effects of cannabinoids on adipose tissue. This constitutes what is referred to as part of the endocannabinoid-gut-adipose tissue axis of physiological events.

A number of studies have focused on the anti-inflammatory effects of cannabinoids in animals with experimentally induced colitis. The outcome of these studies has been quite promising. Recent studies of cannabis in bowel disease in humans (ulcerative colitis and Crohn's disease) have shown positive results. Furthermore, cannabinoids may exert control over cells in the central nervous system and gastrointestinal tract that secrete hormones, which play a role in appetite and overall digestive processes (e.g., vasointestinal peptide [VIP] and the neuropeptide NPY). The role of CB-2 receptors in the control of gastrointestinal functions remains somewhat clouded. That said, animal studies show that CB-2 receptors are present in the stomach and intestines, and they may have a specific role in the act of defecation.

In summary, in studies performed mainly in animals, it has been shown that CB-1 receptor inhibitors cause vomiting and loss of appetite and may increase gut motility. On the other hand, endocannabinoids and certain exogenous cannabinoids (phytocannabinoids) can exert antidiarrheal actions, reduce gut motility, and reduce gastric acid secretion. The stimulation of endocannabinoid receptors may assist in the management of conditions such as cachexia, anorexia, and loss of appetite. In contrast, inhibitors of endocannabinoid receptors may play a role in the treatment of metabolic syndrome X and certain other types of obesity. As stressed in earlier parts of this book, it is recognized that the endocannabinoid receptor systems work in a harmonious manner to create homeostasis in the body. Without this harmony, digestive functions occur without adequate regulation or controls.

The contributions of the endocannabinoid receptor systems to psychosomatic and physical disorders of digestive function have become apparent in several clinical circumstances. The linkage of emotional status and the endocannabinoid receptor system has begun to cast light on psychosomatic causes of gastrointestinal illness, which may figure strongly in functional digestive disorders. These common disorders are associated with abnormal gastrointestinal functions in the absence of clear evidence of the presence of organic gastrointestinal disease (e.g., inflammation or cancer). Table 81 summarizes some of the common clinical circumstances where cannabinoid effects are of major importance (Abramovici, H. et al., ibid. 2014).

Table 81. Clinical circumstances where cannabinoids may find a use in treatment of gastrointestinal disease, based on their summarized effects

Please note that rimonabant is no longer in use.

Condition	Comment
Inflammatory bowel disease	Animal models for the study of inflammatory colitis and Crohn's disease illustrate the potential benefits of cannabinoids in slowing gut motility and helping to control inflammation by direct effects on gut cannabinoid receptors (CB-1).
Peptic ulcer	The role of stress in the peptic ulcer diathesis remains debatable, especially following the common implication of Helicobacter pylori infection in the causation of acid-peptic disease. It is likely that the antistress actions of cannabinoids occur as a consequence of CB-1 receptor stimulation in the gut and brain.
Gastroesophageal reflux disease (GERD)	There are well-defined circumstances that aggravate the reflux of gastric acid backward into the esophagus, such as anxiety, depression, and stress. These influences may be reduced by marijuana.
Vomiting	The value of various cannabinoids in reducing vomiting has been demonstrated conclusively in the use of THC, dronabinol, and nabilone. This antiemetic effect is achieved by actions on the gastric nerve supply (vagus) combined with central nervous system effects.

Secretory diarrhea	A number of studies have attempted to define the role of the endocannabinoid receptor system in water/electrolyte absorption and intestinal motility. Stimulation of CB-1 receptors tends to reduce accumulation of intestinal fluid. In contrast, agents that block CB-1 receptors (e.g., rimonabant) will promote intestinal water secretion. Thus, cannabinoids or analogues may find a role in diarrhea management.

Cannabis and Cystic Fibrosis

The pathophysiology of cystic fibrosis (CF) may be modified by several potential benefits of cannabis treatments. Symptoms of cystic fibrosis resulting from inflammation, lung disease, poor appetite, chronic diarrhea, and pain are variably countered by positive effects of cannabis and selected cannabinoids. Research studies have focused on fatty acid imbalance in CF, which leads to pancreatic and damaging lung inflammation. Many reports describe appetite promoting, analgesic, anti-inflammatory, and bronchodilatory effects of cannabis, which make variable contributions to the apparent progression or favorable outcome of cannabis use (Fride, E., J., *Cann. Ther. 2*, no. 1 (2002): 39–71). Cannabis appears to have some antifibrotic effects.

It is clear that smoking cannabis is to be avoided in cystic fibrosis because of the invariable presence of lung disease due to cystic fibrosis. This has resulted in the use of oral administration of cannabis or its analogues or oro-mucosal sprays in the management of cystic fibrosis, with some reports of the benefits of vaporization techniques.

Some Therapeutic Comments

It seems quite clear that cannabinoids from within the body (endo) or those that are administered (exo or phytocannabinoids or analogues) exert many functions in the gastrointestinal tract.

Alterations in the components of the endocannabinoid system are apparent in several gastrointestinal diseases, both in animal models of digestive disease and in limited clinical investigations in humans. Cannabinoid receptors (CB-1 and CB-2) are well represented in the enteric nervous system. There are regional variations in the concentrations of the endocannabinoids (2-AG and anandamide) with a higher concentration of 2-AG (2-arachidonoylglycerol) in the ileum than the colon. The distribution of CB-1 and CB-2 receptors in the liver and pancreas is different, with the expression of CB-1 receptors in the liver and expression of both CB-1 and CB-2 receptors in the pancreas (Abramovici, H. et al., ibid. 2014).

Laboratory studies in animals with irritable bowel syndrome that are treated with cannabis show reductions in visceral pain experienced in rats and mice that are induced by colorectal distension. Pain responses have been shown to be inhibited with prior mechanical distension and in periods following distension in these animals. There have been promising studies of dronabinol in experimental circumstances of irritable bowel syndrome both in animals and in limited human studies.

Cannabinoid receptor agonists reduce gastric acid secretion, reduce small intestinal and colonic motility in animals, and delay the rate of gastric emptying in humans. With the exception of the latter effect on stomach emptying, these actions may be valuable in the management of irritable bowel syndrome (IBS). In IBS, functional disorders of the gut produce abdominal discomfort, altered bowel habits, and altered gastrointestinal transit. The physiological results of the stimulation of CB-1 receptors or the reduction in the inactivation of endocannabinoids are potentially valuable in the management of IBS because of potent and specific effects on gut motility.

Studies have been undertaken of the effect of dronabinol on several human gastrointestinal functions or outcomes such as transit, satiation, and post-prandial symptoms. While a delay of gastric emptying with cannabis is described in male versus female subjects, there were no observed changes in small or large intestinal transit in some of these studies. Investigations of the effects of dronabinol on colonic sensory and motor events have shown the development of colonic compliance (a measure of colonic contractility in response to colonic distension). Alterations in colonic compliance are important in the cause of abnormal bowel function, where decreased compliance tends to be present in circumstances of bowel urgency and diarrhea. In contrast, increased compliance tends to be associated with constipation. In separate studies of irritable bowel syndrome, a dose of 5 mg of dronabinol was associated with modest increase in colonic compliance (Abramovici, H. et al., ibid. 2014).

Secretory diarrhea results often from a combination of secretion of water and electrolytes, with decreased reabsorption of these fluids. Cannabinoid agonists may cause a reverse effect with actions that oppose this negative circumstance of imbalance of fluid secretion and its reabsorption. Animal studies show that CB-1 receptor stimulation has an antisecretory effect, which is neural in origin. In human experiences, heavy cannabis smoking has been linked to decreases in acid output by the stomach, and it has pain-reducing and anti-inflammatory properties that could be applied to peptic ulcer prevention and treatment. However, smoking, especially tobacco, often makes peptic ulcer worse.

> Changes in the function of the endocannabinoid system are present in ulcerative colitis and Crohn's disease. In common with other circumstances of disorderly endocannabinoid function, there are documented changes in endocannabinoid concentrations in inflammatory bowel disease and notable alterations in cannabinoid receptor distribution and density. These changes occur together with alterations in the functions of endocannabinoid synthesizing and degrading enzymes. In addition, it has been proposed that inflammatory bowel disease would be expected to improve with cannabis use because of the well-defined anti-inflammatory effects of certain cannabinoids (e.g., CBD).

The effects of exogenous cannabinoid administration have been studied in rodents with TNSBA induced colitis (dinitrobenzene-sulfonic acid-induced colitis). Blockade of the CB-1 and CB-2 receptors tends to increase the extent and severity of experimental colitis that can be induced by TNBSA. It is known that the application of CB-2 receptor antagonists aggravate TNBSA-induced colitis. Furthermore, it is noted that the administration of cannabidiol can reduce adverse consequences of colitis induction by TNBSA, with a reduction of histological signs of inflammation and conservation of body weight in the experimental animals. These symptomatic benefits are accompanied by a reduction in biological markers of inflammatory responses. There are several other studies that have shown beneficial effects of CBD in the treatment of experimental colitis in animals (Abramovici, H. et al., ibid. 2014).

In a rodent model of ileitis, the administration of cannabichromene exerted effects on the hypermotility of the distal small bowel, but this effect seems to happen in a manner independent of cannabinoid receptor actions. Many patients with inflammatory bowel disease report benefit of cannabis in the general symptomatic relief of inflammatory bowel disease. A cross-sectional survey of patients with Crohn's disease or ulcerative colitis that used cannabis (Lal, S., et al., *Eur J. Gastroenterol. Hepatol.* 23 (2011): 891–6) revealed common experiences with relief of abdominal pain, improved appetite, and reduced feelings of nausea. Cannabis appears to have a particularly beneficial effect in the reduction of diarrhea in ulcerative colitis, and it causes sleep promotion with reduced stress levels in patients with inflammatory bowel disease. However, side effects in this survey of users were present in about one-third of patients, (e.g., psychoactive changes, dry mouth, memory loss, anxiety, and palpitations).

The systemic and gut symptoms of Crohn's disease are often severe. Underlying this condition is inflammation of regions of the gut (e.g., ileum and colon) or elsewhere, which may be amenable to the anti-inflammatory effects of cannabinoids. Furthermore, cannabis smoking has been reported to improve appetite, reduce nausea, and exert antispasmodic effects in individuals with Crohn's disease. Animal models of inflammatory bowel disease treated with cannabinoid agonists can reduce intestinal motility, and human experiences of benefit are quite promising.

Stephen Holt, MD, DSc

Inflammatory Bowel Disease and Cannabis (Summary)

A useful, easy-to-understand overview of cannabis use in inflammatory bowel disease is available online (www.medical-jane. com/2014/06/28). This summary of cannabis use in inflammatory bowel disease was written by Ariella Gerard, a second-year medical student from New York State. In this medical review, Ms. Gerard draws attention to the relative lack of controlled clinical trials in ulcerative colitis and Crohn's disease but predicts benefits of cannabis in the management of these disorders.

Ms. Gerard refers to a study reported in 2011 that indicated that 51 percent of ulcerative colitis patients and 48 percent of Crohn's disease patients are lifetime users of cannabis. About 50 percent of users with Crohn's disease and 33 percent with ulcerative colitis were applying cannabis for symptom control of their disease.

In patients with Crohn's disease, recent studies of three months' treatment with inhaled cannabis show improvements in quality-of-life measurements, disease activity index, and a rise in body mass index (Lanat, A. et al., *Digestion* 85 (2012): 1–8). In an observational study of the treatment of Crohn's disease with cannabis, several positive effects were reported, with improvements in scores of the Crohn's disease activity index. Apparent success in this study precipitated a recommendation for placebo-controlled trials. This resulted in a small prospective placebo-controlled study of cannabis use in Crohn's disease (Naftali, T. et al., *Clin. Gastroenterol Hepatol* 10 (2013): 1276–80). In this study the induction of remission was not achieved after eight weeks of cannabis smoking treatment, but significant improvements and clinical benefits (symptoms) were observed in ten of eleven patients with active Crohn's disease.

In a small sample (n=30) of patients with Crohn's disease, scores of disease activity improved, with cannabis administration and the use of medications for disease treatment was reduced, with a lower intake of 5-ASA, steroids, thiopurine, methotrexate, and a TNF (tumor necrosis factor) antagonist (Naftali, T. et al., *Isr. Med. Assoc. J* 13 [2011]: 455–58). Other human studies have reinforced these findings with observations of reductions in clinical disease activity indices, enhanced quality of life, and weight gain in patients with Crohn's disease.

There are several potential mechanisms of favorable actions of cannabinoids in the improvement of inflammatory bowel disease. In brief, Cannabinoids work on both CB-1 and CB-2 receptors to regulate epithelial permeability, motility, secretion, leucocyte migration, leucocyte recruitment, and apoptosis. The effects of cannabis on the CB-1 receptors in the brain are relevant in this situation. The central nervous system may alter intestinal motility and the sensation of pain by overall reduction in the inflammatory process (Schicho, R., and Storr, M., *Pharmacology* 93 (2014): 1–3).

Nocioception (pain transmission) from the abdomen can result in protracted inhibition of gastrointestinal motility (paralytic ileus). The hallmarks of this disorder include buildup of gut secretions and gas with distension of the bowel, vomiting, and/ or abdominal pain. It has been shown in animal studies that CB-1 receptor antagonists increase gastrointestinal motility, and this class of compounds (e.g., SR141716A) may have some potential therapeutic applications in these circumstances, when intestinal blockage has been excluded.

Cannabis and Gerd

Relaxation or incompetence of the lower esophageal sphincter permits the reflux of gastric contents into the esophagus (gastroesophageal reflux disease, GERD). Cannabinoid (CB-1) agonists appear to inhibit relaxation of the esophageal sphincter, whereas CB-1 receptor antagonists have an opposing effect. These findings have led to conclusion that cannabis can exert beneficial effects in gastro-esophageal reflux disease (GERD) by reducing episodes of relaxation of the lower esophageal sphincter and inhibition of gastric acid secretion. However, cannabis may slow gastric emptying in some individuals, and this may aggravate GERD.

Pancreatic Disease and Cannabinoids

There is an association between the short-term excessive use of cannabis and pancreatitis, but no clear causal links are defined.

Studies of the disruption of the endocannabinoid system in humans with acute pancreatitis reveal an enhanced activity of CB-1 and CB-2 receptors and an increased concentration of anandamide. In chronic pancreatitis in humans, studies show decreased endocannabinoid levels and increase in the number of CB-1 and CB-2 receptors. Animal studies of the use of cannabinoids in the treatment of acute or chronic pancreatitis show contradictory results. There is a lack of clarity of the potential application of cannabinoids in the therapy of pancreatitis.

Liver Disease and Cannabinoids

There are variable changes in CB-1 and CB-2 receptor activity associated with an increased concentration of endocannabinoids (anandamide and 2-AG) in many patients with liver disease. The variability of changes in levels of endocannabinoids appears to be related to the type of liver disease (e.g., hepatocellular cancer, liver fibrosis, nonalcoholic fatty liver disease, etc.). Overall, it is proposed that CB-1 and CB-2 receptors may have opposite roles in the regulation of aspects of liver function. However, CB-2 receptors are not readily detected in normal liver tissue. Enhanced activity of CB-1 receptors is common in a variety of liver diseases, and it is associated often with disease progression. These CB-1 effects are notable in alcoholic steatosis, cirrhosis, and other circumstances of liver fibrosis. In contrast, CB-2 upregulation exerts benefits in alcoholic steatosis, hepatocellular inflammation, fibrosis, and liver regeneration.

Animal experiments reveal that cannabidiol (CBD) may inhibit liver fibrosis as a consequence of chronic ethanol intake or other types of liver injury. Animal experiments in rodents demonstrate that CBD can protect against hepatic injury resulting from lack of blood supply to the liver (ischemia). In brief, CBD affords protection against acute hepatic/reperfusion injury when administered before and after its experimental induction in the laboratory. Similar results in the attenuation of hepatic/reperfusion injury have been noted in animals that received pre- or post-treatment with delta-8-tetrahydrocannabivarin.

Cannabis and Hepatitis C: Paradox

Reports about the effects of cannabis on the progression of hepatitis C and its treatment appear somewhat confusing. In one study, daily use of cannabis appeared to be associated with progression of moderate to severe liver fibrosis, whereas in another study cannabis has been reported to have very beneficial effects on hepatitis C viral infection.

The effects of cannabis on hepatitis C include assistance with the reduction of hepatitis C treatment side effects and arguable benefits on liver structure and function. Cannabis has been used as a substitute for intravenous drug use in addicted individuals who have hepatitis C. Some studies have implied that liver fibrosis increases with cannabis use in hepatitis C infection. Some studies imply that liver steatosis increases with cannabis use, and others do not. The jury remains out on these issues, but coinfection with HIV virus and hepatitis C virus is associated with a poor prognosis. That said, recent studies indicate that marijuana smoking does not appear to accelerate the progression of liver disease in individuals with HIV infection (Brunet, L. et al., *Clinical Infectious Diseases* 57, No. 5 [June 28, 2013]: 663–70).

Cannabis Hyperemesis Syndrome

Cannabis hyperemesis syndrome is an uncommon condition that results from continuous use of synthetic or natural cannabis. Most of the time, cannabis use results in antiemetic effects and other beneficial actions on disturbed gastrointestinal function, but cannabis hyperemesis syndrome seems to be a paradoxical effect of cannabis. In this disorder symptoms of abdominal pain with pronounced nausea and vomiting dominate the clinical picture.

There is a risk of missing this diagnosis because gastrointestinal investigations may often be noncontributory. The origin of this disorder appears to be mainly due to central nervous system effects of heavy cannabis use. One clue to the diagnosis of this disorder is that the patient may often describe relief of symptoms from hot baths or showers.

Conclusion

The guts are formed by a collection of clever tissues. Cannabis has versatile effects on gastrointestinal and associated metabolic functions. The overall effects of cannabis on digestive function are profound, given the intelligence of the guts. This intelligence is modified by the endocannabinoid system.

Chapter 10

BONES AND JOINTS

Introduction

Most comments on studies of the use of cannabis in arthritis management stem from the results of animal studies. These studies have been performed most often in experimental forms of rheumatoid arthritis and osteoarthritis. The principal symptom of pain in many types of arthritis can be managed to a variable degree by cannabis use, but cannabis may have a special role in the beneficial modulation of immune function in autoimmune types of arthritis (e.g., rheumatoid disease or systemic lupus erythematosus, SLE). Animal studies indicate that cannabidiol (CBD) suppresses immune-related arthritis with some beneficial effects on inhibiting disease progression (Abramovici, H. et al., ibid. 2014).

Several observations or limited studies in humans show benefits of cannabis in the management of rheumatoid disease. The positive effects of cannabis have been noted with increased patient mobility and reduction in morning stiffness of joints. One important observation is the ability of cannabis to exert synergy with painkilling medications that are used in arthritis treatment. These medications commonly include nonsteroidal anti-inflammatory drugs (NSAID) and opioids. In fact, research on metabolites of cannabis has shown therapeutic effects similar to those of the NSAID, indomethacin. Thus, cannabis may serve a major purpose of assisting the actions of drugs used in treatment of arthritis. This may permit the reduction of dosage of certain painkilling drugs. This effect is quite advantageous because high dosages of arthritis medications have many onerous side effects.

The result of the body's metabolism of THC is the production of chemical compounds with different effects on body functions. Researchers have been able to modify selected metabolites of THC and focus on one or more modified metabolites that have pain-relieving and painkilling effects. An example of a modified metabolite is a synthetic form of a carboxylic acid called CT-3 (dimethylheptyl-THC-11-oic acid). This compound is a potent inhibitor of inflammation with demonstrated painkilling actions in animals, making it an attractive candidate for the treatment of arthritis.

The release of certain cytokines (inflammatory compounds) is inhibited by cannabis. Moreover, certain fats contained within cannabis (sterols and sterolins) have been proposed as alternative arthritis medication. Sterols and sterolins may also reduce the production of inflammatory cytokines. The release of these cytokines is controlled by TH2 helper cells, and related mechanisms can result in alterations of controls of antibody secretions by B cells. It is proposed that these immunomodulatory effects of cannabis can be beneficial in control of damaging autoimmune effects on the body. As mentioned earlier, cannabinoid analogues, such as ajulemic acid, can result in relief of experimentally induced arthritis in laboratory animals.

Upon review, it is well known that the endogenous cannabinoid system is a principal factor in maintaining body homeostasis. In this situation it is known to reduce pain perception and increase tolerability to pain. Moreover, cannabis can reduce stress and exert significant effects on sleep. Cannabinoid receptors are present on nerves, immune-competent cells, bone cells, and tissues within the joints of the body. In animal models of arthritis, there are known to be increased endocannabinoids in the spinal cord, together with upregulation of CB-1 and CB-2 receptors (Abramovici, H. et al., ibid. 2014).

Cannabis and Arthritis

Cannabis has been used in different types of arthritis because of its ability to control several joint symptoms, including pain and inflammation, and it can assist in overcoming associated sleep disorders. While pain control and joint mobility are key issues in arthritis management, cannabis has attracted much interest as a potential treatment for autoimmune rheumatoid disease (arthritis) (www.huffingtonpost.com, 011/06/08/can-medicalmarijuana-help-arthritis). However, the safety and effectiveness of the use of cannabis in rheumatoid arthritis and other forms of arthritis are controversial. Concerns exist about the development of drug dependence with cannabis and its unknown effects on the natural history of the disease. There are many anecdotal reports of benefit of cannabis in several studies of rheumatoid disease.

As noted, there have been relatively few studies of cannabis treatments in human cases of arthritis. At the time of writing, there has been one prominent study of cannabis medication in rheumatoid disease, but there have been several trials in fibromyalgia. A couple of studies of the drug nabilone in fibromyalgia have not shown significant overall improvements compared with placebo. However, nabilone may be valuable in correction of sleep problems in patients with fibromyalgia (reported at www.webscape.com).

Some medical reviews of cannabis use in rheumatoid diseases do not provide robust support of efficacy. While pain reduction may be an obvious benefit of marijuana use, this benefit may not be as effective in joint pain present in rheumatoid disease, compared with other causes of pain (e.g., neuropathic pain). Clearly, there are differences in the cause of pain generation in different diseases, and this makes the painkilling actions of cannabis quite variable.

Endocannabinoid concentrations (2-AG and anandamide) are elevated in humans with osteoarthritis (degenerative types of joint disease). In animal experiments cannabis decreases measures of pain with improvements in limb mobility, in association with inhibition of nociceptive activity. This blocking nocioceptive activity can be generated in pain fibers that innervate joints. For these reasons there is a reasonable foundation for the use of cannabis or selected cannabinoids in arthritis treatments, where conventional therapies have not worked effectively or in patients who may not be considered to be able to benefit from conventional therapies (Abramovici, H. et al., ibid. 2014).

Bone Structure

There are several conflicting animal studies on the effects of cannabinoids on the maintenance of bone structure and function. That said, the endocannabinoid system is believed to play an active role in modulating bone deposition, resorption, and growth. Many components of the endocannabinoid receptor systems are present in bone, notably both types of CB receptors and endocannabinoids. How endocannabinoids regulate different types of bone (cancellous versus trabecular) remains underexplored. Studies of receptor stimulation and antagonism have cast light on mechanisms of bone formation in relationship to cannabinoids, which may have a role to play in the management of osteoporosis (thin bones).

The joints and other components of the musculoskeletal system contain an endocannabinoid receptor and control system. However, relatively little is known about the functions of this system in normal and disease circumstances. The relative absence of human clinical trials in the use of cannabis in management of many types of arthritis has not stopped an increasing use of cannabinoids in these circumstances. Cannabinoids are used often in arthritis because of their assumed anti-inflammatory effects. In brief, combinations of troublesome arthritis pain and the negative consequences of immobility are seen as targets for relief by cannabis and cannabinoid drugs in different forms of arthritis.

While moderate and severe rheumatoid arthritis are often accepted as a good reason to use cannabis for symptom control, some reviews of its use indicate that not all methods of administration of cannabis produce convincing benefits. For example, it has been reported that the use of cannabis delivered in an oro-mucosal spray (nabiximols) have not been very effective in global pain control of symptoms in rheumatoid disease, and its adverse psychoactive event profile appears to be an occasional disincentive for its use.

Cannabis and Osteoporosis

Osteoporosis affects about one in three women and one in ten men, usually at advanced stages in life. Animal studies made in mice that lacked CB-1 receptors support a role of cannabis in reducing bone tissue in young animals, with a contrarian effect of increasing bone mass in elderly animals. Moreover, concern has been expressed that marijuana use may inhibit bone healing following breaks of bone. Furthermore, cannabis smoke reduces bone formation around titanium implants in animals (Abramovici, H. et al., ibid. 2014).

Fibromyalgia

There is a lack of controlled trials of cannabis use in the treatment of fibromyalgia. However, the spectrum of disorders found in fibromyalgia helps to predict some beneficial effects of marijuana in this complex disease. Some of the main problems in fibromyalgia are shown in table 82.

Table 82. Some of the main problems encountered in fibromyalgia

Autoimmune factors may contribute to the causation of fibromyalgia.

widespread pain	allodynia and hyperalgesia
fatigue	sleep disorders
cognitive decline	emotional upset
depression	deficits in pain inhibition
altered function of pain processing	alterations in neurotransmitter levels

A significant number of people with fibromyalgia self-medicate with marijuana, using both approved and illicit sources of cannabis. Patients report the amelioration of several problems in fibromyalgia with cannabis use, including pain, sleep problems, mood disorders, muscle and joint stiffness, anxiety, headaches, fatigue, and digestive upset. In addition, smoked or edible cannabis can result in an overall sense of well-being with feelings of relaxation. In keeping with accepted guidelines for medical cannabis use, it is suggested that pharmaceutical preparations of the drug are recommended for fibromyalgia management when there are significant sleep disorders that are not manageable by conventional means. Nabilone and dronabinol have been studied in the management of fibromyalgia, but studies have shown limited or variable benefits.

Nabilone is known to improve sleep disturbances that are common in fibromyalgia, and it results in variable pain relief. Moreover, studies of dronabinol in dosages of 2.5–15 mg in patients with fibromyalgia reported decrease in pain by a factor of 50 percent after three months of treatment. However, adverse effects were common in these studies, resulting in needs for patient discontinuation of the study. These positive results with nabilone were followed by a further study that resulted in pain control with 7.5 mg of dronabinol over a period of several months. Furthermore, it was noted that dronabinol administration often permitted reduction of the need for painkilling medications, and it exhibited a degree of synergistic effects on pain control (Abramovici, H. et al., ibid. 2014).

Failure of Classic Treatment of Fibromyalgia

The National Institutes of Health has indicated that about five million patients in the United States suffer from fibromyalgia. As mentioned earlier, this disorder is associated with pain in deep tissues, headaches, depression, sleep disturbances, and fatigue.

An important online survey of the use of cannabis in 1339 people with fibromyalgia suggested that cannabis is considerably more successful in treatment than three standard (FDA-approved) prescription drugs (duloxetine [Cymbalta], pregabalin [Lyrica], and milnacipan [Savella]) (Anson, P., April 24, 2014, nationalpainreport.com).

There is no doubt that many patients with fibromyalgia lack confidence about their selected drug treatment using FDA-approved medications (Cymbalta, Lyrica, and Savella). The difficulties encountered in fibromyalgia patients were quite disturbing, and survey results (Anson, P., ibid. 2014) implied what follows in table 83:

Table 83. Difficulties encountered by fibromyalgia patients seeking medical care

- Forty-three percent felt that their physician was not knowledgeable about fibromyalgia.
- Thirty-five percent of patients felt that their physician did not take fibromyalgia seriously.
- Forty-five percent of friends and family did not take their fibromyalgia seriously.
- Forty-nine percent had onset of fibromyalgia in the age range of eighteen to thirty-four years.
- Only 11 percent received a diagnosis of fibromyalgia within the first year of symptoms.
- Forty-four percent reported that it took five or more years before a diagnosis of fibromyalgia was made.

The National Pain Report by Pat Anson (editor) indicated that eight out of ten patients with fibromyalgia stopped attending a physician because of their perception of poor treatment (nationalpainreport.com/marijuana-rated-most-effective-for-treating-fibromyalgia-8823638.html). The number of patients with fibromyalgia who self-medicate with cannabis is not clear.

This study of cannabis use in fibromyalgia rings a powerful alarm bell. Patients are highly sensitive to their perception of the knowledge and competence of their attending physicians. It is known that physician education on cannabis use and science requires correction or amplification. However, patients with a lack of confidence about their treatment tend to not get better!

Conclusion

The use of cannabis in arthritis management shows promise, but its effects on bone structure and function present confusing areas of science. Cannabis represents a logical solution to pain and inflammation in arthritis, but human studies are somewhat lacking.

Chapter 11

CANNABIS AND CARDIORESPIRATORY DISORDERS

Association between Cannabis and Cardiorespiratory Disease

There is a clear opinion that much further research is necessary to clarify the potential connection between cannabis use and cardiovascular disorders or lung disease. One balanced opinion is that studies to date have suggested a link between cardiovascular or lung disease and cannabis, but clear causal relationships are not defined. It is quite difficult in many circumstances to separate the specific effects of marijuana smoking on cardiovascular or lung function because many cannabis users engage in multiple substance abuse, especially cigarette smoking and excessive alcohol intake. However, it seems like the evidence is leaning toward a relatively uncommon causal link between cannabis use and cardiovascular or respiratory events in people of all ages.

It has been reported in one study that tobacco smoking increases the risk of lung cancer by up to twenty-three times in men and about thirteen times in women. It is clear that common, dual use of marijuana and tobacco smoking has had a major impact on an inability to define clearly the use of marijuana as a cause of lung cancer. Similar confounding circumstances are present in the dual use of tobacco and cannabis when it comes to the occurrence of coronary artery disease and stroke risk. These cardiorespiratory risks appear to be increased in some studies as a direct consequence of marijuana smoking, but arguments prevail (Abramovici, H. et al., ibid. 2014).

The magnitude of the potential problem of heart attack caused by marijuana may be much greater than reported. This is due, in part, to judgmental opinions of the illicit use of cannabis, which may stand in the way of disclosures about cannabis use by many people. To assess the impact of this potential problem, one may consider data from the 2012 National Survey on Drug Use and Health where it is reported that 18.9 million individuals in the United States had used marijuana in the past month. In addition, it has been estimated that about seventy-seven million people in the European Union have used cannabis at least once in their lifetime, with common usage in people in the age range of eighteen to twenty-five years. Using these numbers to predict the size of the potential problem reveals that even a small prevalence of heart attacks or cardiovascular problems caused by marijuana would result in a few thousand cardiovascular events caused by cannabis.

Cannabis and Vascular Disease

Research suggests that CB-1 and CB-2 receptors play opposite roles in the pathogenesis and progression of arteriosclerosis. In brief and oversimplified statements, CB-1 receptor activity seems to be a factor involved in the occurrence and progression of atherosclerosis, but CB-2 receptor stimulation seems to prevent atherosclerosis. However, the role of CB-2 receptors activity in the prevention of atherosclerosis is debatable (Abramovici, H. et al., ibid. 2014).

Several studies have highlighted the protective effects of CB-2 receptor activity on atheroma development. One proposal is that CB-2 receptor activity may not be a key influence in the initiation of atherosclerosis, but it may exert adverse effects on its progression. It is notable that cannabidiol (CBD) may interfere with the activity of the enzyme lipoxygenase. This enzyme appears to play a significant role in the development of atheroma.

Some early reports of cannabis use in animal studies imply that the presence of low-dose THC or CB-1 receptor antagonists or CB-2 receptor agonists inhibit the progression of atherosclerosis. The actual mechanisms of these effects remain underexplored, but the antiarteriosclerotic effect of low-dose THC has been hypothesized as due to actions on CB-2 receptors. Most of these data are derived from animal studies, and their portability to humans is in question.

A number of cardiovascular diseases have been associated with cannabis use, but causal links may not be clear.

Table 84. Major cardiovascular and cerebrovascular adverse effects with a described temporal relationship to marijuana smoke inhalation. The associations are not always known to be causal, and the etiology of these disorders is sometimes corrupted by simultaneous tobacco and cannabis use (Abramovici, H. et al., ibid. 2014).

Cardiovascular	Peripheral Vascular	Cerebrovascular
• precipitation of angina	• Raynaud's phenomenon	• transient ischemic attacks
• myocardial infarction	• ischemic ulcers	• cerebral flow
• coronary flow	• digital necrosis	• strokes
• cardiac arrhythmias	• angitis	
• cardiomyopathy		

How Does Cannabis Damage Cardiovascular Function?

In healthy individuals, cannabis may cause a rapid, dose-dependent increase in heart rate (tachycardia) and blood pressure (hypertension). This effect is due to stimulation of the sympathetic nervous system, which is typically involved in the fight-and-flight reaction. This reaction is associated with acute stressful events. In contrast, chronic cannabis use often leads to an increase in parasympathetic activity, which tends to slow the heart (bradycardia) and reduce blood pressure (a mellowing effect). This viewpoint of cannabis use and cardiovascular function is simplified.

The medical literature proposes several ways in which cannabis can interfere with cardiac function. These mechanisms of action are shown in table 85.

Table 85. Circumstances that may favor acute and chronic cardiovascular events with cannabis use (summarized by Kyriazou, A. V., online *Aristotle University Medical Journal* 41, no. 1 [February 2014]).

- THC can contribute to poor oxygen supply to heart muscle, associated with production of carboxyhemoglobin. Tachycardia then ensues. THC stimulates the production of catecholamines that can cause abnormalities of heart rhythm, with excessive premature ventricular ectopic beats and the risks of arrhythmias.
- Cannabis smoking leads to the production of free radicals that cause stress responses, which, in turn, increase risks of blood vessel blockage by the precipitation of an inflammatory response, platelet activation, and the enhanced production of oxidized LDL. This hypothesis of action seems to contradict reported favorable effects of low-dose THC that may protect the myocardium from hypoxia (low blood oxygen).
- Falls of blood pressure during the adoption of an upright position (orthostatic hypotension) can cause fainting (syncope). This may be an effect of THC due to a reduction in left ventricular ejection time and lowering of peripheral vascular resistance.
- Sympathic stimulation causes an increase in heart rate and workload of the heart. This may predispose to myocardial ischemia (lack of coronary blood flow). There are several anecdotal reports of myocardial infarction occurring

sometimes in people without significant cardiovascular risks (e.g., young men). This situation may be related to the occurrence of coronary artery spasm.

- Altered pain perception as a consequence of THC may result in a delay of patients seeking acute medical care for heart attacks.

Cardiovascular events with cannabis use in animals may be different from those in humans. In animals, slowing of the heart and lowering of blood pressure may occur, whereas in humans it is noted that THC increases heart rate, and it may result in minor increases in supine blood pressure and sometimes significant degrees of orthostatic hypotension. It is often observed, however, that tolerance to these initial cardiovascular events occurs. Early research (Jones, R. T., *J. of Clinical Pharma* 42, (2002): 58S–63S) has described the acute cardiovascular effects of marijuana, which do not tend to challenge otherwise healthy young people, but as noted, uncommon occurrences of myocardial infarction and stroke have been reported in young adults (see table 77).

More than thirty years ago my colleagues and I described the occurrence of myocardia infarction in the virtual absence of risk factors in a twenty-five-year-old man after marijuana smoking. This individual had normal coronary arteries, as assessed by coronary arteriography (Charles, R., Holt, S., Kirkham, N., *Clinical Toxicology* 14, no. 4 (May 1979): 433–8, doi: 10.3109). Similar findings have been reported subsequently by many physicians. There is an increasingly clear relationship between cannabis use in young people and serious cardiovascular adverse events, but these events are uncommon.

Signals of Risk for Cannabis Induced Cardiovascular Disorders

An important recent study reported that there are signals of increasing risk of serious cardiovascular problems with cannabis use (Juanjous, E. et al., *J. Am. Heart Assoc.* [April 23, 2014]: doi: 10.1161/JAHA. 113.000638). I support the opinion that these recent data associating adverse cardiovascular events with cannabis use do not appear to have occurred by chance alone. In this study in France, information was taken from the national system of the French Addictovigilance Network, between the years 2006 and 2010. This network of reporting constitutes a highly desirable act of vigilance, where serious cases of abuse of or dependence on psychoactive drugs are subject to mandated reporting. There has been a call for a similar national system in the United States, and this would help to track details of adverse effects with cannabis.

In brief, this French study indicated that 1.8 percent (thirty-five out of 1979) of all cannabis-related reports of cardiovascular problems were in men (85.7 percent), with an average age of 34.3 years. Nine of the thirty-five individuals with cardiovascular problems died. The report uncovered twenty-two cardiac events with twenty examples of acute coronary syndromes. In addition, data showed ten peripheral vascular complications of various types. These included juvenile arteriopathies and Buerger's-like diseases (peripheral arteritis). In addition, three examples of cerebral vascular diseases occurred, including transient cortical blindness, spasm of the cerebral artery, and acute cerebral angiopathy. The overall conclusion of this study was that cannabis is a "potential triggering factor" for cardiovascular disorders in young adults.

These contemporary French data do not stand alone. Some scientists have suggested that cannabis use must be considered as a premonitory event in several circumstances of serious cardiovascular problems. As noted earlier, a confounding factor that works against the identification of a clear causal relationship between cannabis use and cardiovascular diseases is simultaneous tobacco and other drug use with marijuana. However, many other studies support the cannabis/cardiovascular disease link. For example, some studies have implied that the combined use of cannabis and tobacco in smoking may be likely to cause coronary artery syndromes in individuals with a history of coronary disease, compared with those who use tobacco alone. In one study of four thousand hospitalized patients with acute myocardial infarction, cannabis was identified as a clear cardiovascular risk factor.

As noted earlier, increased heart rate (tachycardia) occurs in a dose-related manner in most users of cannabis, but tolerance to these effects often occurs in a short time. This tachycardia is best avoided in people with preexisting angina or other types of heart disease. As mentioned earlier, the undesirable combination effects of cannabis on preexisting heart disease present an increased risk of heart attack and cardiac arrhythmias. These cardiovascular effects are mediated most often by 9-delta-THC, which causes an increase in cardiac output and myocardial oxygen requirements. To reiterate, other THC-related effects include raised catecholamine levels (sympathetic drive) and occasional unpredictable falls in blood pressure, resulting from postural hypotension associated with episodes of peripheral vasodilatation.

This book highlights that there are several problems with the interpretation of retrospective, descriptive studies of cannabis use when it comes to the demonstration of causal disease links. While underreporting of cannabis use seems to be a predictable problem, it is recommended that prospective studies of all cardiovascular cases associated with cannabis use are necessary to provide evidence of a causal disease link. These studies could be improved by the application of efficient techniques of interviewing for cannabis use with objective measurements of drug use by urine analysis or other reliable forms of testing. The recording of patterns of clinical signs and symptoms that permit the detection of marijuana abuse with a high degree of diagnostic discrimination would also be valuable in this context.

It is obvious that the expanding use of cannabis with both recreational and medical legalization has prompted safety concerns. Recent reports of adverse cardiovascular events, linked to marijuana use, continue to highlight the continuing lack of existing safety studies (Rezkalla, S., Kloner, R., *J. Am. Heart Assoc.* [2014], doi: 10.1161/JAHA.114.000904). It appears that vascular problems presumed to be caused by marijuana require much further study. Perhaps staunch warnings should be present more often on cannabis products, such as those warnings that are applied to cigarettes.

Basic science and clinical studies show some strong support for a causal link between marijuana smoking and vascular events. In one study, the blood concentrations of a variety of proteins were measured in eighteen heavy users of cannabis and compared with twenty-four volunteers who had not used the drug. This analysis showed significantly higher blood levels of apolipoprotein C-111 in the marijuana consumers. It is known that APO-C111 is a protein that is identified as a risk factor for cardiovascular disease, as a result of its interactions with other fats in the body. Accumulation of fats occurs in the lining of arterial blood vessels, leading ultimately to atherosclerosis. This results in blockage of blood vessels as a consequence of the delay in the breakdown of triglycerides. Studies of the presence of blood protein markers of cannabis use as a predictor of cardiovascular events have attracted criticism, largely because of their inability to define a cause/effect relationship.

Cannabis, Hypertension, and Arrhythmias

Certain cannabinoids can result in an overall reduction in arterial blood pressure and contractility of the heart (e.g., THC). There are, however, relatively few studies on the effects of cannabis in individuals with hypertension. Some observations on cannabis smoking have recorded a prolonged decrease in blood pressure in subjects with hypertension, compared with those who have normal arterial blood pressure recordings. These results were noted as a consequence of an intake from smoking materials that contained 2.8 percent of delta-9-THC, but these results have not been confirmed in a conclusive manner in further controlled studies.

Clearly, cannabis use in the presence of cardiomyopathy should be avoided. There have been several reports of arterial inflammation (arteritis) caused by long-term, heavy cannabis smoking. The use of cannabis by AIDS patients requires special monitoring because of the increased occurrence of cardiovascular disorders, which have been proposed to result from the combined use of some antiretroviral drugs and cannabis (e.g., ritonavir). This drug combination is suspected to be cardiotoxic (Abramovici, H. et al., ibid. 2014).

Physicians have drawn attention to the underreporting of cardiac arrhythmias following cannabis use (Fisher, B. A. et al., *Emerg Med J* 22, 679 [2005], content online at emj.com). A number of abnormalities in heart rhythm have been associated with cannabis use, including occurrences of tachycardia, occasional bradycardia, atrioventricular block (second degree), and atrial flutter or fibrillation. While the timing of episodes of arrhythmia following marijuana use are difficult to predict, estimates show most abnormalities of heartbeats will occur within thirty minutes after cannabis smoking, and they can persist for up to a couple of hours. However, the situation is unpredictable, and sustained or brief episodes of arrhythmia can occur. The propensity for cannabis to cause cardiac arrhythmias is believed to occur as a result of effects on the autonomic nervous system. Cannabis use has been linked with the occurrence of ventricular ectopic beats and a variety of effects on the P, T, and QRS recordings of an EKG.

It is sometimes overlooked that cannabis can increase the symptoms of angina at lower levels of exercise pursuit in some individuals. There is probably an uncommon link between cannabis use and sudden death from acute cardiovascular events, but this latter circumstance has not been clearly documented. Attending physicians should take note of the continuing reluctance of patients to disclose cannabis use. The hidden potaholic (see chapter 18) will emerge increasingly in the future (cf. hidden alcoholic).

Respiratory Disorders and Cannabis

People are tired of the continuing debate about the ability of cannabis smoking to cause pulmonary disease, but smoking anything is not healthy. There are several animal studies that describe the regulation or alteration of airway diameter (bronchoconstriction or bronchodilation) by the endocannabinoid system. Cannabis use or the administration of certain cannabis analogues have been found in preclinical studies to be a potential treatment for asthma as a consequence of bronchodilatory effects. That said, episodes of bronchoconstriction may occur during cannabis smoking, especially in the uninitiated smoker. This may be due to the irritant effect of smoke on the airways, and this effect can limit the use of cannabis smoking in the treatment of asthma. Several human studies, however, have recorded overall reductions in airway resistance and increased airway conductance with cannabis smoking in the short term. As mentioned, these airway changes are likely due to the properties of THC as a bronchodilator. The occasional negative consequences of cannabis smoke on breathing have prompted the study of alternate modes of delivery of cannabis or cannabis analogues with oral or vaporized preparations.

> The results of some limited clinical trials appear promising, with the use of an aerosol of delta-9-THC producing improvements in breathing functions in obstructive airways diseases at modest and well-tolerated dosages of administration. However, results are inconsistent in some other studies of both edible or aerosol preparations of cannabis, where there has been no association with benefit in reversible airways disorders. For example, in some experiences with aerosol use in asthma treatment, negative actions of cannabis were observed, resulting in bronchoconstriction. Cannabis or selected analogues, given in oral dosages of 2 mg (nabilone) or 10 mg (delta-9-THC) have not demonstrated consistent or reliable bronchodilatory effects in asthmatic subjects.

Against this background of the potential treatment of asthma with cannabis, much further study is required to understand changes in lung structure and function in the established cannabis smoker. While debate about the adverse effects of cannabis smoking on the lungs continues, it is useful to repeat the advice that smoking anything can be expected to be detrimental to health. This situation has led to recommendations for the use of vaporized cannabis preparations, but universal safety of vaporized cannabis remains to be demonstrated. Recent data from National Surveys show that vaping is becoming increasingly popular in teenagers and to a lesser degree in adults. In fact, vaporization techniques for both tobacco and cannabis use show a trend for reaching high degrees of popularity.

Smoking cannabis appears to increase the occurrence of respiratory infections with chronic use. Two factors seem to operate in this situation. First, researchers have commented on the potential role of cannabis in depressing immune function. This may increase a person's susceptibility to infection. Second, bacterial, fungal, or other contaminants are sometimes present in poorly processed cannabis smoking material (street cannabis). Street cannabis is not consistently subject to adequate techniques of sterilization.

Different styles or techniques of cannabis smoking play a major role in the delivery of toxic or noxious chemicals into the body. It is reported that tar is delivered in high amounts with extreme smoking conditions. Conditions of extreme smoking are adopted by the cannabis smoker who wishes to maximize the high feelings that can be obtained from a joint (cigarette, reefer, pipe, or bong). The extreme condition of smoking involves deep and frequent inhalation with breath holding, which contrasts with standard types of smoking that occur with tobacco. In brief, compared with tobacco smoke, higher concentrations of carbon monoxide, increases in ammonia, and substantially higher amounts of oxides of nitrogen and hydrogen cyanide are present in cannabis smoke. Thus, concentrated administration of the many components of cannabis smoke occurs with extreme conditions of smoking. The risks of exposure to secondhand cannabis smoke have not been charted in detail, but they are a concern.

Smoking occurs at high burning temperatures of cannabis, in comparison with vaporization, which is a much lower temperature process. The administration of cannabis by vaporization results in less formation of toxic products than are found in smoke. In other words, the amount of carbon monoxide, polycyclic aromatic hydrocarbons, and tar delivery from vaporization can be expected to be significantly less. In addition, a greater extraction of THC occurs with vaporized material. It is misleading to keep reading literature on the web that totally denies harmful effects of cannabis smoking on the lungs. Table 86 summarizes several defined effects of cannabis on lung structure and function.

Table 86. Reported effects of cannabis smoking on lung structure and function (reviewed by Abramovici, H. et al., ibid. 2014)

Effects on Lungs	Comment
Pathologic changes in the lining tissues of the respiratory tract	Many pathologic changes, including basal cell and goblet cell hyperplasia, inflammation, squamous cell metaplasia (a premalignant cellular change). Lung cancer risk is debated.
Changes in lung functions, often mild in severity	Reduction of forced expiratory volume in one second and increased airway resistance occurs with heavy cannabis use.
Symptoms of bronchitis	Wheezing, excessive phlegm production, chronic cough, and later risk of chronic obstructive airways disease, with a risk equivalent to that of tobacco smokers. More chest infections.

There is no doubt that residual arguments on the adverse effects of cannabis smoking on the lungs persist. However, one contemporary study of data collected over a twenty-year period (the CARDIA study) failed to show clear association of marijuana smoking and diminished pulmonary function (Pletcher, M. J. et al., *JAMA* 307 (2012): 173–181). While low levels of marijuana smoking were not associated with major alterations in pulmonary function, heavy and continuous use resulted in reductions of FEV-1 (forced expiratory volume). In summary, it would be healthier to choose alternative cannabis delivery systems to smoking, and systems such as vaping are accepted increasingly as safe and effective. However, smoking is by far the most employed method of cannabis delivery, and its psychoactive and welcome relaxing effects are of rapid onset in many people who smoke cannabis. The rapid onset of the effects of smoking cannabis is perceived as a real advantage for acute symptom management in several circumstances.

Conclusion

Scientific findings continue to cast suspicion on cannabis as a cause of cardiorespiratory diseases, but causal links are often not able to be demonstrated in a conclusive manner.

Chapter 12

NEUROLOGICAL DISORDERS

Endocannabinoids Modulate CNS Function: A Recap

The endocannabinoid system is often viewed in an oversimplified manner. In the classic model of the description of the function of endocannabinoids, signals are given to cannabinoid receptors to provide homeostatic messages that control many body functions. Beyond these processes are elaborate mechanisms that control endocannabinoid synthesis and degradation in the central nervous system (CNS). The main functions of the endocannabinoid system are summarized briefly in table 87.

Table 87. The main functions of the endocannabinoid system

• neuroprotection	• antioxidant functions
• antinociceptive actions	• modulation of immune functions
• anti-inflammatory actions	• endocrine function

The endocannabinoid system has major effects on neuromodulation, which is disrupted in many diseases of the central nervous system. This impaired system of control is encountered in several neurodegenerative diseases, including multiple sclerosis (MS), amyotrophic lateral sclerosis (ALS), Alzheimer's disease (AD), Parkinson's disease, Huntington's disease, and others.

In brief, the endocannabinoid system is comprised of the endocannabinoid ligands, the receptors, and enzymes that synthesize or degrade or catalyze inactivation of endocannabinoids. The main endocannabinoids involved in the signaling system are anandamide (AEA) and 2-arachidoylglycerol (2-AG). The key enzymes involved in degradation of endocannabinoids are fatty acid amide hydrolase (FAAH) and monoglyceride lipase (MAGL). Much ensuing information is found in Abramovici et al. (ibid. 2013 and 2014).

Function of Cannabinoid Receptors: A Review

A review of the many physiological functions of cannabinoid receptors casts much light on the importance of endocannabinoid control systems (see chapter 5). Table 88 summarizes some of the principal functions of cannabinoid receptors that are relevant to this discussion on neurological structure and function.

Table 88. Distribution and some of the main effects of cannabinoid receptors on the CNS and elsewhere (adapted from Abramovici et al., ibid. 2014)

Receptor	Distribution	Function
CB-1	Present on nerve cells in areas of the brain that control motor function and coordination, cognition, judgment, emotions, and memory, notably cerebellum, ba-sal ganglia, substantia nigra, cerebral cortex, amygdala, and hippo-campus.	A clear role in motor function control, acts of hearing and memory, and alterations in emotional states.

CB-2	Present on immune cells and other tissues, including the spleen, tonsils, bone marrow, and pancreas. Occur in smaller amounts in CNS on glial and microglial cells.	Modulate the release of cytokines and various proteins that regulate immune and inflammatory responses.

One can forecast, to some degree, the potential effects of neurodegenerative diseases on endocannabinoid functions in the central nervous system (CNS). These neurodegenerative diseases cause a wide variety of symptoms. Symptom complexes of CNS disease are explained to a significant degree by understanding cannabinoid receptor distribution and function that can alter controls of CNS activities.

The increased occurrence of stroke in young adults who use cannabis is more likely to be caused by stenosis of intracranial blood vessels, rather than due to brain hemorrhage. In this recent research (Wolff V et al. Characteristics and prognosis of Ischemic Stroke in young Cannabis Users Compared with Non-Cannabis Users, Journal of the American College of Cardiology, 2015, 66(18): 2052 DOI: 10.1016/j.jacc 2015.08.867), cannabis users were younger than controls and were more likely to have other risk factors, such as smoking tobacco.

Epilepsy and Cannabis

The majority of cases of epilepsy have no clear cause. In these circumstances, it is often assumed that the cause is some degree of brain damage. There are three main types of epilepsy, including 1) symptomatic epilepsy where a cause has been identified, 2) idiopathic epilepsy where no cause is identified, and 3) cryptogenic epilepsy where no cause is identified, but brain injury is strongly suspected. Marijuana itself is capable of causing symptomatic epilepsy (a paradoxical effect).

Overall, basic science and animal experiments define an anticonvulsant effect of cannabinoids, but the double-edged sword of cannabis is apparent, with the description of uncommon, cannabinoid-precipitated (THC) convulsions. Antiepileptic effects of CB-1 receptors are explained by the presynaptic inhibition of glutamate release. In contrast, proconvulsant effects appear to be related to presynaptic inhibition of GABA release.

The role of cannabinoids in the potential management of patients with epilepsy requires much further definition. A tendency to convulsions has been noted in animals and humans that are associated with changes in the distribution of CB-1 receptors in the hippocampal regions of the brain. In addition, reduced concentrations of anandamide have been found in subjects with a diagnosis of temporal lobe epilepsy. This is perhaps another example of the endocannabinoid deficiency syndrome of Russo.

Causes of Epilepsy

The causes of epilepsy vary significantly by age. The overall prevalence of this disease in the United States is about three million individuals. A number of causes of seizure are presented in table 89.

Table 89. Causes of seizures by age (adapted from Schachter and Shafer, www.epilepsy.com)

Age Group	Causes
Newborns	Hypoxic brain damage, brain malformations, maternal drug use, and metabolic diseases
Infants and children	Infections, brain tumors, and febrile seizures
Children and adults	Congenital diseases (e.g., Down syndrome), genetic factors, and head injury
Seniors (elderly)	Alzheimer's disease, stroke, and head injury

Much attention has been focused on the use of cannabis in the treatment of epilepsy syndromes in children. These syndromes are fortunately quite uncommon, but convulsions may be severe, frequent, and prolonged. Table 90 lists some of these seizure syndromes (epileptic syndromes).

Table 90. A list of epileptic syndromes with special associations and characteristics (www.epilepsy.com, by G. L. Holmes, adapted 2014)

• Dravet syndrome	• Reflex epilepsy
• Rasmussen's syndrome	• Frontal lobe epilepsy
• Temporal lobe epilepsy	• Myoclonic epilepsy
• Lennox-Gestault syndrome	• Landau-Kleffner syndrome

Some medical literature reviews of the use of cannabinoids for epilepsy treatment imply that there is not sufficient evidence to reach firm conclusions about their benefit in epilepsy. Moreover, it has been proposed by some scientists that cannabinoids have no significant antiepileptic actions in many circumstances. The safety of long-term cannabidiol administration in high dosage (often 200–300 mg/day or more) that may be required to control epilepsy has not been proven. Furthermore, the role of cannabinoids alone as therapy (monotherapy) for epilepsy has not been demonstrated in a convincing manner. Cannabis is usually combined with other medications for the control of seizures.

Beyond THC and CBD are the effects of cannabidivarin (CBDV). Studies sponsored by G. W. Pharmaceuticals (UK) were performed in rodents (rats and mice) with several different types of epilepsy. In this research, it was discovered that CBDV is a potent suppressor of seizures, without many overt side effects. Moreover, CBDV may have synergistic effects with selected anticonvulsant drugs. Further research is warranted with CBDV in epilepsy, and it has been speculated that CBDV may be the most effective phytocannabinoid with anticonvulsant actions.

The Double-Edged Sword of Cannabis in Epilepsy

The use of cannabis in the treatment of epilepsy has become an emotive subject, especially related to childhood cases of refractory convulsions. A survey of the use of cannabis with high cannabidiol content for resistant epilepsy in childhood has been reported recently. This survey collected nineteen responses from a Facebook group of parents who used cannabidiol to treat convulsions in their children. In this group of respondents, the following conditions were present: thirteen cases of Dravet syndrome, four cases of Doose syndrome (myoclonic astatic epilepsy), one case of idiopathic epilepsy, and one case of Lennox-Gastault syndrome. In this survey sixteen of nineteen of the patients (84 percent) were reported to have reduction in seizure frequency as a consequence of the administration of cannabidiol-enriched cannabis preparations. These promising results were associated with other reported benefits, including positive alterations in mood, improved sleep, and greater alertness. Side effects in this study included drowsiness and fatigue, but overall positive outcome was experienced (Porter, B. E., Jacobson, C., *Epilepsy Behav* 29, no. 3 [2013]: 574–7).

Epilepsy treatment with cannabinoids presents the double-edged sword of cannabis. This double-edged sword refers to paradoxical effects of cannabis with its propensity to cause both the precipitation and the prevention of convulsions. The British Epilepsy Association has taken a favorable but cautious approach to cannabis use in epilepsy. This association draws attention to many anecdotal reports that suggest that cannabis (cannabidiol) can relieve seizures to a variable degree, but they acknowledge that some reports describe an increase in seizure activity as a consequence of cannabis use.

The position of the American Epilepsy Society stresses the anecdotal nature of reports on cannabidiol use in epilepsy treatment and the current lack of scientific studies. Furthermore, they opine that "use of marijuana for epilepsy may not be advisable due to lack of information on safety and efficacy" (see http://mnepilepsy.org/news/marijuana-for-the-treatment-of-epilepsy-what-do-studies-show/). In a fence-sitting conclusion, the American Epilepsy Society relegates cannabis use to a secondary position in epilepsy management and its use, only after exhausting other treatment options.

A significant number of families with a member afflicted by refractory seizures have relocated to Colorado or Washington State to obtain the perceived benefits of cannabidiol for epilepsy. Until relatively recently, the availability of quality cannabidiol in the United States has been generally poor. Now, a number of companies are selling cannabidiol, despite FDA rulings, as a dietary supplement, but the concentrations of CBD in some of these oil products is quite low or even absent, and their purity is sometimes in question. Little is known about dose response relationships between CBD and the control of convulsions. Furthermore, the costs of treatment in some children are exorbitant. It is reported but not confirmed that some parents of children with seizures have paid as much as five thousand dollars per month for CBD treatments.

Multiple states have approved the use of medical marijuana in epilepsy treatment, but many scientists continue to argue that there is only limited scientific data to support the use of marijuana (or cannabidiol, CBD) for epilepsy treatment. However, in one randomized, controlled clinical trial, cannabis in the form of Epidiolex was found to be effective in cases of human epilepsy. (Epidiolex is a drug used specifically for childhood epilepsy, which has received orphan drug status.)

Some support for the efficacy of THC in epilepsy in animal studies exists, but again the double-edged sword emerges with reports of seizures that have been triggered in animals by THC. This contrarian circumstance may be influenced by unknown effects of marijuana withdrawal that may exacerbate epilepsy. Again, one may conclude that the jury remains out on cannabis and epilepsy control. That said, there are a large number of favorable reports of cannabis use in convulsions, even though such information is anecdotal. The vacillation of opinion about cannabis use in epilepsy is confusing for many people, but it has resulted in approval of CBD (cannabidiol), with orphan drug status in some states of the United States.

Charlotte's Web

The story of Charlotte Figi of Colorado has attracted much attention among protagonists of compassionate-care programs that involve cannabis use. In August 2013, Dr. Sanjay Gupta made a CNN documentary about Charlotte's response to high-CBD-containing cannabis (referred to as Charlotte's Web). Prior to the institution of medical cannabis treatment, Charlotte was experiencing about three hundred grandmal (major) seizures per week. Within a short time following medical cannabis use, Charlotte's seizures were reduced in frequency to two or three convulsions per month. In brief, Charlotte's Web is a strain of high-CBD-containing cannabis that was used in Charlotte's treatment.

These days, the message that there is only limited evidence to support the use of cannabis in epilepsy management is becoming increasingly questioned, especially by parents of afflicted children. This circumstance is an emotive subject. That said, objective data on the benefits of cannabis use in epilepsy remains thin and somewhat anecdotal. Contemporary studies seem to echo uncertainties about the value of cannabis treatments for epilepsy in children, and these findings are apparent in studies at the Children's Hospital of Colorado where a large number of epileptic children have been treated with CBD.

In a retrospective study of fifty-eight children or adolescents with severe forms of epilepsy treated at the Children's Hospital (Colorado), only one third of patients reported a reduction of seizures by about 50 percent with prior cannabis use. It was noted in this study that improvements in seizures did not correlate with improvements in electroencephalogram (EEG) recordings. Of sixteen patients with baseline EEGs, only two showed improvement in EEGs. In this study, 47 percent of patients experienced adverse events, and, notably, 21 percent had increased seizures or new seizures.

Much further research is required to determine the role of cannabis in the treatment of epilepsy. There is a major disparity between positive anecdotal reports of benefit and the reality of valid survey data (prereported abstract number 1.326, Chapman K. et al., American Epilepsy Society (AES, 2014, www.newswise. com). The arguments for (pro) and against (con) cannabis use in epilepsy are summarized at www.medicalmarijuana.procon.org, with more cons than pros.

The Endocannabinoids Control Motor Function

A variety of controls over body motor function (movement) are exerted by the endocannabinoid system. I mention later in this book that many investigations have described alterations of

CB-1 receptor activity and density in several diseases that are characterized by alterations of body movements. The overall effects of activation of the CB1-receptor results in interference with body movements in a complex manner. This situation is illustrated by evidence of endocannabinoid dysregulation or dysfunction in several neurological disorders, including Tourette's syndrome, Dystonia, Huntington's disease, and Parkinson's disease (Abramovici, H. et al., ibid. 2014).

Tourette's Syndrome

Tourette's syndrome produces involuntary verbal tics that may be quite offensive. Surprisingly, there may be more than 100,000 individuals in the United States with this neuropsychiatric disorder, which seems to improve in adults with advancing age. Tourette's syndrome may be linked to obsessive-compulsive disorders. Attacks of Tourette's syndrome are variably responsive to delta-9-tetrahydrocannabinol (THC) administered in a dosage of 10 mg daily, but dosage requirements can vary.

In limited clinical studies, improvements of symptoms associated with Tourette's syndrome have been observed. One randomized clinical trial of THC in a range of dosages (5–10 mg) demonstrated improvements of control in motor and vocal tics together with reductions in obsessive-compulsive behavior. There were no serious adverse events in this study, but some side effects were noted (e.g., anxiety, headache, nausea, fatigue, and ataxia). In the previously mentioned six-week-long, randomized, placebo-controlled trial of 10 mg of THC in Tourette's syndrome, a significant reduction of tics was recorded, and there were no declines in measures of neuropsychological performance. However, some reviews of the use of cannabis in the control of symptoms in Tourette's syndrome have shown an overall lack of evidence of effectiveness.

The benefits of THC in Tourette's syndrome have been observed in several clinical trials including key trials that have used a randomized, double-blind, placebo-controlled, crossover approach. In one recent overview, treatment with THC in Tourette's syndrome has been advised after the use of standard first-line therapies have not produced good outcomes.

Dystonia

Anecdotal reports of improvements in symptoms of dystonia in humans are available in the absence of controlled clinical trials (at the time of writing). Both cannabidiol (CBD) and the administration of CB-1 and CB-2 receptor stimulating compounds can delay the progression of dystonia and improve symptoms overall, but they can sometimes cause severe side effects of catalepsy and spontaneous locomotor occurrences (jerks and tics).

Clinical findings with the use of cannabis in human cases of dystonia have tended to show improvement. In one six-week, open-label observation of five patients taking 100–600 mg of cannabidiol (CBD) per day, there was minor evidence of a dose-dependent improvement in symptoms. However, a study with nabilone in a dose of 0.03 mg/kg failed to show significant reduction in dystonia. Clearly, the jury remains out of the benefit of cannabis treatment in cases of dystonia.

Parkinson's Disease

In a survey of patients with Parkinson's disease receiving cannabis (2004), 45.9 percent of these patients described variable improvement in Parkinsonian symptoms. Moreover, 30.6 percent showed improvements in tremor at rest, 44.7 percent experienced improvement in bradykinesia, and 37 percent had improvements in rigidity, with benefits noted on L-Dopa-induced (treatment) dyskinesia in 14.1 percent of patients.

Parkinson's disease is due to death or dysfunction of dopaminergic neurons in the substantia nigra (basal ganglia). The end result is defective or disordered stimulation of the cerebral cortex. Several studies on the value of cannabinoid agonists or antagonists have resulted in contrarian findings in Parkinson's disease. It is known that activation of CB-1 receptors tends to alleviate dyskinesia in Parkinson's disease. Dyskinesia is usually a relatively long-term adverse effect of levodopa treatment (L-Dopa). It is proposed that this benefit of cannabis may be due to changes in dopamine and glutamate release that are controlled to some degree by the CB-1 receptor.

As mentioned earlier, Parkinson's disease is associated with major degenerative effects on the basal ganglia of the brain, and it has been associated with high cerebrospinal fluid levels of the endocannabinoid ligand, anandamide. These findings in humans are similar to those in other animal models where dopamine-containing cell loss in the brain is associated with elevated concentrations of anandamide. The brain has many cannabinoid receptors that are densely packed in the basal ganglia. These receptors are perceived to be targets for new drug development to use in Parkinson's disease treatment.

Animal studies show CB-receptor agonists may tend to reduce movement (hypokinesia). This effect would be undesirable in the patient with Parkinson's disease who often has rigidity and slow movement (bradykinesia). In fact, this circumstance limits cannabinoid applications in therapy. That said, it has been argued that hypokinesia could have some value in reducing dyskinesia (abnormal movement) that may occur with long-term treatment of Parkinson's disease with L-Dopa. One randomized clinical trial of nabilone (0.03 mg/kg) in a small number of patients with Parkinson's disease has shown a reduction in dyskinesia caused by levodopa (L-Dopa). Whether or not the neuroprotective or antioxidant effects of cannabis can exert benefit in the progression of Parkinson's disease remains unclear. However, the effects of delta-9-THC from cannabis smoking appear to have little effects on tremor in Parkinson's disease.

As noted earlier, there have been several reports that support the use of marijuana in the relief of certain symptoms of Parkinson's disease. However, these reports are largely anecdotal. A few observations in clinical practice indicate that cannabis may not be helpful in tremor or L-Dopa-induced dyskinesia. The American Academy of Neurology has not given much support for cannabis use in Parkinson's disease, but this could change as a consequence of more successful research.

Huntington's Disease

Huntington's disease is a hereditary disorder (autosomal dominant transmission) that results in cognitive impairments and choreiform movements. In this disease, CB-1 receptor density tends to decrease in the brain, which has implications for the potential lack of effectiveness of CB-1 agonist use. The role of CB-2 receptor function in Huntington's disease is far from clear, but it appears that selective CB-2 agonists may reduce neuronal losses in the basal ganglia as a consequence of inhibition of the activation of glial cells.

There is a significant body of evidence that alterations in endocannabinoid function are linked closely with Huntington's disease. In postmortem studies and animal experiments, basal ganglia containing CB-1 receptors are lacking in sensitivity and function as a result of the accumulation of a mutant protein. These changes occur prior to the appearance of symptoms or signs in Huntington's disease, and they have been shown to be present in investigations of brain imaging using PET scanning. These latter studies have revealed marked decreases in CB-1 receptor density in the cerebellum, brain stem, and cerebral regions of the brain in individuals with Huntington's disease.

In contrast, CB-2 receptor levels are increased in several types of nerve cell in Huntington's disease, including glial in cells, astrocytes, and microglial cells. One clinical trial of patients taking cannabidiol (10 mg/day, n=15) reported a lack of improvement in symptoms of Huntington's disease. Furthermore, an investigation of nabilone versus placebo in Huntington's disease showed no real benefit. There are a number of single case reports both showing benefit or lack thereof of cannabis or nabilone treatment of Huntington's disease. The jury remains out on the efficacy of cannabis in Huntington's disease (Abramovici H. et al, ibid, 2013).

Amyotrophic Lateral Sclerosis

Anecdotal reports of cannabis smoking in human cases of amyotrophic lateral sclerosis (ALS) have described a variable reduction in muscle cramps and fasciculations caused by this disease. These observations are supported by the occurrence of some delay in disease progression in mouse models of ALS. In these experiments, delays in disease progression were associated with a longer survival in the animals. The results of human clinical trials of dronabil in patients with ALS, in a dosage range of 2.5–10 mg, revealed better sleep patterns and enhanced appetite, but there were no major effects on muscle fasciculations or cramps caused by ALS. Other studies have failed to show any significant benefit of dronabinol (10 mg/day) on symptom improvement in ALS (Abramovici H., ibid, 2013).

Amyotrophic lateral sclerosis (ALS) is often a devastating disease associated with neuro-inflammation. The ability of cannabinoids to suppress inflammatory responses has attracted much interest in their use for the management of ALS. Cannabinoids can reduce inflammatory mediators such as chemokines and cytokines in individuals with ALS, as projected from detailed animal studies. In humans with ALS, the spinal cord, brain stem, and cerebral cortex show evidence of motor neurone damage. The CB-2 receptor system seems to play a special role in ALS progression in animals and humans. For example, the administration of a CB-2 agonist can reduce disease progression in mouse models of ALS.

The disruption of neurological functions in ALS is related, in part, to altered cannabinoid receptor activity. As mentioned earlier, the occurrence of neuroinflammation in ALS may be inhibited by the reduction in inflammation-provoking chemokine and cytokine production. A treatment of ALS has been proposed using a terpenoid, tamoxifen. This terpenoid may have anti-inflammatory effects that may be shared with cannabinoids. Potential beneficial actions of cannabis may involve alterations of glutamine uptake in the CNS. Moreover, endocannabinoids have been shown to alter glutamatergic neurotransmission by indirect mechanisms that involve NMDA receptors (Abramovici H., et al ibid, 2013).

Human studies of cannabis treatment in ALS have produced mediocre outcomes. It was found in one study that 5 mg of THC had little effect on cramps, fasciculation, quality of life, sleep, or depression. Moreover, a trial of dronabinol in ALS was not universally successful, and the use of this drug was limited by psychoactive effects and excessive sedation. However, some surveys of cannabis use in ALS have produced benefits in motor functions, appetite, mood, and sleep. The neuroprotective effects of CBD (cannabidiol) appear to exceed those of THC. This observation provides promise for the expanded use of oral combined CBD/THC sprays (Sativex) in ALS management.

Spinal Cord Injury or Disease

Animal experimentation that involves the induction of spinal cord injury produces changes in neurological controls that are exerted by the endocannabinoid system. There is a paucity of data in humans on the use of cannabinoids to alleviate symptoms of spinal cord injury. Anecdotal benefits of cannabis smoking in spinal damage have been reported in humans, with some variable improvements in symptoms of pain, muscle spasms, spasticity, and difficulty in sleeping. Several well-controlled studies of cannabis analogues or pharmaceuticals have shown some value in the symptomatic management of spinal cord disorders, notably spasticity. These studies of spasticity treatment have involved the use of several preparations, including Sativex, oral THC (31 mg of delta-9-THC), rectal THC (43 mg of THC), administration of delta-9-THC or nabilone (0.5 mg bid.). In these studies the effects of the drugs on control of spasticity appeared promising (Abramovici H., et al ibid, 2013).

Multiple Sclerosis (MS)

An important approach to MS management is the modulation of immune response in what is considered to be an autoimmune disease. In this disease, myelin coverings of nerves are attacked, resulting in both structural and functional problems of neurones. Animal studies in the presence of experimental demyelination of nerves have shown positive benefits from cannabis use. It has been mentioned repeatedly in the literature that both the activation of CB-1 and CB-2 receptors in MS may reduce symptoms of spasticity, neuropathy, and tremor. Moreover, it is believed that CB-2 receptor activation plays a significant role in reducing advancement of disease as a consequence of its anti-inflammatory effects.

The neurodegeneration present in multiple sclerosis (MS) is due to inflammatory demyelination of areas in both the central and peripheral nervous systems. It is reported that the use of cannabis to attempt to reduce spasticity in patients with multiple sclerosis (MS) has been applied for more than a century with variable beneficial effects. Multiple sclerosis has been associated with regional changes in endocannabinoid concentrations, but results of several studies have been conflicting. In addition, cannabis has been recorded as effective in improving sleep, pain, anxiety, and depression in the patients with MS. Cannabis smoking has been popular among individuals with MS, but recommended dosages for symptomatic improvement are not well defined. The self-titration paradigm using cannabis smoking or vaping for symptom relief in MS has been suggested as a potentially effective approach.

There are conflicting data on the role of CB-1 and CB-2 receptor functions in MS. Animal studies indicate delta-9-THC, but not cannabidiol (CBD), reduce tremor and spasticity with a reduction of the overall severity of the disorder. It is clear that recurrent inflammatory processes in MS alter the natural history of this disease. While some debate exists on the potentially beneficial role of the immunomodulating effects of cannabis in

MS, it is likely that the neuroprotective/antioxidant actions are the most important aspect of the beneficial actions of cannabis in MS treatment.

There have been a significant number of human clinical trials of the oral administration of cannabinoid drugs in MS patients, including cannabis extracts, oral THC, dronabinol, nabilone, and nabiximols. These drugs are well tolerated in MS patients, and, in general, they have positive symptom-relieving effects. A specific area of benefit of cannabis medications in MS is the variable control of abnormal bladder function that is common in MS. Variable urinary symptom control has been noted in about 50 percent of patients with MS in clinical trials of Sativex, delta-9-THC, alone and cannabidiol, CBD, alone.

There is a wealth of clinical trial data on cannabis use in MS management. Table 91 summarizes some of the principal studies in MS (Abramovici H., ibid, 2013).

Table 91. Examples of clinical trials that have shown the use of cannabis-related products in the management of MS. Overall, results are positive. Note trials are rereviewed at end of this section (table 92).

Study	Results
CUPID study, the Cannabis Use in Progressive Inflammatory Brain Disease	A three-year UK study of the ability of orally administered to slow the progression of MS. The CUPID trial found no overall evidence to support an effect of delta-9-THC on the progression (course) of MS. Any observed benefit was restricted to patients with mild disabilities.

MUSEC Study, the Multiple Sclerosis and Extract of Cannabis trial	Twelve weeks of treatment with Cannador (2.5 mg of delta-9-THC with 0.9 mg of CBD per capsule) was associated with a reduction of patient reports of muscle stiffness, muscle spasms, pain, and sleep problems. The daily dosages of medication taken were 10–25 mg of delta-9-THC, with an accompanying 3.6–9 mg CBD.
Smoked Cannabis	Studies in MS have used standardized cannabis cigarettes. Reduction in spasticity and pain without effects on physical performance has been noted. Cognitive function predictably decreased in the short term.
CAMS study, Cannabis in Multiple Sclerosis Study	This examined the effects of cannabis extracts, Cannador in six hundred patients. There were no significant improvements in spasticity (measured by Ashworth Scale), but subjective improvements in patient-reported spasticity were noted.
Other studies	Nabiximols (Sativex) or standardized cannabis extracts have been shown to exert overall positive effects in MS. Nabiximols (Sativex) are marketed in Canada for the adjunctive treatment of spasticity and pain in MS.

Multiple Sclerosis Is an Autoimmune Disorder

There are several common autoimmune diseases, which include multiple sclerosis (MS), systemic lupus erythematosus (SLE), rheumatoid arthritis (RA), muscular dystrophy (MD), and Lou

Gehrig's disease (ALS). Many of these disorders affect the central nervous system in a variable manner. In simplistic terms, autoimmune disease involves the body's immune attack on its own tissues. Multiple sclerosis provides a good example of autoimmunity where damage to the myelin sheath around nerves (demyelination) disrupts nervous system communications.

The value of cannabinoids in MS is due to their interactions with CB-1 and CB-2 receptors that exert controls over nerve injury and apoptosis. These processes determine degrees of central nervous system damage that occur in MS. As implied earlier, the activation of CB-2 receptors appears to be neuroprotective. One mechanism of action of CB-2 receptor stimulation is interference with the function of microglia that cause inflammatory responses. There are favorable responses to THC administration as a consequence of altered expression of microRNAs, which play a role in the regulation of gene expression. These microRNAs are single-stranded forms of noncoding RNAs that can be altered by THC administration in mice.

The actions of microRNAs are complex. These substances are capable of suppressing the expression of genes and even silencing gene expressions. In addition, microRNAs can act to control the occurrence of myeloid cells (specifically myeloid-derived suppressor cells, MDSC). These types of myeloid cells are known to suppress inflammatory responses. These MDSC are more abundant in the presence of THC (Hegde, V. L., et al., *J. Biol Chem*, Nov. 7, 2013).

Multiple Sclerosis: NMSS Review of Trials

The National Multiple Sclerosis Society (NMSS, www.nationalmssociety.org) concedes that "better therapies are needed for distressing symptoms of multiple sclerosis—including pain, tremor, and spasticity—that may not be sufficiently relieved by available treatments."

The NMSS has summarized recent clinical trials of cannabis in multiple sclerosis, which are described in table 92.

Table 92. A review of recent clinical trials on cannabis use in MS, adapted from information available at www.nationalmssociety.org

Note there is some overlap with data shown in table 91.

Study	Result
Neurology: an e-published study ahead of print, April 2014	The effects of cannabis smoking on cognition were studied in patients with MS who smoked cannabis and were compared with noncannabis smoking controls. Individuals who smoked cannabis performed less well on several cognitive tests associated with abnormal patterns of brain activity, measured by functional magnetic resonance imaging.
A British placebo-controlled clinical trial using six hundred patients with different forms of MS	Subjects took capsules containing extracts of marijuana and THC. No objective improvement in spasticity was observed, but subjective improvements were noted in pain and spasticity in the cannabis-treated group. The study was interrupted as a consequence of unpleasant side effects in the active treatment group.
CUPID three-year clinical trial of dronabinol in individuals with primary or secondary progressive MS.	Study published in *Lancet Neurology* (2013) showed no effect of dronabinol on disease progression.

MUSEC study (2013) of oral cannabis extract in four hundred people with different types of MS.	Muscle stiffness improved two-fold in cannabis-treated patients, and improvements were noted in body pain, spasms, and sleep quality. Side effects included dry mouth, dizziness, headache, and urinary tract infections.
Sativex was used in well-controlled clinical trials to examine benefits in MS. *European Journal of Neurology,* March 1, e-pub. 2014)	This Sativex Spasticity Study showed that an oral spray significantly improved spasticity in a proportion of patients with MS who had been identified as likely to respond to therapy.
Impact of cannabis on cognition studied (*Neurology* 76 [2011]: 1153–60)	Twenty-five people with MS who smoked street cannabis were compared with twenty-five people with MS who did not use cannabis. Cannabis users performed worse on measures of information-processing speed, working memory, executive functions, and other cognitive functions. The study concluded that cannabis worsened cognitive problems in patients with MS.

Alzheimer's Disease and Dementia

Between five and six million Americans have Alzheimer's disease, which is the sixth leading cause of death in the United States. Alzheimer's disease (AD) is a common cause of dementia in the elderly (greater than sixty-five years of age). Pathological changes in the CNS of patients with AD involve the atrophy (degeneration) of neuronal tissue that links the cerebral cortex and the hippocampus. Studies on human brains show that CB-1 receptor expression may be sometimes reduced in the brain of people afflicted by AD, but CB-2 expression is upregulated to a significant degree (Abramovici, ibid 2013).

There is reasonable evidence to link dysfunction of the endocannabinoid system with Alzheimer's disease (AD). Memory deficits, cognition issues, and impairments of motor function are hallmarks of AD. The nervous tissue degeneration encountered in AD is believed to be caused by the deposition of amyloid protein (amyloid-beta protein) that causes local inflammatory responses in the brain, with the development of neurofibrillary tangles. Several animal studies show the role of the endocannabinoid system in general neuroprotection. It has been proposed that delta-9-THC may alter the function of acetylcholinesterase (ACHE) in AD. Changes in ACHE contribute to the formation of amyloid fibrils. In addition, cannabidiol (CBD) has some versatile neuroprotective actions in AD. These actions include antioxidant effects and inhibition of apoptosis.

Researchers have proposed that neuroprotective approaches to the management of AD may include the use of low doses of CB-1 and CB-2 receptor agonists or attempts to alter endocannabinoid degradation. The possibility of altering the function of the endocannabinoid system in AD with low-dose cannabinoid treatments may assist in the production of positive effects on the disease. These beneficial effects of cannabis could be mediated by anti-inflammatory effects, neuroprotective actions, retention of neurogenic activity, and inhibition of memory loss.

How does marijuana exert positive effects in MS? The favorable outcomes of cannabis use are most likely contributed by the well-described antioxidant and neuroprotective effects of cannabis (David Downs, online review, sfgate.com/smellthetruth/2014, 11, 29) and interference with the deposition of beta amyloid in the brain. A number of basic scientific observations support the proposal that delta-9-THC can lower the levels of amyloid-beta protein deposited in the brain. The presence of this protein is correlated with symptoms and signs of AD. Moreover, THC seems to exert its beneficial effects by positive actions on mitochondrial functions and inhibition of amyloid-beta aggregation.

An important finding in basic science studies is that THC works in a dose-dependent manner. Whether or not cannabis smoking or ingestion of cannabis prevents AD is not clear, but some experts have proposed that smoking in young adults could be a preventive measure against the development of AD in later years (in the elderly). In addition, it has been speculated that cannabis may slow the aging of nervous tissue. Cannabinoids are fat-loving chemicals (lipophilic agents) that are stored in adipose tissue and released at a slow rate over a period of one to three days. This slow release of THC is believed to help to prevent abrupt withdrawal symptoms after discontinuation of the drug.

There is only limited clinical research of cannabis compounds in the treatment of AD. It is reported that 5 mg/day of dronabinol (delta-9-THC) may have benefits in reducing behavioral disturbances in patients with AD, but its use is associated with a significant number of side effects (e.g., euphoria and fatigue). Trials of dronabinol in patients with severe dementia and AD imply that 2.5 mg at night of this drug has a calming effect on nocturnal agitation. It is not clear if the positive effects observed in AD are related to specific treatment effects of cannabinoids or if they are related to general sedative effects of delta-9-THC or cannabis analogues (e.g., nabilone). While the jury remains out on cannabis benefits in AD, it is generally accepted that insufficient evidence exists to support the general or routine use of cannabis in dementia management.

Pain Syndromes

The classification of pain syndromes into acute, subacute, and chronic types serves mixed purposes. The transition of acute to chronic pain is characterized by pain that remains for longer than the normal course of the illness or for more than three months. The prevalence of chronic pain in US adults is at least one in five people. There are many types and causes of chronic pain, some of which are summarized below in table 93.

Table 93. Some of the more common causes of chronic pain. All of these disorders have been treated with cannabis to a variable degree.

• headache	• nerve entrapment
• back pain	• neuropathy
• arthritis	• neuralgia
• tendonitis	• temporomandibular pain
• fibromyalgia	• complex regional pain syndromes

A number of clinical trials demonstrate the ability of marijuana smoking to ease neuropathic pain. Many of these trials have been of high quality and good outcome, with reports of the reduction of neuropathic pain in HIV patients by greater than 30 percent compared with placebo. Other studies using vaporized cannabis have shown promise in the management of chronic pain. Moreover, the role of cannabis inhalation, by both heavy and light smoking, has been found to reduce neuropathic pain of various causes in subjects who did not respond to other pain therapies. Many physicians who are treating chronic pain are prescribing cannabis in order to reduce opioid drug usage. This is an example of harm reduction by cannabis use (Collen, M.C., *Harm Reduction Journal*, 9, no. 1 [2012]).

The usual management of chronic pain involves the combination use of different analgesics and other specific classes of drugs, including antidepressants, anxiolytics, antiepileptics, muscle relaxants, sedatives, and opioids. However, drug use in many circumstances is not safe, as illustrated by a 425 percent increase in deaths from pain-relieving drugs (opioids) in a decade (approximately in the years 2000–2010). In contrast, medical cannabis prescriptions or smoking cannabis have been reported often to be associated with pain relief and secondary benefits such as reduction in muscle spasms, anxiety relief, reversal of depression, and improved sleep patterns.

Cannabis users often claim that pain is more bearable during a cannabis high or in states of lesser psychoactive effects. In one study, inhalations of 25 mg of 9.4 percent THC three times daily for five days' duration reduced intensity of chronic neuropathic pain and improved sleep (Ware, M. A. et al., *CMAJ*. 182, no. 14 [Oct. 5, 2010]: E694–E701, doi: 10.1503/cmaj.091414). In addition, the use of cannabinoids in analgesia has been reinforced in several other studies of chronic pain control. General advice on options to control chronic pain include recommendations for adjunctive use of topical pain killers, natural physical therapies, stress-reduction techniques, and a healthy lifestyle (Holt, S. et al., *The Topical Pain Control Revolution*, CreateSpace, Amazon 2013).

Headache, Migraine, and Cannabis

The hypothesis that headaches are a consequence of endocannabinoid deficiency has limited scientific support but strong positive speculation. Migraines, however, are believed in some circumstances to be precipitated by nitric oxide and calcitonin-gene-related peptide, which are inhibited by anandamide. In contrast, it appears that concentrations of anandamide are reduced in the cerebrospinal fluid of people with migraines. This latter finding supports the theory of Ethan Russo, MD, that migraines are an example of an endocannabinoid deficiency disorder that can be helped by cannabis.

The positive recommendations for cannabis use in headache treatment are not consistent with the knowledge that cerebrovascular spasm (vasoconstriction), and severe headaches have been associated on occasion with cannabis use. Up pops the paradox again! A headache is a well-documented adverse effect of the use of whole herbal cannabis or cannabis-derived pharmaceuticals, and it is sometimes a prominent symptom during cannabis withdrawal. Again, we see the double-edged sword of cannabis use.

Clinical studies of cannabis treatment of headaches are mixed, and many are quite anecdotal. Favorable reports of headache relief in cluster headaches and the uncommon condition of pseudotumour cerebi are not definitive. In one study, the use of cannabis was found to be quite frequent in patients with chronic or episodic cluster headaches, but its efficacy has been noted to be highly variable, ranging from modest benefit to occasional negative effects.

The Chatter between Cannabinoid and Opioid Systems

There is a body of evidence that supports the presence of bidirectional cross talk between opioid and cannabinoid systems in the brain and body. This evidence draws upon several observations of opioid and cannabinoid function. Animal studies show a degree of overlapping distribution of opioid and cannabinoid receptors in a variety of tissues. Both types of receptors process information that is transmitted during the processing of painful stimuli. Moreover, the two different receptor types play a role in the regulation of neurotransmitter release.

In preclinical studies, the administration of cannabinoid receptor agonists results in endogenous (from within) opioid peptide release. The evidence for communication (chatter) between opioid and cannabinoid systems is increasingly clear, and it is recognized that cannabinoids and opioids exert similar physiological effects, such as sedation, lowering of body temperature, lowering of blood pressure, reductions of gastrointestinal motility, inhibition of locomotor actions, and, of course, properties of antinociception.

It is often stated that cannabinoids have opioid-sparing effects, and there is a general opinion and evidence that cannabinoid/ opioid synergy (actions together) can increase the analgesic effects of opioids. Cannabinoids may contribute to a reduction in the tolerance that can develop to opioids. In simple terms, synergy acts to reduce the dosage of opioids required for a given pain-relief effect. This finding is very important for the potential to reduce opioid intake (dosage), which is a cause of much preventable death and disability. These inferences are supported by limited evidence from clinical trials (Abramovici, H, ibid 2013).

Studies in humans that rate differences between sensory responses to painful heat stimuli have failed to any significant difference in response between low-dose THC, morphine, and combined morphine/THC administration. That said, the use of a combination of THC and morphine may act in a synergistic manner in affective responses to painful thermal stimuli. A significant improvement in pain relief has been reported following inhalation of vaporized cannabis. Add to these findings the positive effects of 10 or 20 mg of dronabinol/per day on pain control, and it is concluded that opiate-induced analgesia is magnified by the coadministration of cannabinoids. These observations of synergistic effects are consistent with reports of reductions in fatal opioid overdose in some locations of cannabis legalization in the United States.

Cannabis and Sleep

Clinical trials have identified a beneficial effect of smoked cannabis, cannabis extracts, and several cannabinoid-type pharmaceuticals on sleep in a variety of circumstances. Table 94 summarizes diseases in which sleep benefits have occurred with cannabis use.

Table 94. Diseases in which beneficial effects on sleep have been observed. Information derived from use of smoked cannabis, dronabinol, nabilone, and nabixinols in various circumstances. Outcomes are variable and are considered in aggregate. Restoration of good sleep improves the well-being of many patients.

neuropathy	diabetic neuropathy
cancer pain	multiple sclerosis
noncancer pain	spinal cord injury
HIV wasting syndromes	amyotrophic lateral sclerosis
rheumatoid disease	fibromyalgia
inflammatory bowel disease	neurological bladder dysfunction
PTSD	anorexia in cancer

Benefits of Correcting Sleep Disorders

Cannabis use can assist in correcting poor sleep patterns, but it can cause sleep disturbances. It appears that chronic heavy use of cannabis can cause sleep disorders as a consequence of tolerance and withdrawal effects. Evidence exists that psychiatric and substance-abuse disorders are often associated with sleep problems, and normalization of sleep patterns can often improve disease symptoms.

The role of stress or stress-related diseases, such as post-traumatic stress disorder (PTSD), affect sleep in an adverse manner. Moreover, sleep disturbances play a significant role in generating negative symptomatology in substance-abuse problems or addiction. In summary, correction of sleep problems may play a versatile role in improving disabilities resulting from substance abuse, psychiatric disorders, and PTSD (and other diseases).

Cannabis has been shown to be valuable in correcting sleeplessness in several circumstances, and it is best applied where the benefits outweigh risks. However, caution is required because cannabis may exacerbate psychiatric disorders and exert a negative paradoxical effect on sleep when used in a chronic and heavy manner (Vandrey, R., et al., 26, no. 2 [2014]: 237–247, doi: 10.3109/095).

Sleep Apnea

Sleep apnea results in frequent breathing cessation of up to ten seconds or more. Individuals with sleep apnea have a greater incidence of fatigue, hypertension, headaches, stroke, and cardiac arrhythmias. Some studies have shown an increased prevalence of myocardial infarction (heart attack) in some sleep apnea patients.

Studies in animals have indicated that 9-delta-tetrahydrocannibol THC reduces disorders of breathing during sleep. In humans, the use of dronabinol (Marinol, a CB-1 and CB-2 receptor agonist) in dosages of 2.5–10 mg/day had positive effects scores of a baseline of hypopnea (reduced breathing). These promising effects of cannabis or cannabis analogues have not been fully confirmed in humans.

Conclusion

Cannabis has been used in a beneficial manner in many neurological disorders. While disease cures have not been experienced, cannabis forms a promising basis for the management of neurological diseases of diverse cause. For a comprehensive review of cannabis and neurological disorders, see Abramovici, H. et al., ibid. 2014.

Chapter 13

DIABETES MELLITUS

The prevalence of diabetes mellitus has reached epidemic proportions, and it is the third principal cause of death in the United States. A number of clinical studies or surveys indicate a lower prevalence of diabetes mellitus (type II), metabolic syndrome X, obesity, and insulin resistance in cannabis users. Cannabis users seem to have a lower chance of developing diabetes mellitus, even in the presence of greater caloric intake, which can occur as a consequence of appetite stimulation by cannabis. This protective effect of cannabis against diabetes is found in both cannabis users with modest and heavy intake of cannabis, but those with smaller intakes of cannabis appear to have even a lower prevalence of diabetes mellitus.

Data that demonstrates this positive trend of a lower occurrence of disturbed carbohydrate metabolism with cannabis use are apparent in repeated analysis of the National Health and Nutrition Survey Data (NHANES data) in the years 2005 to 2010. In these studies of more than 4,500 males and females, 12 percent were currently using cannabis, and 48 percent had experienced marijuana use. Marijuana consumers had lower fasting blood-insulin levels and increased blood concentrations of high-density lipoprotein (cholesterol associated with lower risks of heart disease). The reason for the association of cannabis use with better carbohydrate metabolism remains somewhat unclear.

Investigations using islet cells (insulin-secreting cells) of human origin show the presence of both CB-1 and CB-2 receptors. Stimulation of these receptors reveals a consistent positive effect of the CB-1 receptor on insulin and glucagon release, but the effects of CB-2 receptor stimulation results in some conflicting findings of both decreased and increased insulin secretion. Human studies of glucose metabolism, following the intravenous administration of delta-9-THC (6 mg) in healthy male subjects, show significant reductions in glucose tolerance following glucose challenge. These findings seem to be inconsistent with observations of favorable effects on diabetes that have been noted in survey studies (e.g., NHANES data). Experiments in dogs reveal increases in blood glucose with intramuscular administration of cannabis resin and in rats with the administration of a CB-1 receptor agonist. Clearly, much more human research is required (Abramovici H., ibid 2013).

Cannabis and Energy Controls in the Body

The endocannabinoid system appears to control energy balance by both central (CNS) and peripheral actions. The main central nervous system controls of energy balance are present in the hypothalamus and other areas of the brain that have substantial endocannabinoid receptor density. A large amount of experimental data collected in animals suggests that CB-1 receptor stimulation results in enhanced energy storage with lipogenesis. The effects of CB-1 receptor stimulation with cannabis and its prescription analogues form a basis for the treatment of cachexia and appetite loss in the presence of HIV, AIDS, cancer, and some neurodegenerative diseases.

> The cannabinoid receptors in the brain are known to regulate appetite and general body metabolism in complex ways. This has stimulated studies of what could be described as an axis of energy controls involving appetite, caloric intake, and insulin or glucagon responses (carbohydrate metabolism). Several studies have described the importance of endocannabinoid control in the overall regulation of energy balance. It is postulated that increased endocannabinoid tone exists in several tissues or organs in obese animals or humans. As noted earlier, impaired controls of the endocannabinoid system are associated in humans with obesity, metabolic syndrome, atherosclerosis, and type II diabetes mellitus.

Endocannabinoids play a pivotal role in altering the release of several neurotransmitter substances and a variety of neuropeptides with hormonal effects. These substances include opioids, serotonin, and GABA, all of which alter appetite. The endocannabinoids also affect the actions of hormones, such as leptin, ghrelin, and corticosteroids. The sum total of the overactivity of the endocannabinoid system may result in reduced expenditure of energy, increased nutrient uptake, and storage of energy, with or without consequential weight gain. The reader should not lose sight of many other factors that could alter outcome in these circumstances.

The role of cannabis in reducing the effects and production of stress hormones, such as glucocorticoids and catecholamines, may have favorable effects on stabilization of blood sugar. There is an emerging description of the role of CBD (cannabidiol) in diabetes management. The recognition that stimulation of the endocannabinoid system causes weight gain, resistance to actions of the hormone insulin, and abnormal blood lipids has prompted research with substances that can inhibit endocannabinoid functions. This research involved the use of rimonabant, which is an endocannabinoid receptor inhibitory drug. This drug has been removed from use following the occurrence of cases of severe depression that sometimes resulted in suicide.

Rimonabant, however, had several beneficial effects on blood glucose and cardiovascular parameters that are worthy of review. The SERENADE study was performed comparing the administration of 20 mg of rimonabant daily in combination with diet and exercise. In brief, the drug was found to decrease body weight, lower elevated blood pressure, improve insulin sensitivity, lower hemoglobin A1C levels, and reduce the occurrence of metabolic syndrome X. Some of these outcomes have been also noted with the use of CBD in animal and limited human observations. The benefits of CBD in diabetes mellitus are listed in table 95.

Table 95. A list of the proposed benefits of CBD (cannabidiol) in diabetes mellitus, based on animal and limited human studies or observations (adapted from Abramovici, H. et al., ibid. 2014)

- positive role in diabetic neurological complications (e.g., neuropathy)
- general anti-inflammatory effects
- neuroprotective activity
- protection against diabetic retinopathy in animals
- attenuation beta cell damage in type I diabetes
- decreased clot formation
- reversal of obesity with several secondary benefits
- favorable effects in metabolic syndrome X

Preliminary clinical trials with THC combined with CBD in humans have suggested that this combination may improve fasting blood-glucose levels in individuals with type II diabetes. This combination of cannabinoids reduces blood pressure and enhances pancreatic function. However, these outcomes require confirmation in further clinical trials. Moreover, recent research by GW Pharmaceutical (London, UK) has examined the potential benefits of tetrahydrocannabivarin (THCV) in preserving islet cell function with promising results.

Overall, anecdotal reports of the benefits of cannabis use in diabetic individuals stress improvements in blood-glucose control and general improvements in regional blood flow. The entity of diabetic gastroparesis (characterized by substantial delays in the emptying of the stomach) has been treated by cannabis with variable outcome. This work is confusing because cannabis seems to delay gastric emptying (in men), which would make gastroparesis worse. Secondary benefits of cannabis use in diabetic patients include improvement in sleep patterns and reductions of symptoms of diabetic peripheral neuropathy. Relaxation and improved sleep function from cannabis use is believed to benefit blood pressure control in diabetes. Furthermore, there are emerging reports of the ability of topical cannabinoids to reduce symptoms of neuropathy. Cannabinoid-containing creams may help reduce the pain and tingling found in diabetic neuropathy. This area of research involving topical cannabis is worthy of much further attention.

It is estimated that at the present time 18.1 million Americans use marijuana (7 percent of the US population). This use is increasing quite rapidly. Leading scientists have cautioned, and this book has indicated, that evidence used for supporting the benefits of cannabis is sometimes corrupted, or it varies in quality. That said, cannabinoids seem to alter the metabolic activity in diabetic individuals in a favorable manner, but risks and benefits of cannabis therapy in diabetes mellitus require further clarification. Table 96 describes the potential benefit of cannabis use in diabetes mellitus.

Table 96. The potential use of cannabis as therapy in diabetes mellitus. Much evidence of benefit remains anecdotal or is derived from animal studies.

- may help in blood sugar stabilization
- reduces catecholamines and glucocorticoids (stress hormones)
- neuroprotective

- reduction of inflammation with protection of myelin sheath around nerves
- reduction of pain by activation of CB-1 and CB-2 receptors
- reduction of muscle cramps and spasms
- reduction of intestinal spasms
- vasodilator effects with improved blood flow
- may reduce blood pressure in a variable manner
- cannabis or hemp oil in food products as a source of valuable unsaturated fats that are heart healthy (omega-6:omega-3 in a 3:1 ratio)
- topical cannabis for use in pain and tingling of neuropathy.
- improves restless leg syndrome (RLS) and poor sleep
- antioxidant effects

An excellent review of the role of cannabis and cannabinoids in diabetes management is found in Fisher, M. et al., *Br. J. of Diabetes and Vascular Disease* 10, no. 6 (2010): 267–273.

Endocannabinoids and Obesity

As discussed earlier, endocannabinoids and selected cannabinoids (or some of their analogues) have been shown to increase weight gain associated with increased food intake in experiments in animals. This circumstance occurs as a consequence of interactions of cannabinoids with cannabis receptors in the brain or peripheral nervous system. Moreover, there is a growing interest in what has been termed "the endocannabinoid deficiency syndrome" (of Russo). I believe that there is a condition of endocannabinoid excess (hyperendocannabinoidism) that has not been described in any detail but may be present in several diseases. Some measurements of endocannabinoids in different diseases have shown increased concentrations of these ligands. How other factors, such as increased density of CB receptors, fit in this picture and confound the situation remains to be defined.

It should be noted that there is variable activation of the peripheral endocannabinoid system in human obesity. Obese people have evidence of upregulation of their endocannabinoid system that is revealed by increase in concentrations of anandamide (AEA) and 2-arachidonoylglycerol (2-AG). This activity, involving the increase in AEA and 2-AG endocannabinoid ligands, occurs with changes in cannabinoid receptor expression. The end results of this activity include orexigenic effects, altered fatty acid synthesis, insulin sensitivity, glucose uptake, and utilization, with increased energy storage in fatty tissues of the body.

In an excellent review article entitled "Care and Feeding of the Endocannabinoid System," J. McPortland and his colleagues (2014) describe many interventions that modify the actions of the endocannabinoid systems in a variety of ways. Examples of these ways of modifying endocannabinoid systems include increases in ligand production, ligand inhibition, ligand removal or actions, alteration of cannabinoid receptor functions, and so forth.

The work of McPortland et al. (ibid. 2014) describes many ways to upregulate the endocannabinoid system. Some of these regulatory pathways that modify body functions are listed below (table 97).

Table 97. Examples of various factors that modulate the endocannabinoid system

• pharmaceuticals, including analgesics, antidepressants, anxiolytics, and anticonvulsants	• lifestyle interventions with massage, acupuncture, and botanical supplements
• diet and weight control	• exercise

The complexity and amount of accrued information on the functions of the endocannabinoid system cannot be summarized easily in this book. For a very valuable and comprehensive review on this subject of modification of endocannabinoid system functions, please refer to McPortland, J., (ibid. 2014) (published online, *PLOS One* 9, no. 3 (2014): 895–66).

Negative and Positive Effects of Cannabinoids in Diabetes Mellitus

While cannabis is known to have blood-glucose stabilizing effects, there are a number of negative effects of cannabis on blood-sugar control. Table 98 summarizes some of these issues.

Table 98. Negative effects on cannabis on blood glucose control

These suggested effects require further substantiation. Most changes refer to type II diabetes, but effects on type I diabetes may be favorable due to beneficial actions of CBD in autoimmune disease and some degree of inhibition of beta cell damage in the pancreas.

- Poor memory and lack of attentiveness in cannabis users can influence behavior and secondarily alter blood-sugar control.
- Increased appetite with cravings for sweet food caused by cannabis can cause high blood sugar (the munchies).
- Heavy use of cannabis has been associated with poor glucose tolerance and masking of low blood sugar by occasional confusion of diabetic symptoms with effects of the drug (cannabis).

Animal experiments have shown that THCV and cannabidiol can reduce cholesterol in the blood and liver. A series of observations reveal several potential benefits of cannabis in diabetic individuals. These benefits are summarized below and complement information listed in earlier tables (table 99).

Table 99. Potential benefits of cannabis in diabetes mellitus

Not all of these benefits have been shown to occur in an unequivocal or consistent manner in diabetic patients.

- stabilization of blood sugar
- reduction of arterial inflammation
- reduction of symptoms in neuropathy
- lowering of blood pressure with long-term use
- improved circulation
- reduction of intraocular pressure
- relief of muscle cramps and certain causes of abdominal pain

Endocannabinoids, Inflammasomes, and Diabetes

A pivotal study on the role of endocannabinoids that can act as triggers of inflammation has been performed by NIH scientists. Research in animals has demonstrated the ability of endocannabinoids to activate macrophages, which are associated with loss of beta cells (insulin-secreting cells) in the pancreas. The researchers showed that endocannabinoid activation results in the presence of an inflammasome protein complex in macrophages called Nrp3 inflammasome. This protein complex causes beta cell death and contributes to the progression of type II diabetes mellitus.

There are known differences between the natural history of certain diseases in animal models compared with humans' experiences. This situation of mismatch of observations has led scientists to focus their attention on the clinical effects of standardized cannabis-related drugs on type II diabetes (table 100), but results have been variable.

Table 100. Three randomized, controlled clinical trials with cannabinoids or analogues in type II diabetes

Note: Rimonabant has been removed from the market because of depression and suicide risk.

Stephen Holt, MD, DSc

Cannabinoid or Drug Activity	Clinical Effects	Clinical Protocol
Rimonabant (CB-1 antagonist) (withdrawn)	Decrease fasting glucose and insulin with reductions of insulin resistance.	RIO—Europe study of 20 mg of Rimonabant in 1507 obese patients.
Rimonabant (CB-1 antagonist (withdrawn)	Reduction of hemoglobin A1C in overweight diabetics.	RIO—Diabetes Rimonabant (5 or 20 mg/day) versus placebo in obese diabetics.
Sativex	Inconsistent analgesia in diabetic peripheral neuropathy.	Sativex compared with placebo in peripheral neuropathy. Mixed results.

Treating Complications of Diabetes

The potential treatment of common complications of diabetes mellitus has prompted much animal and human research. These common complications include cardiovascular disease, neuropathy, retinopathy, and nephropathy. Principal underlying causes of these diabetic complications are related often to the presence of vascular disorders and oxidative damage to tissues. Diabetic retinopathy has been treated in experimental animals with CBD (cannabidiol). This cannabinoid appears to have specific protective effects by reducing the expression of inflammatory and adhesion molecules (e.g., TNF and ICAM-1).

Cannabidiol (CBD) reduces the blood levels of VEGF (vascular endothelial growth factor), which is one of a group of inflammatory cytokines that is involved in the development of new blood vessel growth in body tissues. This reduction of VEGF induced by CBD is associated with an improvement in cardiovascular symptoms and a reduction in serum levels of other inflammatory cytokines (e.g., TNF-alpha and IFN-gamma). Cannabidiol (CBD) causes both anti-inflammatory effects and effects on the modulation of immune function. These observations are consistent with theories underlying the treatment and causation of type I diabetes that are considered to be autoimmune phenomena.

Neuropathy may be reduced in cannabis users by antioxidant actions derived from cannabis (reduction of oxidative stress). Extracts of cannabis are known to increase the levels of reduced glutathione in the liver—a powerful antioxidant effect. One may predict from these studies that Sativex, which combines THC and CBD, would be valuable in the management of neuropathy. However, some controlled clinical studies of Sativex have shown little advantages over placebos in circumstances of neuropathic pain. The reasons for this disappointing outcome have not been explained in a satisfactory manner (Abramovici, H., ibid. 2014).

Cannabis and Diabetes (Summary)

Cannabis has many actual and potential effects on the body that may be helpful in the management of diabetes mellitus. While the main application of cannabis in diabetes has been mostly for type II diabetics, some of the beneficial effects may be applicable to the management of type I diabetes. Foundations of knowledge to support cannabis use in diabetes are mainly anecdotal and often derived from animal experiments. Much further research is required in this area. Potential benefits of cannabis in diabetes are reiterated in line-item statements below (Abramovici, H., ibid, 2013).

- Cannabis may stabilize blood glucose by reducing catecholamine and stress-response hormones such as glucocorticoids (other mechanisms may operate).
- Cannabis posses clear anti-inflammatory properties by inhibiting effects of certain prostaglandins and cyclooxygenase (COX-2) enzymes. Cannabis is a free radical scavenger (antioxidant) that inhibits aspects of white cell function in macrophages and the production of tumor necrosis factor (TNF).
- Cannabis acts as a vascular relaxant (vasodilator) with some variable antihypertensive effects. It may enhance blood flow to tissues.
- Cannabis protects nervous tissue from damage (neuroprotective). In particular, cannabis could reduce

pain in diabetic neuropathy and prevent glycoprotein damage to myelin sheaths of nerves.

- Cannabis can improve sleep patterns, and it has a muscle-relaxing effect that can help to combat restless leg syndrome.
- Cannabis use has been associated with less obesity, improved carbohydrate metabolism, lower fasting insulin levels, less insulin resistance, and increases in blood levels of HDL (good cholesterol).
- Tetrahydrocannavarin (TCHV) has shown benefits by preserving islet cells (insulin-producing cells) in the pancreas. This circumstance is being investigated by G. W. Pharmaceuticals in the United Kingdom. The promise of this drug-development program is for the management of metabolic syndrome X and type II diabetes.
- Animal studies with CBD cannabidiol show prevention of diabetes, diabetic retinopathy (eye damage), and cardiomyopathy.
- Cannabinoids of selected types may be valuable in the management of several diabetic complications, but further research is required.
- In a study of cross-sectional data from NHANES111, marijuana use was independently associated with a lower prevalence of diabetes mellitus.
- Cannabis is neurogenic—causes growth of neurones in the brain.

Conclusion

There are several reports and websites that promote cannabis use for diabetes treatment in a zealous manner. The claims of benefits of cannabis in the management of diabetes mellitus are sometimes so pronounced that some scientists have protested the validity of such claims (Fisher, M. et al., ibid. 2010). One major problem is the inappropriate attempt to project results of experiments in cell cultures and animals to human circumstances. This situation continues to impact conclusions about much research on cannabis.

Chapter 14

INFECTIONS, HIV DISEASE, AND INFLAMMATION

The Association of Illicit Drug Use and Infection

Many studies demonstrate that the use of illegal drugs is associated with several types of infectious disease. Debility is caused by drug addiction, but other factors operate to increase rates of infection, including risky behavior, such as sharing utensils or needles used in drug delivery. Many scientists have acknowledged the effects of substance abuse and drug addiction on reducing immune function. Sometimes drug addicts engage in poor nutritional practices that further lower immune function. The emergence of HIV infection and the development of AIDS have focused much attention on the role of illicit drug use in the cause of increased susceptibility to opportunistic infections, largely because of immunodeficiency, which is the hallmark of AIDS. It is known that a large number of AIDS patients are intravenous drug abusers, and drugs of abuse have been considered often to make a contribution to the progression of HIV infection to full-blown AIDS, but opinions differ. In summary, the collapse of immune function in the patient with AIDS leads to a susceptibility to opportunistic infections with weaker pathogens that otherwise have a tendency not to infect the healthy individual.

Cannabinoids exert immunomodulating and immuno-suppressive effects by both receptor and nonreceptor interactions. Cannabinoids alter the function of several immune cells, including natural killer cells, T- and B-lymphocytes, and macrophages in animals and humans. Most information has accrued on the negative effects of THC on immune function, where reductions in host resistance to various bacteria and viruses may be observed. It has been recognized for more than twenty years that the administration of 9-delta-THC has a common effect on the suppression of certain specific immune functions in humans. These suppressive effects have also been noted in preclinical studies in animals or in vitro. Table 101 summarizes some of these effects.

Table 101. Suppression of immune activities by delta-9-THC (Abramovici, H., ibid. 2014)

- reduced antibody production
- impaired lymphocyte blastogenic transformation by mitogens
- reduction in the abilities of NK cells (natural killer cells) to exert cytotoxic effects on cancer cells
- diminished cytokine and chemokine production
- monocyte/macrophage function impaired by THC in a dose-related manner

Cannabis and Immune Phenomena

The role of cannabis or cannabinoids on changes in immune function is quite clouded, and there is still a dearth of research on this subject in humans. The net effects of cannabis on immune functions depend on several factors that are listed below (table 102).

Table 102. Factors that alter measures of immune function in the cannabis user

- route or method of drug delivery
- length of exposure to cannabinoids

- dosage and type of cannabis used
- specific receptor targeting
- experimental protocols
- investigator bias
- types of outcome measures
- patient or users health status

The endocannabinoid and immune systems appear to operate with some degree of coordination. That said, the effect of endocannabinoids or phytocannabinoids on immune functions are not readily predictable (table 103).

Table 103. These described effects of cannabis on immune function and some mechanisms of action are adapted from Abramovici, H. et al., ibid. Feb. 2013

- CB-1 and CB-2 receptors are present on immune competent cells.
- Immune cells metabolize endocannabinoids in a comprehensive manner.
- CB-2 receptor stimulation appears to be generally immunosuppressive, and CB-1 stimulation is a variable stimulus to promote immune activity.
- Cannabinoids affect the release of proinflammatory or anti-inflammatory cytokines, which affect the functions of the endocannabinoid system by upregulating receptor expression.
- Low doses of THC appear to be immunostimulatory with proinflammatory effects, but higher dosages appear to be immunosuppressive.
- THC and CBD alter cell-mediated and humoral immunity.
- Cannabinoids may stimulate or inhibit proinflammatory cytokine release.
- CBD causes a shift in TH1/TH2 balance.
- Immunosuppressive and anti-inflammatory actions of cannabinoids may diminish host defenses to infection.

The suppression of resistance to infections by the combination of AIDS and cannabis use has been demonstrated in both animal models and humans. For example, HIV-positive smokers of cannabis appear to be prone to develop herpes virus infections. Moreover, smokers of marijuana have abnormal function of alveolar macrophages. These abnormal functions result in decreased bacteriocidal and phagocytic activity in pulmonary macrophages. Cannabinoid receptors (especially of the CB-2 type) are expressed to a major degree on cells involved in immune processes, and these receptors control cytokine or chemokine production (e.g., tumor necrosis factors, TNF). In addition, it is important to reiterate that many ancillary factors operate in providing optimum host defenses (e.g., hormonal controls and good nutrition).

A Note on Bacterial Infection

Methicillin-resistant staphylococcus aureus (MRSA) is sensitive to the antibacterial actions of marijuana. This antibacterial action of cannabinoids was demonstrated in six different strains of MRSA that are associated with human infection. MRSA infections cause 18,000 deaths (perhaps 23K) in the United States, and it affects approximately 94,000 individuals. Mortality from this cause of infection is increasing.

While CBD and CBG are strong inhibitors of methicillin-resistant staphylococcus aureus (MRSA), certain terpenoids in cannabis have similar effects. Pinene appears to be particularly effective against MSRA, and it shares the common benefit of many monoterpenoids. For example, pinene can enhance permeability of the skin to other drugs. Thus, one may be able to enhance the transdermal delivery of antibiotics or certain drugs with several different types of terpenes. An exciting recent discovery is the antibiotic teixobactin that appears to have versatile and potent effects against superbugs. Would this new antibiotic benefit from the addition of cannabis?

Lyme Disease

Lyme disease is caused by infection with the bacterium Borrelia burgdorferi, which is transmitted by the bite of a tick. Three stages of Lyme disease are recognized: stage 1, primary Lyme disease; stage 2, secondary Lyme disease (disseminated Lyme disease); stage 3, tertiary Lyme disease (chronic persistent Lyme disease). Despite many anecdotal reports of the value of cannabis in Lyme disease, controlled studies have not been performed to any significant degree and are long overdue.

Prions

Cannabidiol has been shown to inhibit prion accumulation in preclinical studies. Prions are proteins that can cause spongiform encephalopathy, such as mad cow disease and Creutzfeld-Jakob disease. Researchers in France and the United States have shown that CBD can inhibit prion infections of neurons and protect neurons against prion toxicity.

Antiviral Actions

Many studies on immune function in animals and humans indicate antiviral actions of cannabis, but paradoxical effects have occurred with worsening of viral disease in some cases. Cannabinoids are capable of modulating immune function by direct actions on immune-competent cells. In addition, cannabinoids have been shown to play a role in increasing host resistance to several infectious agents by actions on secondary immune responses.

Resistance to infections with murine retroviruses, herpes simplex virus, and modification of several different types of bacterial infections has been studied with cannabis use (e.g., Staphylococcus, Listeria, Treponema, and Legionella). In several animal experiments, cannabinoids alter the production and functions of cytokine networks. The overall actions of cannabinoids on immune function are complex, and they involve immunomodulatory effects. Under certain circumstances, cannabinoids may have immunodepressant effects, which could act to enhance disease progression. It appears that cannabis can inhibit the progression of HIV and perhaps hepatitis C viral infections to some degree. Of major interest are recent suggestions that certain cannabinoids could play a role in the management of Ebola virus infection, but this hypothesis has not been tested.

Cannabis and Ebola Virus

There are claims that compounds with antiretroviral properties are contained within cannabis. These compounds could exert beneficial effects on Ebola virus infection (Brad Morehouse, www.newcure.com). The favorable effects of cannabis use on HIV spread and Lyme disease have encouraged some individuals to believe in potential benefits of cannabis in Ebola virus infection, but these diseases have different characteristics.

The rational for using cannabis to fight Ebola virus comes from observations that Ebola kills by the induction of an inflammatory "cytokine storm." This storm is alleged to be amenable to interruption by cannabis, but objective evidence is lacking.

Cannabinoids and the Immune System: Focus on HIV/AIDS

There are many described effects of cannabinoids on immune function. These effects occur notably as a consequence of the suppression of cellular, cytokine, and chemokine actions. Much interest has focused on the ability of cannabis to contribute to the management of HIV infection and AIDS. Several relevant findings are summarized in table 104.

Table 104. Cannabinoids and the immune system with special reference to HIV disease and AIDS (adapted from Abramovici H. et al., ibid, 2014)

Action	Comment
Cellular effects	Cannabinoids alter the functions of T cells and B cells. They can interfere with the proliferation and cytolytic activity of natural killer cells (NK), theeby reducing defenses against cancer and microbes.

Cytokine/hormone effects	Cytokines provide instructions to macrophages and Th cells. These actions are modulated by cannabinoids. Immune functions may be altered by changes in hormone release with overall inhibitory effects on immunity.
Cannabinoid use in AIDS or HIV infection	Cannabinoids may induce apoptosis in immune cells with a resulting decrease in inflammatory responses, but they do not appear to adversely effect HIV disease, as measured by HIV-RNA levels and CD4 or CD8 cell counts.
Therapeutic actions of cannabis	Improvements in mood, creativity, sensory experiences, appetite and socialization are noted with cannabis use in patients with AIDS/HIV. Cannabinoids may treat pain, nausea, vomiting, muscle spasms and other general symptoms in AIDS/HIV disease. Marijuana is used by a large number of individuals with HIV infection (up to about 60 percent of patients).
Pain management in AIDS	Neuropathic pain affects one in three individuals with AIDS. Animal and human studies confirm pain relief in a reasonably consistent manner in the short term. There appears to be a lessening of pain intensity and an increased ability to tolerate pain with cannabis use in HIV disease.

Wasting syndrome (cachexia)	This unpleasant stage of disease may herald the death of HIV patients. It results from a combination of reduced food intake, specific nutritional deficiencies, and catabolic events. Cannabis has favorable effects on weight gain in this condition.
Antiemetic action and appetite improvement	The ability of cannabis to reduce vomiting is complex. Both THC and CBD can exert favorable antiemetic effects. The analysis of collected data from several published clinical trials confirm the valuable antiemetic affects of cannabis. Cannabinoids have been shown to increase food intake and appetite in several studies. Dronabinol and cannabis have both been shown to increase weight gain.
Mood and emotion	Psychiatric and psychological disorders are increased in HIV disease. Depression is common and it may increase disease progression from HIV disease to AIDS. Cannabinoids (CBD and THC) can help alleviate depression, reduce stress and improve sleep by modulation of serotonergic transmission in the CNS.

Reviewing Effects of Cannabis in HIV and AIDS

Immune function and the activity of cannabinoid receptors are inextricably linked. As noted earlier, cannabinoid receptors of the CB-1 type are found mainly in tissues of the nervous system, and CB-2 receptors are present mainly in immune tissues, with specific concentrations on lymphocytes and macrophages. Both CB-1 and CB-2 receptors are proteins with seven regions that span the cell membrane. The portion of these receptors present within the cell differs, and this accounts for differences in receptor response to ligands (endocannabinoids). Cannabinoids can alter immune reactions in the brain and tissues of the body by both direct and indirect actions on immune-competent cells.

Cannabis can reduce the actions of cytotoxic leucocytes and can compromise natural killer (NK) cell function. NK cell functions have a pivotal role in defenses against cancer and microbial infections. Moreover, cannabinoids alter the actions of certain cytokines by affecting their production from macrophages or other immune cells. In addition, the effects of cannabinoids on hormone release can result in changes in immunity. For example, it has been shown in animals that THC administration can increase corticosteroid levels and levels of adrenocorticotropic hormones, with consequential secondary depression of certain immune functions.

It has to be appreciated that there has been much research that implicates cannabis in the suppression of immune function. One notable study from the University of South Carolina shows that cannabis can stimulate the production of myeloid-derived suppressor cells (MDSCs), which work to inhibit immune functions (studies reviewed in ScienceDaily.com/releases/2010/11.). It is believed that this may make cannabis users more susceptible to infections and cancer. The proposals that MDSCs can actually promote cancer growth as an indirect effect of cannabis use are quite worrisome. Other studies have shown increases in MDSCs due to the actions of interleukin-1 beta that is produced by certain tumors. The end result is weakening of immune function that favors interference with the actions of cancer-killing immune cells.

With cannabis use, about one in three patients with HIV or AIDS may experience variable relief of pain, nausea, loss of appetite, and wasting (cachexia). Immunodeficiency leaves the HIV/AIDS patient vulnerable to a host of opportunistic infections, resulting sometimes in the development of tuberculosis, infectious diarrhea, meningitis, pneumonia, and encephalitis. It is the presence of a low CD4 plus T cell count with development of infections that often defines the progression of HIV infection to AIDS.

Cannabis use improves the tolerance of patients to antiretroviral therapy for AIDS, such that individuals are 3.3 times more likely to continue high-dosage administration of antiretroviral therapy. In addition, certain components of cannabis may have direct antiviral effects against HIV. As mentioned earlier, a compound found in cannabis called denbinobin has been shown to slow HIV replication. It is notable that while Marinol is a common drug used in HIV/AIDS therapy, many afflicted patients prefer whole herbal cannabis.

Cannabis (cannabinoids) has been used widely in the management of AIDS with reasonable safety and without much evidence of interference with the efficacy of antiretroviral therapy (e.g., indinavir or nelfinavir, examples of protease inhibitor drugs). However, drug treatment (chemotherapy) for HIV disease can have notoriously unpleasant side effects, such as nausea, vomiting, reduced appetite, weight loss, headaches, and other mixed symptoms of gastrointestinal upset. Favorable reduction in unpleasant side effects caused by antiretroviral therapy has been reported with cannabis use in many surveys of patients with HIV disease or AIDS.

Pain in HIV Disease

Despite the application of various common treatments, neuropathic or muscular pain reduces quality of life in one-third of patients with HIV disease. In well-controlled clinical trials, cannabis smoking has been shown to ease neuropathic pain in many patients with sensory neuropathy due to HIV disease. Research has also shown beneficial outcomes with cannabis in the control of muscular and other types of chronic pain. As discussed earlier, a number of scientists have pointed to the synergistic (additive or helper effects) of cannabinoids and opioids in pain control. Furthermore, recent studies imply a significant reduction in opioid dosage is possible in AIDS patients, with the addition of cannabis to treatment regimens. This circumstance is advantageous in the presence of a need for protracted palliative treatment in AIDS, and it is a safer treatment approach than the use of opioid painkilling drugs alone.

Wasting syndromes are a common result of advanced AIDS. The syndromes are recognized by a loss of greater than 10 percent of body weight and at least thirty days of diarrhea, fever, or general weakness. In AIDS wasting, reduced food intake, nutrient malabsorption, and altered body metabolism with dominant catabolism are often present. These circumstances are often partially correctable with the use of cannabis. The antiemetic actions of cannabinoids are due to their binding on CB-1 receptors. While CB-1 agonist drugs suppress nausea and vomiting, the reverse occurs as a consequence of CB-1 antagonist administration. In recent research, the benefits of cannabidiol CBD as an antiemetic in AIDS patients have been demonstrated.

In summary, a number of medical reviews and studies of the antiemetic properties of cannabis show that cannabinoids are active and effective, often with a degree of superiority to other drugs that are used to prevent vomiting. As mentioned, in addition to antiemetic effects, cannabis smoking can improve appetite and increase weight gain in HIV-positive individuals. Management of symptoms of HIV disease is a very common reason for illicit or legal cannabis use. In brief, cannabis seems to be quite effective in HIV-related symptoms, such as nausea, vomiting, appetite loss, pain, anxiety, and depression. Sometimes troublesome psychoactive effects can be experienced that limit dosage or acceptance of treatment (Abramovici, H. et al., ibid. 2014).

Psychiatric disorders are common in patients with AIDS or HIV infection. The most common mental disorders in AIDS patients include depression, dysthymia, anxiety disorders, and panic attacks. There are several possible causes or contributory factors to psychiatric disease in HIV patients, including life situations, effects of HIV on the brain, nutrient deficiencies, and side effects of drugs. Overall, cannabis use and dronabinol treatments have positive effects on the mood of individuals with HIV disease. Depression can have a negative effect on the clinical course of the HIV-infected patient. Depressed mood limits healthy behavior, and, as stressed earlier, it has been reported that depression can accelerate the course of HIV infection to the development of AIDS. In many clinical observations, however, cannabis is credited with reducing stress and improving sleep in the AIDS patient. Furthermore, cannabis appears to have valuable and specific antidepressant effects in some people, but THC can cause anxiety.

Inflammation

There are many anti-inflammatory actions of cannabis, which are summarized in table 105. These anti-inflammatory actions of cannabis can contribute to pain control in HIV or AIDS or other diseases that are associated with active inflammation.

Table 105. Anti-inflammatory actions of cannabis contents, summarized from Russo, E. B., *Pain Management*, sixth edition (2002): 357–375

- THC inhibits prostaglandin E-2 synthesis.
- Cannabis smoking may decrease platelet stickiness.
- Cannabichromene is more effective than phenylbutazone in reducing experimentally induced edema in a rat's paw.

- Cannabidiol may function as both a cyclooxygenase and lipo-oxygenase inhibitor in laboratory assays.
- THC has variable effects on the production of tumor necrosis factor (TNF).
- Delta-9-THC inhibits the conversion of arachidonic acid into metabolites derived from cyclo-oxygenase activity.
- Cannabidiol may be useful in the treatment of collagen-induced arthritis (demonstrated in animal models of rheumatoid disease).
- Nutritional benefits of hemp seed or hemp oil are apparent as a consequence of the presence of linolenic acid, which promotes the presence of anti-inflammatory metabolites and reduces the production of proinflammatory compounds from arachidonic acid.
- Flavonoids and terpenoid compounds in cannabis have anti-inflammatory effects.
- Apigenin is a flavonoid that inhibits the expression of cytokine-induced genes and exerts anti-inflammatory actions, and quercetin is a highly active free-radical scavenger (antioxidant).
- Eugenol and Cannflavin A and B inhibit prostaglandin function.

Conclusion

An expanding role of cannabis use or cannabis-related drug use is present in infectious diseases. The anti-inflammatory effects of cannabis have broad uses.

Chapter 15

SKIN DISEASE AND REPRODUCTIVE HEALTH

Cannabis and Skin Disease

On the one hand, cannabis has been reported to increase the severity of some skin problems, and on the other, cannabinoids have been reported to form a basis for the development of therapeutic agents for skin disease. The presence of a well-developed endocannabinoid system in the skin implies that certain cannabis components (notably phytocannabinoids) can have a major impact on skin physiology. It has been demonstrated that anandamide can regulate genes that control skin differentiation through actions on DNA methylation (an epigenetic effect).

Investigations into the response of skin differentiation genes to cannabinoids show significant effects on DNA methylation in preclinical laboratory studies. These studies showed that cannabidiol and cannabigerol act as transcriptional repressors that control cell proliferation and differentiation by mechanisms of epigenetic control. These compounds form a basis for the treatment of certain skin diseases (Pucci, M. et al., *BJP*, doi: 10.111/bph 12309).

There are several properties of cannabis that support its healing benefits in skin diseases. Cannabis is believed to combat inflammation, reduce pain, modulate the immune system, exert some antibacterial or antiviral actions, and produce a status of body relaxation by reducing anxiety and stress. While rigorous controlled trials of cannabis in various skin diseases have not been performed, cannabis has shown increase promise in the management of several skin disorders (table 106).

Table 106. Skin disorders that may or may not benefit from topical or oral cannabis use (adapted from www.unitedpatientsgroup.com blog 2014/04/08).

Skin Disease	Comment
Acne	Most reports support the use of cannabis in acne treatment, but smoking marijuana has been reported to aggravate acne (see text).

Eczema	Eczema may be precipitated by stress or environmental issues (e.g., contact with allergens, including cannabis itself). Topical THC has been reported to be variably effective in eczema management, and it has a specific role in managing allergic inflammation due to contact sensitivities.
Psoriasis	Sometimes referred to as an autoimmune disorder, cannabis has shown anecdotal evidence of the relief of psoriasis (see text).
Rosacea	This skin disease causes reddening and dry skin on the face, cheeks, and chin. The effects of cannabinoids on rosacea are thought to be due to control of inflammation. Topical cannabinoid (CBD) use appears to be more effective than cannabis smoking.
Skin cancer	Cannabis is not able to be defined as a skin-cancer cure, but it has several antitumor actions.
Shingles, herpes, warts, and skin infections	Cannabis (CBD) is described as variably effective in anecdotal circumstances.

There appears to be a move away from the management of skin disease by cannabis smoking. Vaporization or oral sprays and topical preparations seem to be favored.

Cannabis Effects on Skin

Many studies confirm the immune-modulating, anti-inflammatory, or antibacterial properties of cannabis on the skin. Cannabis components may exert benefits when applied topically or in some cases when administered by the oral route (vapor, sprays, edibles, pills, tinctures, etc.). Unfortunately, much of the effects of cannabis on the skin have been demonstrated in preclinical or animal studies, sometimes with questionable relevance to humans.

Early observations on the use of cannabis in skin-disease treatment were made from experiences with smoking. These studies were complicated by the fact that smoking causes skin damage via several different mechanisms of action, especially if tobacco is used in a mix with marijuana. Smoking generates free radicals that cause oxidative damage and premature skin aging. Cannabis use has been associated with increases in testosterone concentrations that arguably may make certain skin disorders worse (e.g., acne). The exacerbation of acne by cannabis has been countered by strong opinions that cannabis can be effective treatment for acne. The reasons for these apparent paradoxical effects are not known.

Studies have shown beneficial effects of cannabis on itching (pruritus). In one study performed in Germany, there was reduction of itching with the topical use of the N-palmitoylethanolamine. The role of cannabis in both causing and treating contact allergic dermatitis is not entirely clear, but studies in mice show a benefit of topical cannabinoids for the reduction of inflammatory skin lesions.

Transdermal Delivery of Cannabis Compounds

The permeation of cannabinoid into the skin is under active investigation. Not only does the skin absorption of cannabis have relevance for the therapy of skin disease, it may be important in the management of soft-tissue injury or local joint pain or peripheral neuropathy. It seems clear that cannabinoids may be more effective and bioavailable when given by topical means, containing carrier substances (e.g., fatty acids or emu oil or DMSO or liposomes).

There are several patents that have been filed on the transdermal delivery of cannabis. The application of cannabis compounds by patches has been favored because of the opportunity to provide a focused and controlled delivery of cannabinoids. Skin patches can be created with reservoirs that may be filled with pain-control agents or cooling additives such as menthol and camphor. There does not seem to be much evidence that topical cannabis can relieve headache, but the scalp may be a favorable place for cannabinoid absorption because of its density of sebaceous glands and hair follicles (Smith, C.K., www.compassioncenter.net/topical-cannabispreparations).

In summary, the hydrophobic properties of cannabis interfere with its ability to transport across the aqueous layer of the skin. This circumstance may be assisted by transdermal carriers that can be used in creams, ointments, gels, and on dermal patches. It appears that cannabidiol (CBD) and cannabinol (CBN) permeate in concentrations ten-fold higher than delta-8-tetrahydrocannabinol. The local absorption of cannabinoids may be advantageous in eliminating the psychoactive effects of THC and accessing specific types of pain by local application to joints and cutaneous nerves.

Acne

The Internet provides confusing information about the role of cannabis in the causation and progression of acne. This information either alleges that acne is caused by cannabis smoking, or it can be prevented and treated by cannabis administration. This circumstance is perhaps due to paradoxical or other effects such as difference in dosages of medications. There is convincing evidence that cannabinoids may modulate lipid synthesis in sebaceous glands in humans and dose-dependent effects on sebum secretion seem to operate. The role of excessive sebum production in acne is unquestionable. While low dosages of cannabidiol (CBD) have little effect on sebum production, it is reported that higher dosages of CBD induce cell death (apoptosis) in sebocytes. These data seem to support the use of CBD in acne treatment by modulating sebum production (Russo, E. B., "Taming THC," *Br J of Pharmacol* 163 (2011): 1344–1364).

The role of the endocannabinoid system in the control of skin differentiation and growth has been elucidated in recent research (www.jci.org/articles view 64628, Olah, A. et al., 2014). Most attention has focused on the sebostatic value of cannabidiol (CBD) on sebum secretion and its anti-inflammatory actions on sebocytes. Complex experiments in cultured sebocytes and human skin show inhibition of sebocyte lipogenesis by CBD. In addition, CBD has definitive anti-inflammatory actions. These findings provide support for the potential value of CBD in the treatment of acne.

The mechanisms of the effects of CBD involve a so-called trinity of cellular actions (Olah, A. et al., ibid. 2014), which include a reduction in lipogenesis (a lipostatic effect). In addition, the trinity includes an antiproliferative effect associated with reduction in proinflammatory mediators. Other factors may account for the favorable effects of CBD on acne treatment, such as interference with comedone formation as a consequence of hyperkeratinisation and interference with the overgrowth of strains of bacteria that cause acne (e.g., Proprionibacterium acnes).

The entourage effect of cannabis is relevant to acne management, especially in relationship to the terpenoid content of cannabis. The terpenoids limonene and linalool inhibit the growth of Propionibacterium acnes, which is a well-defined pathogen in acne. These essential oils (linalool and limonene) have added anti-inflammatory effects in acne by reducing the production of tumor necrosis factor (TNF) that is generated as a consequence of infection with Proprionibacterium acnes. The adjunctive actions of linalool and limonene with CBD appear to offer the possibility of the transdermal application of safe antiacne therapies (Russo, E. B., ibid. 2011).

Skin Esthetics with Cannabis

There is increasing popularity of hemp-seed oil formulated in topical products for both medicinal and aesthetic use. Some of these products are attempting to be "all natural" by the elimination of parabens, sulfates, and other artificial ingredients. There are now several brands of cannabis-containing lotions, creams, shampoos, soap products, and conditioners. Essential oils with desirable smells are added to these products. These products are often focused for sale to women consumers who purchase more than three-quarters of these types of product. The combination of aromatherapy and topical cannabis products are forecast to become increasingly popular. Unfortunately, many types of dried herbal cannabis have a bad smell.

Psoriasis

Cannabinoids have several properties that may be helpful in the management of psoriasis. Cannabinoids inhibit keratinocyte proliferation, have anti-inflammatory effects, and regulate several aspects of immune function. The study of four different cannabinoids (THC, CBD, CBN, and CBG) on rapidly proliferating keratinocytes showed inhibition of growth. These data imply a role for cannabis in psoriasis management and support the anecdotal findings of improvement in psoriatic skin lesions with cannabis.

Cannabis and Pruritus

Cannabis has shown promise in the treatment of itching (pruritus) in both clinical trials and anecdotal studies. Early studies have shown the benefit of cannabis (THC, 5 mg per day) in persistent itching due to cholestatic jaundice. Some benefits of cannabinoid agonists have been reported in pruritus (e.g., Sativex and HU-210). Cannabis-related products can be effective by both systemic and topical use. The use of cannabis-containing creams was shown to reduce dry skin and itching in a substantial proportion of patients with uremia. These potential benefits of cannabis on the relief of itching seem to be underutilized in clinical practice.

Stephen Holt, MD, DSc

Sexual Health and Function

Studies on the effects of cannabis on sexual function and behavior have produced a number of conflicting results. There is no doubt that CB-1 receptor function plays a role in many aspects of sexual function by acting on the central nervous system. These actions are associated with a variety of changes in sex hormone profiles or other hormonal changes that are involved in the hypothalamic-pituitary-axis. There is a general perception that cannabis promotes sexual behavior in women, but the reverse appears to be more likely in men.

The effects of cannabis on human sexual function and behavior are usually dose-dependent. At high dosages, negative effects on sexual behavior are to be expected, but these effects are not experienced consistently in women. However, at modest dosages in women, cannabis may exert beneficial effects on sexual activity, with increased sensitivity to tactile stimuli and general increases in sexual desire and responses. In men, effects are not so clear, but heavy, long-term use of cannabis can dampen sexual drive and possibly contribute to erectile dysfunction (ED). Low-dose cannabis use has been reported to improve sexual desire in an inconsistent manner. These effects on sexual function in men and women have been assumed (perhaps erroneously) to be consequences of the psychoactive effects of cannabis caused by THC.

Reports of the effects of cannabis on testosterone levels in men are confusing. It would appear that long-term, heavy use of cannabis lowers testosterone levels. Studies of men who smoked up to twenty joints per day have shown declines in the function of spermatozoa and abnormal structure of sperm. These changes on sperm function are proposed to be significant in men who have borderline infertility problems. One alarming association between cannabis use and reproductive organ health is a reported two-fold increased risk of developing testicular germ-cell tumors. This association of cannabis and cancer requires further study, but it has been questioned.

Reproduction and Sex

Endocannabinoids play a major role in the controls of human reproduction (Moccarone, M. et al., *Prog. Lip. Res.* 48 (2009): 344–54). These ligands are known to control implantation of the embryo and fetal development in females and spermatogenesis in males (sperm survival, motility, and acrosome reactions). The role of the endocannabinoid anandamide in reproductive processes has been demonstrated to occur as a result of significant CB-1 receptor interactions. However, there is a role of the CB-2 receptors in spermatogenesis that has been demonstrated by studies of the endocannabinoid 2-arachidonoylglycerol (2-AG).

Long-term, heavy use of cannabis alters levels of reproductive hormones, and it may impair normal sexual function, at least by causing occasional aberrant behavior. While some studies or surveys have shown the promotion of sexual activity or promiscuous behavior as a consequence of cannabis use in young females, males can tend to experience low libido, reduced sperm counts, and diminished testosterone levels. As reported earlier, these changes can result in infertility in men and lack of sexual drive. There are suggestions that cannabis can increase testosterone production in females, with resulting reductions in ovulation and interference with the regulation of menstrual cycles. This seems to be more common in teenagers.

There is a common occurrence of infertility in advanced nations (about one in five to seven couples). The endocannabinoid systems of control play a role in sexual function and fertility by actions on both CB-1 and CB-2 receptors. The main functions of delta-9-THC on the regulation of human reproduction are summarized in table 107.

Table 107. A summary of delta-9-THC effects on reproductive function in men and women

FEMALES	MALES
• Interference with oviductal transport of embryo	• Sperm survival diminished
• Interference with embroyo implantation	• Motility of sperm diminished
• Interference with fetal development	• Acrosome reaction diminished

Many of the actions listed in table 106 can be explained by the effects of anandamide with perhaps other changes in the endocannabinoid system. Of major relevance is the function of the anandamide-degrading enzyme fatty acid amide hydrolase (FAAH). Interference with FAAH increases anandamide. High levels of anandamide are believed to be predictors of miscarriage in some women.

The CB-2 receptor is believed to exert variable control over reproductive functions, including placentation, communications between mother and fetus, interactions between sperm and oocytes, and embryo development. CB-2 receptor function is stimulated by 2-arachidonoylglycerol (2-AG). Clearly, a well-orchestrated balance between CB-1 and CB-2 receptor activity is an important determinant of fertility. Disruption of this balance alters fertility by complex actions.

Endocannabinoids and the Fetus or Newborn

Several studies have demonstrated the presence of endocannabinoids or phytocannabinoids in breast milk. As defined earlier, endocannabinoids are lipid-ligands that have properties of neuromodulation. It has been proposed that endocannabinoids teach or guide suckling processes in newborns. The activation of CB1 receptors by endocannabinoids seems to be critical in the breast-feeding infant, perhaps by exerting effects on the motor muscles in the mouth of a baby. It has been suggested that cannabinoids of specific types may have important beneficial applications in newborns who exhibit failure to thrive or who are born with metabolic diseases such as cystic fibrosis, but further research is required.

Population studies that have examined the short-term effects of cannabis use in women during pregnancy have often been inconclusive in their outcome. Some studies, however, have associated cannabis use in pregnancy with small babies, increased occurrence of sudden death in babies, and failure to thrive. Of major concern is the association of cannabis use in pregnancy with the later occurrence of attention-deficit disorders (ADD and ADHD) and disordered cognitive function in children.

Thus, cannabis exposure in pregnancy appears to have some distinct long-term effects on offspring that require further definition, but cannabis use should be avoided in pregnancy. The administration of THC in the perinatal period seems to be quite problematic. Animal studies indicate that the endocannabinoid system exerts controls over brain maturation in the fetus. Observations of babies with a history of THC exposure have been reported to exhibit occasional signs suggestive of compromise of neurological development and function. Marijuana exposure in pregnancy is associated in some infants with increased tremor, high-pitched crying, and altered responses to visual stimuli. Some of these problems persist to a variable degree in babies or in young children who may exhibit poor memory, diminished attention, and impaired problem solving. However, controversy exists on the reports of some described problems with human offspring as a consequence of exposure to marijuana.

Two main reasons have been proposed to explain the development of marijuana-related problems in babies and youngsters. One hypothesis suggests that the adverse lifestyle of drug abusers contributes to problems experienced in infants. Another hypothesis attributes the infant's problems to cannabis use. The other option to consider is the likelihood that both mechanisms contribute to these problems.

Information pertaining to the use of cannabis in pregnancy is debated, but overall risks to mother and child should be avoided by not using cannabis or related compounds in pregnancy without further research. Table 108 summarizes information about marijuana use in relationship to pregnancy, fertility, and reproductive health.

Table 108. Issues that are relevant to the health and well-being of the mother and child. The marijuana-using mother requires special follow-up and monitoring (adapted from NCPIC website).

Issues	Comment
Uses	Cannabis is the most frequently used illicit drug in pregnancy, and it has been proposed that its adverse effects can be exacerbated by alcohol intake. Avoid both in pregnancy.
Fertility	Heavy use of cannabis is linked to decreased fertility in men and women, by exerting adverse effects on hormonal controls and reproductive functions. It should not be used in cases of infertility if couples are trying to have a baby.
Use in pregnancy	Delta-9-THC crosses the placenta into the fetus with many undetermined effects. Passive smoke inhalation from cannabis has potential adverse effects on the fetus, which require more study. Smoking tobacco or cannabis could alter nutrient and oxygen supply to the fetus.

Effect on fetus	Some evidence of adverse effects, including low birth weight, increased startle responses, poor eyesight, poor adaptation, and possible cardiac defects. There appears to be a greater risk of pulmonary disease (asthma and chest infection) for the first six months of life. When three to four years old, some children may have cognitive disorders, hyperactivity, and reduced motor skills. Some links to cannabis use in pregnancy and childhood cancer exist (e.g., leukemia, sarcomas, and brain tumors), but arguments prevail. Please note that arguments about the safety of cannabis in pregnancy are quite common.
Breast-Feeding	Delta-9-THC passes into breast milk and can be absorbed by the baby. Marijuana use affects the behavior of the baby and interferes with feeding.
Health-Care implications	The personality of the heavy cannabis user may lead to failure to report information relative to health in pregnancy and general health. Complex interpersonal issues can develop with health care workers. Pregnant mothers should be counseled to quit cannabis use.

Neonatal Suckling

Evidence has been presented that CB-1 receptor actions in newborns are required for the development of sucking reflexes. These reflexes are highly dependent on the development of the motor function of the mouth. These animal observations have been further investigated by the administration of rimonabant (a CB-1 receptor antagonist) in newborn animals. Rimonabant administration in neonatal animals often causes death and immediate growth failure from lack of feeding. Extended treatments of mature animals with rimonabant can cause pronounced reduction in body weight, but this drug has been withdrawn from use because of serious side effects. Studying the effects of rimonabant on the body assists in the understanding of the actions of cannabinoid receptors.

A Summary of Cannabis Use in Pregnancy

Several review articles have covered the risks of cannabis use in the disruption of maternal or fetal well-being. The negative data on cannabis use and pregnancy have been used to advise pregnant and nursing mothers not to use cannabis. The potential negative outcomes of cannabis use in pregnancy are summarized in table 109.

Table 109. The consequences of cannabis use in pregnancy

This list of putative problems resulting from smoking cannabis in pregnancy is incomplete (adapted from cssmun.weebly.com/ uploads/1/6/6/2/16623356).

- There may be interference with fetal growth and development, with occurrence of low birth weight.
- Delta-9-THC can alter fetal heart rates with bradycardia (slowing effects).
- It has an association with cancer risk (controversial).
- Children of cannabis-using mothers in pregnancy may have lower verbal and memory scores than controls.
- Nursing mothers secrete cannabinoids, most notably THC, in their breast milk, which can slow motor developments in children.

While cannabis use in pregnancy most likely causes harm to the fetus, there are many confounding variables that can skew perceptions. Cannabis-using mothers are more likely to have an adverse lifestyle, use other substances of abuse, have compromised nutritional status, and engage in less prenatal care, compared with nonusers.

As noted earlier, children exposed to cannabis in utero show other developmental problems (e.g., tremors and altered vision). Worrisome observations include the reports of the occasional presence of deficits in important higher brain functions, such as operational planning, in older children who have experienced cannabis exposure in utero.

Cannabis, Menstrual Problems, and Menopause

It is often stated that Queen Victoria of Britain used cannabis to treat her menstrual cramps. It appears as though she was well advised. Several contemporary studies suggest a benefit of cannabis in the treatment of premenopausal and menopausal syndrome as a consequence of its variable ability to inhibit vasomotor abnormalities (hot flashes), cramps, and altered emotions. A variety of delivery systems of cannabis have been utilized for menopausal symptom management, including smoking, oral tinctures, vaporized products, and oro-mucosal sprays. Anal suppositories of cannabis (in hemisuccinate form) are expected to be active, but vaginal administration is illogical and best avoided.

There are many anecdotal reports of the benefit of cannabis in common symptoms of premenstrual syndrome (PMS) or premenstrual dysphoric disorder (PMDD). However, several authors have complained about the lack of information to support cannabis use in menstrual disorders, even though physicians and dispensary staff give advice that promotes this activity. In a variety of weed blogs, several effective strains of cannabis for use in menstrual problems or menopause have been highlighted, but evidence to support these claims require more research (www.simonefischertheweedblog/.com/top-five-marijuana-strains-for-pms/).

Cannabis and PMS

The symptoms of PMS may be classified as behavioral, physical, and psychological. The symptoms are summarized in table 110.

Table 110. The many symptoms of PMS. Note many, but not all, of these symptoms are known to improve with cannabis. The knowledge that many of these individual symptoms are responsive to cannabis treatments reinforces its use in PMS.

• headache	• abdominal cramps
• bowel upset	• mood swings
• cravings	• episodic confusion
• change in sex drive	• hostility
• insomnia	• anger
• excessive sleep	• negative thoughts
• fatigue	• pain

The use of cannabis in premenstrual syndrome (PMS) has precipitated significant debate. There seems to be little doubt that many women can use cannabis to relieve several symptoms of PMS when symptoms are at their peak. That said, other opinions about the lack of benefit of cannabis sometimes stress the risk of the development of marijuana dependence. This can be avoided by using CBD only, but many women claim a need for the added psychoactive effects of THC.

In the second part of the nineteenth century, marijuana was used by physicians to relieve physical symptoms such as menstrual cramps and associated psychological changes in women who had problematic menstrual cycles. Several drugs with antidepressant, anxiolytic, and analgesic actions have been used to treat troublesome menstrual periods, but drug side effects and slow onset of action have limited their use. This has led to increasing use of cannabis smoking in the control of PMS symptomatology and other conditions of disturbed menstruation.

Conclusion

The effects of cannabis use on skin disorders are begging to be further researched. Reproductive function is influenced by cannabinoids, but data are conflicting, with an overall negative perception of its effects in the short and long term.

Chapter 16

MISCELLANEOUS ISSUES

Actions of Cannabis

It is useful to get an overall picture of the effects of cannabis. This information is summarized below in table 111, and it has formed a basis for discussions in several areas that have been covered by this book.

Table 111. An overview of the effects of cannabis to provide information at a glance

This valuable table is adapted from the work of Hana Abramovici et al., "Information for healthcare practitioners," Feb. 2013 (www.hc-scgcca/dhp-mps/marihuana/med/infoprof-eng.php#fig 1). Please note that conflicting evidence exists on the effects of cannabis on certain body systems or organs. A significant number of published studies on cannabis or prescription cannabis medication has included individuals taking other medications or drugs (alcohol or tobacco).

Central Nervous System

- **psychological**—causes: anxiety, psychosis, depersonalization, euphoria, and so forth
- **perception**—misperceptions, increased or distorted intensity of perceptions, hallucinations, altered sense of time, and so forth
- **sedation**—drowsiness and additive effects with other CNS depressants
- **cognition**—impairment of performance, clouded thoughts, memory problems, and so forth
- **motor function**—can cause ataxia, lack of coordination, weakness, and altered speech
- **analgesia**—variably effective in different types of pain, overall more effective in noncancer pain.
- **antinausea/antiemetic**—an effect of acute dosing with uncommon paradoxical effects with chronic heavy use causing hyperemesis
- **appetite**—increased appetite in normal individuals and people with chronic diseases (e.g., AIDS, cancer, multiple sclerosis, etc.)
- **tolerance**—may occur quite quickly (a couple of weeks) with need to increase dosage for the same effect
- **dependence**—more likely with chronic, heavy cannabis use, with occurrence of withdrawal symptoms (e.g., anger, sleep problems, weight loss, etc.)

Cardiovascular System

- **tachycardia**—with acute dosing, and may precipitate abnormal heart rhythms (e.g., premature ventricular beats, atrial fibrillation, etc.)
- **peripheral circulation**—increased oxygen demand by heart and increased cardiac output
- **cerebral blood flow**—variable effects, but acute dosing tends to cause increased blood flow, and chronic dosing causes decreased flow
- **myocardial infarction**—increased risk in the young and elderly; Higher risk in individuals with heart disease

- **stroke**—increased risk with cannabis smoking, arguable

Respiratory System

- **carcinogenesis**—conflicting evidence for cannabis smoking as a defined cause of lung cancer (cannabis smoke contains many carcinogens.)
- **lung changes**—associated with chronic cough, wheezing, and excessive production of sputum. (Precancerous changes in lung tissues are noted.)
- **bronchodilation**—occurs with acute smoking but not often with chronic smoking (may be negative changes (often minor) in lung function with chronic heavy cannabis use.)

Gastrointestinal System

- **general actions**—decreased motility, reduced secretion, constipation (or diarrhea)
- **liver**—increases in hepatic steatosis and fibrosis, arguable; helps with hepatitis C treatment compliance
- **pancreas**—acute pancreatitis associated with chronic heavy cannabis use

Musculoskeletal System

- **pain control**—in arthritis, rheumatoid disease and fibromyalgia; reduces spasticity in multiple sclerosis and spinal cord injury; interference with bone healing

Miscellaneous

- **eye**—decreases intraocular pressure and used to treat glaucoma
- **immune system**—variable effects, but overall depressant effects on immunity; has immune modulating ability and may be valuable in autoimmune disease
- **reproduction**—altered sperm function and decreased libido in men; in women, changes in menstrual cycle, alterations in ovulatory function, and reduced or increased sexual activity

Cannabis and Glaucoma

A raise in pressure within the eye is a key factor in the cause of glaucoma. Glaucoma is a disease with complex pathophysiology, including the development of a reduction of blood supply to the optic nerve, oxidative damage to the eye, and apoptosis of nerve cells in the retina. Severe compromise of eyesight and even blindness may occur as a result of glaucoma. Decreased levels of endocannabinoids are found in tissues of the eye in patients with glaucoma. It is known that cannabinoids delivered by ocular dosing (and systemic means) lower pressure within the eye up to a level of 30 percent, by several mechanisms. In addition, sublingual doses of THC and CBD are able to reduce intraocular pressure alone when used in sufficient dosages or with combined administration. However, some patients have shown tolerance to the reductions of intraocular pressure with THC or CBD eye treatments. This development of tolerance has been reported to decrease the therapeutic benefit of cannabinoids in glaucoma as a consequence of a short duration of action and some degree of psychoactive (THC) effects.

Current popular literature discusses the role of cannabis in lowering pressure with the eyes (intraocular pressure, 10P), but its desirability for this use has been questioned by some experts (K. Shen, "Therapeutics Update," *Glaucoma Today* May/June 2014). Cannabinoids can variably lower 10P when administered by different routes. The peak effect of inhaled THC on 10P occurs at approximately two hours following its administration and lasts up to four hours. This short duration of cannabis actions lowers 10P in approximately two-thirds of individuals, but a sustained effect requires multiple dosing (about six joints per day when used as smoking delivery). The mechanism of action of cannabis on 10P is likely to be due to CB-1 receptor activation in the eye, which exerts control over the production of aqueous humor. These (CB-1) receptors are located in choroidal blood vessels and nonpigmented epitheluim of the ciliary body.

Cannabinoids have antioxidant and vascular relaxing effects, and they can preserve neurone survival in some circumstances. It is believed that glaucoma produces optic nerve damage mainly by interference with blood flow to the optic nerve. This circumstance is associated with cell death (apoptosis in the nerve). How important these described mechanisms are in reducing optic nerve damage by the use of selected cannabinoids is not clear.

For the development of effective treatments, optimal modes of cannabis delivery require further development, but topical therapies present problems. Topical applications of cannabis components or drugs can cause local irritation of ocular tissues, and there is lack of solubility of the lipophilic, active ingredients derived from cannabis in an aqueous medium. In conclusion, opinion is divided on the relative benefits of cannabis in the treatment of glaucoma because of disadvantages and limitations that result from its use.

Cannabis and Urinary Problems

Several studies have indicated that cannabis may be of use in the management of an overactive bladder, urinary incontinence, and other urinary problems (e.g., urinary retention). A clear role of the endocannabinoid system is apparent in human and animal experiments of mapping of CB-receptor activity in the urinary tract (Bakali et al., *Int. Urognecology J.* 24, no. 5 (2013): 855–63). Research has demonstrated improvement in the control of urinary incontinence in patients with multiple sclerosis and spinal cord injury after the administration of extracts of cannabis or Marinol.

The use of cannabinoids in the treatment of painful bladder disorders is quite promising. Such disorders are associated with several circumstances, including urinary frequency, urgency and pelvic pain of variable severity. One major factor in the benefits of cannabis use appears to be anti-inflammatory actions on the bladder (beneficial in interstitial cystitis).

Research on bladder pain disorders is progressing with

Sativex (an oromucosal, sublingual spray of cannabis extracts, GW Pharmaceuticals, UK). Psychoactive effects of cannabis-related products may interfere with treatment of some patients, and alternatives are being sought (e.g., ajulemic acid). This cannabinoid analogue has shown some positive effects in the treatment of interstitial cystitis. Again, many studies are preclinical (in animals), but human experiences are expanding with signs of therapeutic promise.

Cannabis and the Kidney

Some animal studies imply that cannabis can cause renal disease, and others describe potential benefits of cannabis in the treatment of renal disease. A recent prevalence study of acute renal failure associated with cannabis use indicated that only eight out of 1,044 people (0.77 percent) who had adverse effects of marijuana also had renal failure (www.ehealthme.com/ds/marijuana/renal-failure; accessed December 25, 2014). This study of disease correlation suffers from the common lack of demonstration of a causal link in such studies.

Early studies linking acute kidney injury (AKI) to synthetic cannabis use were described by Bhanushali, G., et al., *Clin. J. Amer. Soc. Nephrology* 202, doi: 10.2015/CJN.05690612. The role of the use of synthetic cannabis in the cause of renal failure has been reported to be a result of the development of acute tubular necrosis. Synthetic cannabinoids are not detected by routine blood tests, and diagnosis is often problematic. It is important to consider synthetic cannabis use in young individuals as a cause of acute renal failure because the use of synthetic pot is the second most commonly used illicit drug in adolescents and teenagers, (second only to cannabis itself!). The management of this circumstance is compounded by lack of knowledge about what has actually been consumed by the victim.

Cannabis has been reported to be useful in the management of symptoms related to chronic renal failure. Treatments that can reduce the progression of chronic renal failure often rely on dialysis methods, which can have major adverse effects on quality of life. However, cannabis has found a role in the symptomatic management of chronic renal failure. These potentially beneficial effects include reversal of poor appetite and weight loss, chronic pain relief, control of muscular spasms, and antipruritic effects.

There are many attractive actions of cannabis that can be used in the management of a variety of renal disease. For example, the benefits of cannabis on the progression of autoimmune kidney disease (e.g., lupus) and the common occurrence of renal failure caused by diabetic nephropathy are the focus of current research. In a recent study published online by the US National Institutes of Health, experimentally induced diabetic nephropathy was shown to be exacerbated by endocannabinoid deficiency. In brief, these elaborate animal studies showed that absence of CB-2 receptors on glomerular cells reduced their function. These data by Russo provide support for implicating the endocannabinoid deficiency syndrome in certain types of renal disease.

Cannabis and Endocrine Function

Much information about the effects of cannabis use on hormonal controls in the body is limited to the detection of relatively short-term changes in hormonal profiles. Endocrine functions are key factors in body homeostasis, which are controlled by the endocannabinoid system. Delta-9-tetrahydrocannabinol alters hormonal controls of gonadal, adrenal, thyroid, prolactin, oxytocin, and hormones involved in appetite/energy controls. The effects of cannabis on endocrine function have been noted with some differences between males and females (in animals and humans). These differences in effect seem to be linked to the activity (fluctuations) of estrogenic actions in premenopausal subjects.

Several studies have implied that THC effects are different depending on prevailing estrogen levels. For example, pain control by the use of cannabis in rats seems to be amplified at times of high-circulating estrogen levels. With estrogenic dominance, it appears that THC may be converted to potent metabolites, and cannabinoid receptors (CB-1) may increase in number. Cannabis receptor excitability may also depend on estrogen availability. Thus, estrogen seems to be important in effects of cannabis that are altered by gender, but this area of research remains underexplored in humans.

Cannabis (THC) has effects on appetite-stimulating hormones. In controlled studies, cannabis consumption was associated with significant increases in ghrelin and leptin, with decreases in PYY, without significant effects on blood glucose. These findings support the link between THC use and appetite improvement by action on CB receptors (Sorkin, L. S., www.researchgate.net. publications/51845657).

Interference with estrogen dominance occurs with cannabis use. For example, hormonal imbalance in men can result in gynecomastia, impotence, and negative effects on sperm production, perhaps due in part to changes in estrogenic status. In addition, women who are chronic, heavy users of cannabis may have irregular menstrual cycles. In females, cannabis has been implicated in causing raised testosterone levels. Many details of cannabis/hormonal links require further study, and data in studies pertaining to hormonal changes and influences with cannabis have been conflicting.

Cannabis and Biological Rhythms

Alteration of time zones affects circadian rhythms and results in jet lag. This phenomenon has been related to disturbance of the body clock, which is located in the brain. However, the human body is now known to have multiple regional body clocks, which may be influenced by the "master brain clock" (Summa, K. C., Turek, F. W., "The Clocks within Us," *Scientific American*, Feb. 2015, 51–55). If the master clock is not in synchrony with the peripheral clocks, then several diseases or disorders can emerge. The actions of clocks in the body are summarized in table 112.

Table 112. The clocks of the body, which have many effects on body functions. Disruption of timekeeping or synchronization of these clocks can cause disease (e.g., depression, diabetes, etc.) (adapted from Summa, K. C., and Turek, F.W., "The Clocks within Us," *Scientific American*, Feb. 2015, 5–55).

Site of Clock	Actions on Body
Brain	The suprachiasmatic nucleus acts as a timekeeper and is responsive to environmental changes (e.g., light and dark).
Liver	The liver clock plays a role in fat and carbohydrate metabolism.
Adipose tissue	Release of components (e.g., fatty acids) occurs out of sync.
Heart	Genes that control heart function prime the body for activity during waking.
Pancreas	Synchronized actions occur with insulin secretion.
Kidneys	Clock genes control mineral and chemical metabolism (e.g., sodium, potassium, and chloride) that are involved in blood pressure control.

The concepts that have been highlighted recently by Summa and Turek (ibid. 2015) led to proposals for further development of circadian medicine or the medicine of biological rhythms, which is closely linked to sleep medicine. This is highly fertile ground for future cannabis research.

It is now clear that marijuana affects the body clock (or clocks?) to a significant degree. These effects include the sensation of a time warp with sensations of slow or fast passage of time. This situation of changes in the sense of time occurs with marijuana and other drugs.

Exposure to light plays a major role in the maintenance of a circadian rhythm due to effects on the suprachiasmatic nucleus of the brain. Research has demonstrated the presence of cannabinoid receptors on nerves of the suprachiasmic nucleus. These nerves have 50 percent more activity when exposed to cannabis (Latefi, N., quoting Avanden Pol, www.newsciencemag.org).

There has been much research on the effect of cannabinoids on sleep patterns. As early as 1975, the effects of THC on sleep patterns in humans were studied in a controlled manner (Feinberg, I., et al., "Effects of high-dosage delta-9-tetrahydrocannabinol on sleep patters in man," *Clin. Pharmacol. Ther.* 17, no. 4 (1975): 458–66). The importance of the research by Feinberg et al. (ibid. 1975) was the demonstration of a reduction in rapid eye movement (REM) sleep in cannabis users, followed by a rebound effect associated with dreaming, when THC was withdrawn. Most users of cannabis report the absence of dreaming, which is consistent with loss of REM sleep (Gumbiner, J., *Psychology Today*, www.psychologytoday.com/blog/the teenage mind).

In a pivotal article, the occurrence of endocannabinoid signaling in a rhythmic manner was proposed by Dr. Linda K. Vaughn and her colleagues (Vaughn, L. K. et al., "Endocannabinoid Signaling: Has It Got Rhythm?" *Br. J. Pharmacol* 160, no. 3 (June 2010): 538–43). There are a variety of patterns of sleep disorders in marijuana users. Using polysomnographic (PSG) measurements, sleep disturbances can be readily detected in cannabis users during discontinuation of the drug (Bolla, K., et al., 2008, www.ncbi.nim.nih.gov/pmc/articles PMC 244 2418).

Cannabis in Palliative Care

I believe in seizing the opportunity to provide improved palliative care in individuals by symptom relief of all forms of discomfort. However, it has been argued in a responsible manner that further research on the safety and efficacy of cannabis is required in the palliative care setting. Disease palliation is necessary in many disease states, and attempts should be made to support individual choices of patients, empowerment of patients, and improvements in quality of life. Much discussion has arisen about the negative effects of the psychoactive properties of cannabis, but sometimes such effects can often be considered a welcome blessing.

Many physicians have experienced the ability to decrease concomitant use of several medications in chronically ill patients by cannabis administration. Furthermore, cannabis has strong support for the alleviation of many symptoms of chronic disease that may be physical or psychological. One must applaud the potential and defined ability of cannabis for increasing quality of life in many patients with chronic disease.

Cannabis and Anesthesia

Cannabis use may be encountered in patients requiring anesthesia, but systematic studies of potential problems of interactions have been few. Cannabinoids are eliminated from the body in a relatively slow manner. This means that drug-drug interactions may occur, especially as a result of enhanced sedative and hypnotic actions of various drugs that are administered in pre- and perioperative circumstances.

Arguably, lung disorders are often present in chronic cannabis smokers (who often use tobacco). These disorders may contribute to pulmonary complications of anesthesia (e.g., postoperative chest infections). Cardiovascular effects of cannabis may interact with vasoactive drugs, and adverse psychiatric or autonomic effects of cannabis may affect the induction of anesthesia or postoperative recovery. The patient's history of marijuana consumption should result in increased clinical vigilance at times of surgery and anesthesia (Bryson, E. O., Frost, A. M., "The Perioperative Implications of Tobacco, Marijuana, and Other Inhaled Toxins," *International Anesthesiology Clinics 49*, no. 1 [2011]: 103–18) (Ashton, C. H., Br *J Anesthesia* 83, no. 4 [1999]: 637–49).

Cannabis and Hearing

Cannabis use has been associated with hearing loss, improved hearing, or tinnitus precipitation, or relief in fragmented, medical, anecdotal literature. In a group of people with side effects while taking marijuana, only eight (0.76 percent) of 1050 reported hearing loss. Marijuana appears to be potentially ototoxic, in common with several illegal drugs of abuse. Many drugs may alter multisensory functions, including the auditory system, spatial perceptions, memory (including speech discrimination), and goal-orientated logic (jdsde.oxfordjournals.org/content/ 13/3/336.full, author Titus, H. C. et al., *J. of Deaf Studies and Deaf Education* 13, no. 3 [2008]: 336, doi: 10.1093/deafed/enm068–50).

Cannabis and Performance

The role of cannabis in the impairment of short-term memory, judgment, and perceptions results in impaired performance in a variety of tasks. The pundits who argue against these outcomes may feel overwhelmed by the supporting evidence for this circumstance, or they may perhaps join the flat-earth society. Of increasing concern is the potential effect of cannabis use on brain development in youngsters that may pave the way for long-term cognitive disabilities.

Evidence exists that cannabis use is a cause of cognitive impairment in college students and the increasing use of regular cannabis or synthetic pot is a growing problem in high school students. It seems that cannabis is more addictive in teenagers than adults, and young people are recorded to have difficulty in registering information and shifting attention from one task or issue to another, compared with adult cannabis users. While such impairments are known to continue for up to four weeks, after cessation of cannabis use, other cognitive disorders may persist (e.g., verbal expression and mathematical skills).

The cause of the cognitive problems resulting from cannabis use may be the result of neuron loss in the hippocampus and other areas of the brain, due to effects of THC. Furthermore, chronic, heavy cannabis use may accelerate the loss of age-related reductions of neurones involved in the memory registration in the brain (hippocampus).

Cannabis and Exercise

There is much confusing information about the relationship between cannabis and exercise. Putative health benefits of cannabis combined with exercise are summarized in table 113.

Table 113. Effects of cannabis on exercise (adapted from wellspring-collective.com/marijuana-and-exercise/)

Please note that this information is quite controversial.

Effect	Comment
Increase the potency of cannabis psychoactive effects	One study showed that delta-9-THC levels were about 15 percent higher after subjects had engaged in exercise (thirty-five minutes of exercise on a stationary bike).
Activation of endocannabinoid system in the brain	It appears that cannabis and exercise activate the endocannabinoid system in the CNS, which complements the effects of endorphin release.
Staying balanced?	Stress and other challenges of sports can be assisted by cannabis smoking. Athletes claim that they can remain focused, despite the monotony of some exercise routines.
Weight control	Certain cannabinoids can play a role in the combat against metabolic syndrome (obesity, high blood cholesterol, hypertension, and insulin resistance). Cannabinoids can help overcome insulin resistance. Pot smokers tend to have higher fasting insulin levels and lower measures of insulin resistance, thereby improving glucose handling by the body.

Anandamide has been implicated in the exercise-induced high (runner's high), and researchers have suggested that endocannabinoid release may be a body response to pain or stress resulting from exercise, especially running (www.davidwolfe.com/invasion-of-the-cannabinoids/).

Cannabis and Children

There are an increasing number of reports of children with accidental exposure to cannabis in the United States (Borgelt, L. M. et al., *Pharmacotherapy* 33, no. 2 (2013): 195–209). In locations with legalized cannabis, there is worrisome documentation of children or adolescents who attend emergency rooms with various degrees of physical and mental impairment from cannabis. There are obvious risk factors for these circumstances, which appear to be most often due to cannabis edibles, such as candies or brownies (baked goods). Sometimes information on potential cannabis exposure is not disclosed, and children may undergo extensive medical investigations without useful outcome.

There is still only limited information on the prevalence of cannabis exposures in children. In 2011, the National Poison Data Center received more than five thousand contacts concerning cannabis exposures, and 358 (out of 5371 contacts, 7 percent) were present in children aged twelve years or younger. The risks of accidental exposure in children appear substantial, but many cannabis products are not labeled consistently with adequate warning statements. Packaging on cannabis products is often appealing to youngsters with the frequent use of cartoon-like designs. Thus, many factors contribute to what is a growing public health concern in children. Greater medical problems can be anticipated in children with more toxic forms of cannabis (e.g., synthetic pot).

Cannabis and Chocolate

Some individuals may be critical of any advice that is given to amplify the effects of cannabis, but much of this knowledge is available on the Internet. Of course, I do not endorse this knowledge because of safety concerns. Chocolate is allegedly a somewhat surprising source of anandamide, certain cannabinoid breakdown inhibitors (e.g., N-oleolethanolamine, OEA, an antiobesity factor, and N-linoeoylethanolamine, an anti-inflammatory agent). This latter compound exerts its effects by actions on TRPVI receptors. It is suggested that these latter two compounds can reduce the breakdown of anandamide and perhaps other cannabinoids, including THC. This situation may prolong the acute effects of cannabis. Furthermore, theobromine (a xanthine alkaloid) present in chocolate may amplify the effects of cannabinoid receptor agonists (e.g., THC and anandamide). This information is highly relevant for the use of cannabis jollies (edibles), which are often given in chocolate-containing snacks or foods. Beware of the chocolate munchies!

Cannabis and Stem Cells

Recent studies confirm that the neuromodulatory and neurogenic properties of cannabis are linked with stem-cell growth. Not only does cannabis exert neuroprotective effects on the brain, it can influence the development and fate of neural stem cells (NSC) in the central nervous system. These effects of cannabis have been attributed to a proliferation of NSC by signaling through IL-1 pathways. The implications of this and other research are the discovery of a foundation to consider the potential role of cannabis in brain repair following injury or damage. In other words, cannabis seems to facilitate the new growth of functioning brain cells.

There is clear evidence that the brain does not cease its growth, and it engages in continuing neurogenesis. However, the brain's capabilities of neurogenesis do seem to decline with age. Interest has focused on defining the actual cannabis components that exert major influences on this new brain growth (neurogenesis). Recent studies have defined the important role of cannbichromene in supporting NSC (neural stem cells). Also, this positive effect has been shown with THC and CBD administration in experimental animals, but these cannabinoids do not possess the same neurogenic potency as CBC (cannabichromene).

It is of notable interest that many drugs of abuse interfere with new brain-cell growth, in contrast with cannabis (reported at Shinyo, N., DiMarzo, V., *Neurochemistry International*, doi: 10.1016/ J, euint, 2013, 08 002 and Jiang W et al *J Clin. Invest*, 2005; 115,11,doi 10.1172/JCI2 5509). One important conclusion in this latter study was the suggestion that the candidate drug HU210 decreases anxiety and depression by causing neurogenesis in the hippocampal regions of the brain. Of parallel interest is the suggestion that the drug fluoxetine (Prozac) reduces anxiety by neurogenesis.

Neurogenesis induced by cannabis, or other factors, occurs in the hippocampus (dentate gyrus) and subventricular parts of the brain. Alterations of neurogenesis in adults may be implicated or associated in many circumstances, including learning, neurodegenerative disease (e.g., Alzheimer's disease), schizophrenia, depression, stress, anxiety, sleep deprivation, Parkinson's disease, aging, and exercise (positive and negative neurogenic effects).

There are applications of cannabinoids that provide versatile ways of manipulating stem-cell mobilization and functions. These actions are relevant to controlling the activity of cancer stem cells. For example, research performed at the Pacific Medical Center Research Institute 2012 has shown that selected cannabinoids can decrease the growth of both breast cancer and serious malignant types of brain cancer. Of significant importance is the finding that these anticancer effects are mediated by CBD (cannabidiol) by downregulating Id-1 gene. The future of stem-cell therapy modulated by the use of cannabis-based drugs seems very promising.

Cannabis and Organ Transplantation

The CB-2 receptor has been identified as playing a key role in causing effects on immune functions. A measure of tendencies to graft rejection of skin and organ transplants is the mixed murine leukocyte response (MLR). This MLR has been investigated in mice. Two selective antagonists of CB-2 receptors have been shown to decrease the mixed murine leukocyte response (MLR) to cannabis in a dose-dependent manner. It was found in recent studies that CB-2 agonists decreased T cell function, which are important mediators of graft rejection. These findings imply that certain cannabinoids (selective CB-2 agonists) may have value in prolonging graft survival. The significance of these findings requires further study in humans (Robinson, R. H. et al., *J. Neuroimmune Pharmacology* 8, no. 5 [2013]: 1239–1250).

Cannabis and Oral Health

Recent studies indicate a relationship between poor dental health (oral health) and smoking marijuana. However, some counterarguments exist on the Internet with the opinion that this alleged relationship is merely another example of "antipot quack science." That said, there are several explanations of the risks of cannabis smoking on oral health that have scientific validity.

Table 114. Some oral health problems that are or may be associated with cannabis smoking

Effect on Oral Health	Comment
Dry mouth and throat	Contributes to bad breath and tooth decay.
Immune suppression	May contribute to mouth infections, cavities, and oral cancer. Cannabis causes yellow teeth, poor aesthetics, and bad breath.
THC	THC alters calcium transport and has secondary negative effects on calcification of teeth.
Oral cancer risk	Marijuana smoking may cause a higher delivery of cancer-causing chemicals (carcinogens) than cigarettes. Tar taken from cannabis can cause skin tumors when directly applied to the skin of animals.

Genetics and Cannabis
Comorbidity with Cannabis

A number of genetic influences may overlap to explain the association of early-onset cannabis use and comorbidities (disorders or diseases). These comorbidities include other illicit drug use, psychosis, depression, and suicide (Agrawal, A., Lynskey, M. T., *Addiction* 109 [2014]: 360–70). For example, there is convincing evidence that cannabis use and the entity of cannabis use disorder are inherited to some degree. In this circumstance, about 40–48 percent of cannabis use is related to genetic influences and about 51–59 percent of cannabis use disorders are genetically linked. The role of epigenetics in this situation has not been explored in any detail.

Using a selective review of medical literature, Agrawal, A., and Lynskey, M. T. (ibid. 2014) concluded that genetic determinants underlie a correlation between early cannabis use and other illicit drug use. Moreover, genetics may explain in part the significant link between cannabis use and depression and/or suicide. Differing genetic mechanisms determine associations of comorbidities with cannabis use. However, factors other than genetic influences play a major role.

More on Cannabis and Antiaging

Cannabis may have beneficial effects on several diseases that often affect the elderly, but this does not mean conclusively that cannabis has antiaging properties. That said, a number of recent reports support the notion that cannabis has general antiaging properties. One area to examine is what appears to be a paradoxical effect of cannabis use on mental abilities. In this book, I have reviewed convincing evidence of the negative short-term effects of cannabis on cognition and memory, but animal experiments imply that degenerative brain changes, such as present in Alzheimer's disease, may be somewhat reversed or prevented by cannabinoids. It appears that THC-induced protection against neurotransmitter degradation in Alzheimer's disease can assist in the maintenance of cognitive function by inhibition of the acetylcholinesterase enzyme.

Among the most important antiaging actions of marijuana on the brain involve antioxidant functions and neuroprotective effects of cannabis on nervous tissue. It has been stressed earlier that cannabis can stimulate neurogenesis or growth of new brain cells in certain brain locations (e.g., the hippocampus). Experiments in mice strongly support the existence of these neuroprotective actions of cannabis, where injections of cannabidiol results in improved recognition and memory.

Several studies have described the ability of certain cannabinoids to stimulate the synthesis of brain derived neurotrophic factor (BDNF). This substance protects neurones and has neurogenic properties. These properties of BDNF amplify the demonstrated effects of cannabis on neurogenesis. Some experts continue to express doubts that cannabis can be used to inhibit brain aging and focus on the inability of many elderly people to tolerate the psychoactive effects of cannabis, but cannabidiol has several favorable neurological effects without psychoactive functions.

A principle protagonist of the antiaging benefits of cannabis is Dr. Robert Melamede, who is the president of the company Cannabis Science Inc. (and an associate professor at the University of Colorado). His recent testimony as a defense expert in a cannabis prosecution is widely quoted on the Internet. In brief, Dr. Melamede has referred to cannabis as "an essential nutrient" with antiaging properties that can counter free radical damage to tissues (an antioxidant effect). Dr. Melamede went further in his reported statements to suggest that "a puff or two a day (of cannabis) can improve longevity." These statements have some plausibility, but they are quite arguable.

Of course many of the protagonistic statements about cannabinoids are informed speculations, but one must look at balanced opinions. As discussed earlier, it has been stated that cannabis is a "cancer cure" in the absence of "proof of cure." This information has been repeated in this book because overstatements or understatements about the beneficial effects of cannabis are a root cause of major differences of opinion and emotive responses. These clashes of opinion destroy rational dialogue in some circumstances.

Cannabis and Hair Loss

There is evidence that smoking pot interferes with normal hair growth. Delta-9-THC is deposited in hair shafts. Laboratory studies imply that THC can inhibit hair shaft development and suppress the proliferation of keratinocytes in hair follicles. It is suggested that these effects tend to place the hair in a state of catogen.

The occurrence of testosterone increases in marijuana smokers is believed to be quite modest, of the order of 3 to 5 percent. This small increase in testosterone is not likely to account for substantial hair loss. In brief, the effect of cannabis on hair loss remains unclear, but opinions do lean toward a negative effect on hair growth. That said, a number of cannabis-based shampoos tout their ability to improve hair health. The effects of cannabis on scalp hair, body hair, or beard growth are not clear.

Cannabis and Retinal Degeneration

Cannabinoids exert documented neuroprotective effects in a variety of circumstances. These protective effects are apparent in animal models of retinitis pigmentosa, where the synthetic cannabinoid HU210 has been shown to increase photoreceptor density in the retina, together with preservation of cone and rod structure and function. Whether or not these improvements in retinal degeneration are present in other degenerative or inflammatory eye diseases requires further investigation (Laz, P., et al., *Experimental Eye Research* 120 [2014]: 175–85).

Cannabis and Acupuncture

Chinese scientists have suggested that the pain-control effects of acupuncture are due in part to the actions of cannabinoid receptors, which can be activated by delta-9-THC. One may expect cannabis to be synergistic with acupuncture.

Cannabis and Epigenetics

Cannabis is believed to play a role in epigenetics, as discussed earlier. Epigenetics involves the reversible regulation of various genomic functions that are mediated mainly through DNA methylation and chromatin structure. These mechanisms of regulation do not involve changes in DNA sequence. Epigenetics incorporates the idea that the actions or the environment of parents create genetic responses that can be passed down through generations without any change in the genetic code (DNA sequences).

These circumstances of a role of epigenetic influences of cannabis have been confirmed in rat studies where THC administration has been shown to result in neurobiological alterations that persist for three generations. Earlier studies have shown that THC exposure during adolescence ("teen rats") increased efforts by the rodents to obtain heroin. Epigenetics appears to play an important role in some comorbidities associated with cannabis use.

Cannabis and Pets

To state that cannabis use in pets is controversial constitutes an understatement. Most cases of marijuana use with beneficial or adverse effects are reported in dogs and cats. Some individuals and veterinarians are of the opinion that cannabis is of considerable value in the palliative care of sick animals, whereas others ring the alarm bell of its potential toxicity. Clinical manifestations of cannabis toxicity are most often attributed to the THC content of the ingested cannabis material, which has an onset of actions usually in about thirty to ninety minutes, but effects have been noted to last for up to three days. Table 115 lists some of the main signs of cannabis toxicity that have been noted in dogs and cats.

Table 115. Common clinical signs of cannabis toxicity in dogs. Similar signs have been noted in cats. (Adapted from www. critterology.com/marijuana_toxicity_ in/author S. M. Esneault.)

• Depression	• Ataxia
• Bradycardia	• Hypothermia
• Vocalization	• Mydriasis
• Incoordination	• Respiratory depression
• Hypersalivation	• Vomiting
• Diarrhea	• Urinary incontinence
• Seizures	• Coma
• Hyperreflexia	• Hyperesthesia
• Nystagmus	• Death secondary to inhalation of vomit

The diagnosis of cannabis toxicity in animals is made by history and physical examination, with testing for THC. Symptoms of toxicity occur on a spectrum, and secondhand cannabis smoke is believed to affect pets.

There are many descriptions of benefits for ailing dogs and cats on the internet, but observations have been mainly anecdotal. Cannabis has been used for many disorders in dogs and cats (table 116).

Table 116. Cannabis use in several disorders or diseases. The efficacy and safety of cannabis is *not* clear in animals in many circumstances.

• anxiety	• aggression
• cancer	• cognitive disorders
• diabetes	• digestive diseases
• feline marking	• seizures
• pain modulation	• inflammatory disease
• cachexia	• appetite loss

The American Veterinary Medical Association has taken a conservative position on cannabis therapy for pets with a call for more research studies before it is used in clinical practice. The main cannabis products available for use in pet supplements contain hemp-based derivatives, and much emphasis has been placed on the value of CBD contents (cannabidiol). While there may be growing enthusiasm for cannabis use in specific diseases in dogs and cats, much information used to support claims of benefit is extrapolated from human experiences (www.skepvet.com/Blog/medical_use_of_marijuana_for_pets, posted Nov. 19, 2013).

Several veterinarians and pet owners have reported their success with the use of cannabis in various medical disorders. These reports refer to dogs, cats, and horses. Often, pet owners have decided to treat their pets as a therapeutic trial after conventional therapies have failed (Nolen, R. S., JAVMA news, June 15, 2013, posted May 13, 2013). In brief, the following conditions have shown anecdotal evidence of improvement with cannabis (Nolen, R. S., ibid. 2013).

- Splenic neoplasia with metastases in a Labrador retriever dog with loss of appetite and vomiting. Symptom improvement was excellent.
- Back pain relief in a geriatric cat with resolution.
- Degenerative ligament disease unresponsive to dietary supplements or NSAIDs with post wrist surgery, spurs, and arthritis. Good pain relief noted.

On the other hand, Dawn Boothe, director of the Clinical Pharmacology Laboratory at Auburn University, has referred to risks of cannabis use and associated occasional deaths following its administration. These occurrences were reported in the *Journal of Veterinary Emergency Medicine* in 2012 (ibid. Nolen, R. S., 2013). The deaths were in dogs that ate marijuana-containing baked goods. Dr. Boothe recommends that veterinarians be kept in the "translational medicine" loop concerning cannabis use (switch from human cannabis use to animal use) (Nolen, R. S., ibid. 2013).

Recently, the DEA warned of the possibility of "stoned rabbits" in testimony to a Utah state panel. Rabbits can apparently develop a taste for marijuana. These rabbits may be high all the time, and some lose their fear of humans. Nevertheless, the panel in question approved the legislation for the treatment of certain illnesses with edibles!

Conclusion

Cannabis has many effects on body structure and function in humans and animals. Specific effects in many diseases are unraveling, and safety cannot always be assumed.

Chapter 17

SOME SOCIAL PERSPECTIVES

Introduction

For some readers, the retention of information on the potential application of cannabis use for disease treatment may seem to be a daunting task. Medical and social opinions about cannabis vary greatly. It is the comprehensive and complex effects of the endocannabinoid system that account for the many versatile effects of cannabis on body structures and function. These effects have many mechanisms of action in the control of body homeostasis (harmonious function). We have learned that practically all body functions are affected to a variable degree by cannabis.

The manner in which certain diseases or disorders alter the harmony of body functions may have common root causes or contributory factors. For example appetite loss and vomiting are common companions of many types of acute and chronic disease or disorders. These problems may be amenable to correction variably by cannabis use, regardless of their specific cause. Thus, understanding the physiological and psychological actions of cannabis form a good basis to predict some of its potentially beneficial treatment effects. In nature, there is always an action that can be modified in a beneficial or adverse manner by a reaction. These are the yin and yang of cannabis effects, which may be often reproducible and sometimes unpredictable. Cannabis can be viewed as body adaptogen, which is a term that is often applied to a natural substance in herbal medicine that can be used to normalize and regulate the systems of the body (*Collins English Dictionary* 2012, digital edition).

Examples of cannabis use in medical treatments can be inferred from known generic actions of cannabis in an oversimplified but helpful manner. These circumstances include pain control in the presence of different types of pain generation, suppression of inflammatory responses in disease, and multiple psychological actions to benefit disease symptoms. There is importance in identifying or predicting target pathways of disease mechanisms that may be corrected to some degree by cannabis.

As knowledge about the various corrective actions of cannabis-related medicinal agents increases, the medical application of this drug mixture broadens. In summary, the range of beneficial corrections of body function by using cannabis in disease states are legion, and they can often be inferred by defining abnormalities in specific disease and their propensity to be positively influenced by components of cannabis.

The Cannabis Industry

The respected blogger and cannabis activist Johnny Green (2013) has provided an excellent and succinct discussion on the future of the marijuana Industry (www.theweedblog.com/what-will-the-future-of-the-marijuana-industry-look-like). Green agrees with most experts that the cannabis industry will grow at a fast pace. Table 117 summarizes some of the key predictions or potential consequences of cannabis use that have been described by Green.

Table 117. Adapted from John Green (2013), "What Will the Future of the Marijuana Industry Look Like?" (www.theweedblog.com/what-will-the-future-of-the-marijuana-inustry-look-like). Some statements are partially verbatim to maintain the fidelity of the work by Green.

- The taboo on marijuana has softened.
- Marijuana is easy to obtain—especially on the West Coast.

- Ancillary businesses are going to be much larger than otherwise predicted.
- Competition will grow to have the largest growing or dispensary or collective organizations.
- Consumers will seek the best growing equipment.
- Increasing ordinances will limit where cannabis gardens or outlets can be located.
- Overflow from the industry may occur (e.g., increased cannabis snack food sales, edibles).
- Significant population shifts could occur to fill expanding job markets in specific locations of the cannabis industry.
- Local economies will benefit.
- There are no signs that trends for expansion of use are going to slow down.
- As the cannabis industry grows, large corporate interests are likely to infiltrate.
- Economic issues will dominate industry decisions.
- Conflict will occur from competition.
- Small companies will get pushed out.
- Dispensary businesses may diversify.
- The marijuana industry will have to find new marketing pathways to remain competitive.

It is clear that there are many potential outcomes of marijuana legalization with far-reaching effects on society. An excellent account of what to expect is presented by Jon Walker (*After Legalization: Understanding the Future of Marijuana Policy*, Jan. 12, 2014, ISBN 0991239717). This book is highly recommended to expand knowledge about the shaping of business, politics, and disputes concerning cannabis.

American Indian Tribes and Marijuana

In December 2014, J. Barnard and G. Wozniaka of the Associated Press reported on the US Justice Department's declaration that Indian tribes can grown and sell marijuana on their lands (www.dallasnews.com/news/local-news/2014-12-11). The Department has made it clear that the tribes must follow the same conditions that have been proposed by states that have legalized cannabis.

For a few years some groups of North American Indian businessmen have explored options for the development of marijuana growth and commerce, but it seems clear that many tribes have opposition to legalization. It appears that only a few tribes have openly expressed interest in cannabis business in California, Washington State, and some locations in the Midwest.

Indian tribes have high rates of prevalence of alcohol and drug use, creating a fear that marijuana legalization could only make matters worse. These matters are highly complex given the perception of the lack of defined boundaries of Indian nations and the existence of different law enforcement groups that serve the Indian sovereign nations.

The consumption of marijuana by North American Indians is subject to special rules and exemptions that permit its use. The US Department of Justice issued policy statements in 2014 regarding marijuana issues in Indian Country—a list of actions to be taken that are necessary for law enforcement. The eight federal law enforcement priorities have been discussed earlier in this book and are listed (verbatim) below:

- preventing the distribution of marijuana to minors
- preventing revenue from the sale of marijuana from going to criminal enterprises, gangs, and cartels
- preventing the diversion of marijuana from states where it is legal under state law in some form to other states
- preventing state-authorized marijuana activity from being used as a cover or pretext for the trafficking of other illegal drugs or other illegal activity
- preventing violence and the use of firearms in the cultivation and distribution of marijuana
- preventing drugged driving and the exacerbation of other adverse public health consequences associated with marijuana use

- preventing the growing of marijuana on public lands and the attendant public safety and environmental dangers posed by marijuana production on public lands
- preventing marijuana possession or use on federal property

The above list is part of what is called the Cole Memorandum that does not alter the authority of the federal government to enforce law in Indian Country. Moreover, the eight priorities, as noted above, will guide United States attorneys' marijuana enforcement efforts in Indian Country.

Most Indian reservations are located in the west of the country, and some are present in states that have not legalized cannabis for medical or recreational use. New policies will allow American Indian tribes to cultivate and sell cannabis on reservation lands. It appears that all states have the responsibility to regulate recreational and medical use of cannabis, but what may happen in states that have no legalization is difficult to predict. However, it is anticipated that the Department of Justice will not move to enforce federal laws for the strict control of cannabis use on American Indian reservations. A well-written synopsis of the marijuana cultivation and debates about sales of cannabis on Indian reservations is found at www.azcentral.com/story/news/arizona/politics/2014/12/22.

Cannabis, African Americans, and Latinos

The American Civil Liberties Union (ACLU) has drawn attention to the great expense of marijuana arrests in the African American population. While arguments prevail that marijuana use has not been controlled by law enforcement interventions, it is disturbing that a black person is 3.73 times more likely to be arrested for cannabis possession, compared with a white person. That said, the use of marijuana is approximately equal in black and white individuals (www.aclu.org/billions dollars-wasted-racially-biased-arrests). Furthermore, money expended on enforcing cannabis laws cost US $42,072,288, which has been described as time and money wasted.

The Drug Policy Alliance has stated the following: "the drug policy war has produced profoundly unequal outcomes across racial groups (in the United States), manifested through racial discrimination by law enforcement and disproportionate drug war misery suffered by communities of color" (www.drugpolicy.org/ race-and-drug war, accessed March 2015).

Theodore Thornhill, writing in the *Journal of Ethnicity in Criminal Justice* (9 [2011]: 110–35), has given a thoughtful analysis of the paradox of the African American people and cannabis legalization. One reason proposed for this circumstance is the urban frustration argument. The analysis of data from several sources between the years 1990 and 2000 indicates that blacks' level of support for cannabis legalization is greatest in cities with the highest black drug arrest rates. These results do not support the notion that the urban frustration argument is operative in accounting for the circumstances (Thornhill, T., ibid. 2011). Clearly, other factors operate in these complex social phenomena surrounding cannabis use.

Detailed information about US Latinos and cannabis use is not widely available. However, according to the Pew Research Center, 51 percent of Latinos now support the legalization of cannabis compared with about the same number of Americans, overall (52 percent). The recent legalization of cannabis use in Uruguay was not universally approved by the electorate, with only approximately 32 percent support in some surveys. Moreover, across Latin America, legalization of pot does not seem to be a dominant preference among the public.

Cannabis Testing

Testing for cannabis use is a subject of major interest, but it is handicapped by an inability to correlate results with time of cannabis intake together with its long residence time in the body. There is interindividual and intraindividual variation in the distribution of cannabis caused by a variety of factors, including differences in metabolism and modes of delivery.

One valuable source of technical information on cannabis detection windows following smoking has had application in law enforcement work and guidance for courts involved in drug offenses (www.ndci.org/sites/default/files/indci/THC/ Detection_Window, author Paul L. Cary).

As mentioned earlier, the long elimination half-life of cannabis makes the drug(s) detectable for a long period of time. There has been debate about positive limits using different types of testing on urine or blood samples, but most THC drug tests will give a positive result when cannabis blood concentrations exceed 50 ng/ml. Cannabis screening is included in NIDA-approved drug tests, which often involve screening for at least five drugs (e.g., SAMHSA-5). Unfortunately, a number of commonly used drugs and perhaps some dietary supplements could result in false positive testing for cannabis in body fluids. These days, there are many cannabis-testing laboratories that can measure different components of cannabis with accuracy. A valuable overview of drug testing for cannabis is present online at www.canorma.org/healthfacts/drugtestguide.

Cannabis and Religion

In different religions and cultures, cannabis has been used in spiritual and religious activities for many years. While the role of cannabis in the practice of Hinduism is commonly recognized, several other religions have embraced the use of the plant, ranging from Christianity and Judaism in a variable manner to Rastafarianism in a complete manner. In recent times, the religious philosophy of cantheism has evolved. The word "cantheism" is a neologism that signifies any and all attitudes toward the cannabis plant as a religious experience (www.masscan.org/education/ religious-use-of-cannabis).

Protagonists of cannabis use argue that cannabis should be legalized for many reasons, but to date no states have moved forward in regard to religious legalization of cannabis use. However, a federal court judge in 2013 ruled that religion could be used as a defense in a cannabis distribution charge. Other legal cases have supported the sacramental use of cannabis, but legalization for such purposes is only the subject of discussion or pending among politicians.

Cannabis and Economics

The legalization of cannabis has major impacts on a wide range of economic issues. The complexity of this subject cannot be covered in detail in this book, but a thumbnail sketch of the economic issues pertaining to cannabis legalization is in order. Legalization of cannabis appeals to many politicians or public officials who see the taxation dollars that can be collected. It is suggested that regulated sales of the drug would result in lower retail costs of marijuana and stimulate its sales that generate tax revenues.

While cannabis is a gateway drug that leads to the use of hard drugs in some people, savings in legal enforcement costs pertaining to marijuana use will be realized. Furthermore, law enforcement agencies would be able to focus on controlling hard-drug use (cocaine and heroin) that is more damaging to society. However, a circular argument arises because of the gateway phenomenon that may push hard-drug use. Further complexities involving several factors include legal issues that arise due to different laws in different states and alteration of demands or behavior of buyers and sellers. Overall, it has been projected that complete legalization of cannabis in the United States would result in lowering the costs of cannabis by a factor of up to 90 percent, but this estimate is questionable.

It appears that current levels of taxation will amount to a combined wholesale and retail tax of about 25 percent (add-on state retail taxes). The prevailing cost of cannabis is up to about four hundred dollars per ounce in the United States, but these costs will be reduced over time. At present, the cost of black market cannabis and illegal cannabis is about the same, but many believe that a drastic fall in the cost of illicit cannabis will occur in the future (about five years?). This has happened to a small degree in Colorado. Moreover, the combination of savings in law enforcement combined with taxation revenue could save $17.4 billion if production and sale of cannabis was legal nationwide (reported by the Libertarian Cato Institute). Thus, the economic incentives for legalization of pot seem to be very attractive to many people, including government agencies.

Cannabis, Violence, and Crime

A study performed by the staff of the Office of National Drug Control Policy has revealed a strong association between illicit drug use and crime (Hotakainen, R., McClatchey Washington Bureau, May 23, 2013, www.mclatchey.com). The notable findings in this study (2013) showed that 80 percent of all males arrested for a crime in Sacramento, California, tested positive for one or more illegal drugs. Marijuana use was commonly detected by drug testing in 54 percent of the arrested men.

This California study produced similar results to information gathered from arrests in four other cities (Denver, New York, Atlanta, and Chicago). The range of positive drugs tests for cannabis ranged from 37 to 58 percent among the subjects. Chicago had the most positive test results. This study attracted predictable criticism from the political director of the Marijuana Policy Project and others who doubted (and continue to doubt) the evidence for a link between cannabis use and crime.

There has been much interest in some recent studies that followed cannabis legalization in Colorado. These studies found no escalation in crime rates, including violent crimes and a variety of other offenses. A study published in March 2014 (Morris. R., PLOS one, doi: 10, 1371-75) examined national findings derived from US state panel data. Apparent links between state medical marijuana laws and serious offenses documented by the FBI did not show that crimes increased with the presence of medical marijuana legislation. The data showed a reduction in homicide and assault rates. These results imply that medical marijuana legalization does not result in increases in violent and property crimes. Clearly, these studies linking cannabis use and crime have many confounding factors that interfere with conclusions about a causal link.

An analysis of medical marijuana legalization shows that this policy may or may not increase crime rates. That said, the evidence is leaning toward a lack of general effect on crime rates involving property, violence, and homicide. However, under federal law the possession and use of cannabis remains illegal in many jurisdictions. Matters are confusing given the several studies that report an association of cannabis use with an increase in violent or aggressive behaviors.

Caution should be exercised in assessing the presence of causal links between the use of pot and crime. A weakness of the data gathered in some studies is that it is sometimes based on arrest records, which are not influenced by nonreported crimes to law enforcement. The assessment of medical marijuana laws on state crime rates reveals that these laws do not appear to have much effect on crime rates. Of course, further studies are required and many factors can blur the picture.

Repealing Cannabis Laws?

Antagonism to cannabis legalization has not gone away. Politicians and the general public could change their mind overall on efforts to legalize cannabis, but this seems an unpredictable possibility. While much attention is given to the potential clash of federal and state laws on marijuana use, little attention has been paid to opinions that are emerging to modify certain state laws or even repeal existing specific legislation. It appears that only about 30 percent of Republican government members support cannabis legalization, compared with more than 50 percent of Democrats. A change of federal government will occur within a couple of years (at the time of writing), with a good chance of a Republican majority.

Laws at the state level are somewhat liberal in their freedoms and allowances, such as growing, using, and selling the drug. Some opposition to cannabis laws are growing in certain states, where the original vote to legalize medical cannabis may have been passed with a relatively narrow margin of votes. For example, Colorado has reexamined its position on hashish. How many politicians have a current change of heart about marijuana legislation cannot be estimated with any accuracy. There are still many groups of individuals or organizations that continue to protest cannabis legalization initiatives.

Is Cannabis Addictive?

One major worry about cannabis legalization is that the prevalence of drug addiction will increase. This may occur both as a consequence of its use and the use of other drugs of abuse, due to the gateway phenomenon. A number of protagonists of marijuana use still protest suggestions that cannabis is addictive. However, reality must set in when it is recognized that cannabis can be used in a manner that conforms with the diagnostic criteria for substance abuse, laid down by the American Psychiatric Association and contained within the Diagnostic Manual of Mental Disorders (DSM-IV). If something walks and talks like a duck, it is usually a duck!

Accepting that cannabis can cause physical and psychological addiction, the last person to recognize these circumstances may be the cannabis users themselves. To recognize addiction or the progression of the pathway to dependence and to intervene is likely to become of major importance with more widespread use of the cannabis drug(s). A diagnosis of cannabis use with dependence is defined as present when three of the following seven criteria occur at anytime in a twelve-month period of time (table 118).

Table 118. Adapted from DSM-IV and recommendations of several organizations, including the American Psychiatric Association. This information can facilitate the recognition of dependence on cannabis use (some verbatim quotes).

- Tolerance. A circumstance where more of the substance is required to achieve the same effects, or diminished effect with the same amount of substance. Heavy cannabis users are often not aware of the development of tolerance.
- Withdrawal symptoms. Marijuana use can cause several symptoms when it is withdrawn, including irritability, restlessness, appetite loss, sleep problems, weight loss,

419

shaky hands (tremor), loss of motivation, and more. Symptoms may be delayed in onset after cessation of the use of cannabis, but they are sometimes noted in a delayed occurrence after a one-week period.

- Stubborn continuation of use despite the presence of adverse effects. In this circumstance, a person continues to use despite self-harm or harm to others. Persistence with use after a relationship breakup or suicidal thoughts and so forth are sometimes present.
- Social isolation or change in social activities with a tendency to share the company of cannabis users.
- Individuals withdraw from family activities or hobbies to focus on cannabis use.
- Cannabis is consumed in large amounts over a protracted period of time.
- There is a persistent desire to cut down or stop cannabis use.

To assist in an early diagnosis of progression to cannabis dependence, the following factors should be considered as chronological events (table 119). (Source: oade.nd.edu/ educate-yourself-drugs/marijuana).

Table 119. Progression of cannabis use to dependence or addiction

- experimentation
- social use—with no real impact on lifestyle
- habituation
- abuse—use despite negative outcome
- addiction—compulsion to use, loss of control, frequent relapses

Cannabis Caregivers

Certain state laws describe cannabis or marijuana caregivers as individuals that are registered with a state to provide assistance to medical marijuana patients in accessing medical cannabis. The range of allowable activity of a caregiver does vary state by state, with some states allowing assistance to be given to five patients (or more with a waiver, e.g., Colorado). Some states allow assistance to only one patient (e.g., Massachusetts), and warnings about these restrictions have been sent recently to both caregivers and patients in 2014 in Massachusetts. Caregivers serve a purpose of cannabis supply without the need for an individual to visit a dispensary or grow it him or herself.

Different states permit caregivers to purchase, transport (within the state), cultivate, and dispense limited quantities of cannabis. The caregiver must be licensed and registered by the state in question. Safety issues are very important for the patient and caregiver who must have a good, comprehensive education about cannabis. Those caregivers who grow marijuana must be knowledgeable about good growing practices and the biological activities of the cannabis that they handle. This information about cannabis caregiving is summarized at www.marijuana-caregiver.com/about_marijuana_caregivers.htm.

It is variably estimated that the medical markets for cannabis will double or more within the next five years. About twenty-four million people in the United States may benefit from medical marijuana use, but only about 730,000 individuals (at the time of writing) have received bona fide permission for its use. Different state rules and regulations governing cannabis use and new regulations may continue to foster consumer confusion. Readers are strongly advised to check up on the details of cannabis legislation in their state, because lack of compliance with laws may result in arrest and penalties.

There are different standards for obtaining an approved caregiver's status in different states. For example, reasonable standards for education and eligibility are provided by the Medical Cannabis Caregivers Institute in California (mccdirectory.org/certification_medical_cannabis-caregivers-primary-caregiver-certification.lasso). This pathway of education is approved by the California Department of Social Services and is highlighted in table 120.

Table 120. Highlights of the requirements for medical caregiver certification provided by the Medical Cannabis Caregivers Institute, California. This program is a continuing-education program for licensees and administrators of state-licensed residential care facilities (full details from Liz McDuffie, liz@mccdirectory.org).

- approved acceptance of the application of certification
- background check
- completion of six classes of four hours' duration held at the Medical Caregivers Institute in Pasadena
- internship—optional
- use HIPAA-compliant medical record software

I stress that there is variation in requirements for caregiver licensing. A useful source of information is found at michiganmedical- marijuana.org/page/ articles/caregivers/ what-cg-do.

Cannabis and Public Opinion

Clearly, public opinion about many aspects of cannabis use has changed dramatically in recent times. Data have accumulated from many survey sources that illustrate shifting viewpoints that have rapidly gained momentum. A reliable source of this information is the Pew Research Center, which has reported several recent key areas of consumer or public opinions.

Table 121. Public opinions and legalization in states of the Union (adapted from Motel, S., at www.pewresearch.org/ fact-tank,2014/11/05/6-facts-about-marijuana/).

- The majority of public opinion now supports marijuana legalization for medical purposes, but this preference is present in only 52 percent of the population (perhaps recorded at 58 percent).
- Support is quite variable. About 39 percent of Hispanics support legalization, but Caucasians and African Americans are more supportive. Baby boomers appear more likely to support legalization by a narrow margin. The elderly, age

range sixty-nine to eighty-six years, show the least support, with 29 percent in favor.

- The American public considers that alcohol is more harmful to health, even if cannabis became widely available.
- Most Americans (63 percent) would be bothered if marijuana smoking occurred in public settings.
- About 47 percent of Americans have tried marijuana. A government survey indicated that about 18 million Americans (7.3 percent) age twelve years or older had used cannabis in the prior month.
- Nearly one half of the states of the United States (twenty-three and DC) have approved the use of medical marijuana.

WHO Estimates of Cannabis Use

The World health Organization (WHO) has performed a relatively recent mental health survey of more than 54,000 individuals aged sixteen years and older in seventeen nations. This survey estimated that cannabis had been used by 160 million people (age range fifteen to sixty-five), but remarkable differences in use were apparent in different countries. The highest use of cannabis was reported in the United States at 42.4 percent.

Conclusion

Future increases in cannabis use or abuse are inevitable with many social consequences. Arguments prevail about putative causal links between cannabis use and social problems. This chapter addresses a limited number of social consequences of present or future marijuana use.

Chapter 18

THE HIDDEN POTAHOLIC

The Hidden Pot User—The Hidden Potaholic

The stigma associated with the use of cannabis (marijuana) in society is variably persistent. This results in a reluctance to disclose cannabis use, especially among young people who have to face penalties or negative reactions from many individuals. These reactions range from upset family members to disciplinary actions by authorities. The concealment of marijuana use is part of the "Hawthorne effect" of underreporting of socially undesirable or illegal behavior. The most common use of pot occurs between the ages of eighteen and twenty-five years, at a time when physical, mental, and social maturation occurs. These circumstances create a compelling need for many users of marijuana to hide their use of this complex drug concoction. Welcome to the hidden cannabis user whom I have elected to call the "hidden potaholic." This term is derived from the use of pot in a surreptitious manner, and it bears some resemblance to the characteristics of the hidden alcoholic.

Marijuana use starts often with occasional recreational dabbling in many circumstances. However, there may be a common sequence of events in the development of cannabis dependence (addiction). These events may progress from regular

425

use to increasing chronic heavy use that may lead to a status of substance abuse or addiction. Substance abuse has its own variable components with episodic binging or regular episodes of substantial intake. The individual pot user may teeter on the brink of frank addiction for a while, but in some cases addiction occurs more rapidly, with it hallmarks of compulsive use and craving. Attempts to mask this progression are often present in the socialized individual. Moreover, attempts to hide the problem of abuse and addiction become established, often with a major degree of sophistication. This circumstance evolves often to form the hidden potaholic in society.

A Substance-Abuse Vignette: Alice

Alice is a twenty-year-old, attractive, and bright university student from New York. Every attempt is made to cover up the identity of Alice in this dialogue. She entered her higher education as an accomplished student. In her second term of studies, her divorced mother received a panicked phone call from Alice, who was pleading to leave school because she felt tired, washed out, and depressed. With her usual caring attitude, her mother jumped into her car and went to the rescue of her impending dropout daughter.

On the way home, her mother arranged for her to be seen by a physician friend who had extensive training in the medicine of addictions. The visit had not been planned, and the mother was convinced that her daughter had some form of medical or physical problem. During an interview with this physician, thorough questioning uncovered details of extensive cannabis use by Alice. In the interview, it was clear that Alice had been bursting to discuss her own perceived problems with a third party.

Alice spilled the beans during her medical interview. She described episodes of panic and anxiety that were interspersed with protracted periods of depression. She had seen a psychiatrist on several occasions but had failed to disclose her marijuana habits. Alice had recently spent three continuous weeks huddled in her bedroom in her off-campus apartment with the company of only her pet cat. She had not emerged except to engage in regular cannabis-smoking rituals with her friends who also engaged in pronounced intakes of cannabis or alcohol. In fact, many of Alice's friends were regular pot smokers or pill poppers or heavy drinkers.

On several occasions, Alice had popped a few pills of opioid painkillers, which, like cannabis, were freely available from on-campus dealers. These dealers were often mature, affluent students. Alice remarked that obtaining weed or pills was as easy as shopping at her local grocery store. While Alice had not graduated to pills or harder drugs, she had sampled both, with an admitted degree of pleasure and satisfaction.

Things had been difficult at university for Alice, with frequently skipped classes and episodic needs to buckle down and play catch-up with academic studies. Alice pined for her boyfriend, who was left behind when she went to university. Her unemployed boyfriend had been a heavy cannabis user and had graduated to intermittent use of cocaine.

During an interview with Alice, it became apparent that she had experienced intrusive thoughts of suicide that she had turned into well-kept secrets. The signs of brewing problems with pot had surfaced on occasion in Alice's teens, with her occasional use of pot that had been noted by both her father and mother. Alice's father remained adamant that her behavior was little more than a passing fancy. Reflecting further on conversations with the physician friend, Alice was clearly in a state of denial herself, and she projected her problem on the pressures of being at university.

Dominant in Alice's rhetoric was rationalization where she protested that she could readily quit marijuana. This was accompanied by an admission that on about half a dozen occasions of trying to quit, she had failed within a couple of weeks. It was clear that Alice's attraction to marijuana was very strong and enduring. Welcome to the uncovered world of the hidden potaholic.

Approaching the Edge of Addiction

Alice seemed to be at the edge of developing frank addiction with a transition through a stage of substance abuse. Alice could see through the unpleasant nature of her disability and its potentially destructive influence on her family, but she persisted with her habits or habituation. The point at which an addiction to marijuana exists is arguable, and a questionable body of opinion exists that cannabis is not addictive. Clinging to this false notion that cannabis is not addictive reinforced Alice's cannabis lifestyle.

These circumstances raise the issue that Alice was suffering from a substance-abuse syndrome. A syndrome is best defined as a collection of signs and symptoms that constitute a definable or recognizable disease entity. Alice was indeed a potaholic. Certainly, cannabis use disorder is a classified disease status, but its recognition is often difficult, especially in the hidden potaholic.

Parallel studies on alcoholism show similar problems that occur in the alcohol or pot abuser. It was E. M. Jellineck, in the 1960s, who labeled alcoholism as a disease. Jellineck asserted that hereditary tendencies to physical dependence on a substance affected the brain. This occurred by psychoactive effect of drugs on the brain (e.g., cannabis), which cause withdrawal symptoms when the drug is discontinued. As mentioned earlier, this situation is comparable to the circumstances of the hidden alcoholic who may often avoid detection in a manner similar to the hidden potaholic.

Developing Addiction

Addiction involves often an enduring desire to continue to use a substance to gain gratification (Pearsall, P., *The Last Self-Help Book You'll Ever Need* [New York, NY: Basic Books, 2005], 44–8). Addiction is a disorder with many potential causes, including genetic tendencies, traumatic past experiences, mental disorders, and adverse environmental factors. Addiction often occurs at the end of a continuum of occasional drug use and substance abuse. More than thirty million people try illicit substances, and about eight million or so may become addicted after passing through a stage of substance abuse.

It is clear that the potency of modern marijuana, as measured by its content of 9-delta-tetrahydrocannabinol (THC), is much more powerful than it was in the mid-1970s. The Office of National Drug Control Policy remarks on the increase in marijuana THC concentration from about 1 percent in the 1970s to more than 6 percent in 2002. Moreover, sinsemilla—or skunk types of weed—has been introduced with its increased potency. Over the past twenty years or so, cannabis strength has increased to more than 14 percent, with occasional samples measured at 33 percent. Recent studies imply that this increase in THC content of available cannabis is associated with a greater prevalence of mental disorders, including schizophrenia or schizophrenic manifestations, and depression.

Marijuana is eliminated from the body approximately seven days after smoking one joint, but chronic, heavy use can be associated with persistent THC levels for up to forty-two days. A hallmark of advanced substance abuse or addiction to pot is the occurrence of withdrawal symptoms upon cessation of the drug concoction. These withdrawal symptoms may generally commence about three weeks after significant levels of cannabis smoking. The withdrawal symptoms from pot are highly diagnostic and include a litany of events, including physiological problems, such as nausea, sweating, or tremors, and behavioral manifestations, such as restlessness, agitation, or depressed mood, and so forth. A key problem occurring with marijuana withdrawal is alterations of sleep patterns.

It seems clear that adolescent use of cannabis may cause a three-times greater prevalence of dependence compared with dependence occurring with use in adults, variably estimated. Furthermore, the younger the onset of marijuana use in childhood the greater the occurrence of abuse and dependence on the drug and other drugs. The potential dangers of cannabis use in adolescents continue to be debated. The position of the American Academy of Child and Adolescent Psychiatry (www.aacap.org) is quite clear with expressions of concern about the overall negative impact of medical cannabis use in youngsters. The AACP emphasizes that teenagers and pubertal users of cannabis are very vulnerable to adverse developmental, cognitive, medical, psychiatric, and addictive properties of cannabis (Schneider, MD, *Addiction Biology*, 13, no. 2 [2008]: 253–63). It is believed by many that marijuana may have long-lasting negative effects on brain development, and it may precipitate psychiatric problems (e.g., mood disorders, anxiety, and psychotic reactions).

These days, adolescents appear to be using medical marijuana increasingly for recreational purposes (Thurstone, C., et al., *Drug and Alcohol Dependence* 118, no. 2–3 [2011]: 489–92). Moreover, its legalization for medical use has sent a message to many young people that marijuana is quite safe. Of course, concerns are highlighted about cannabis use, which has resulted in the following decree: "AACAP thus opposes medical marijuana dispensing to adolescents" (AACAP Medical Marijuana Policy Statement, June 11, 2012, www.aacap.org).

Marijuana Use and Short-Term Acute Brain Syndrome

While addiction to drugs has multifactorial causes, there are many reasons why addiction evolves. These reasons include prescription of addictive medications for a disease (e.g., opioid painkillers), peer pressure, and stressful life circumstances or events. A large proportion of patients with different types of mental disorders may self-medicate, and addiction to the chosen alleviating substance ensues. About more than one half of all patients in the United States have used a prescription drug within the last month, but about one in five individuals may use a prescription drug for nonmedical reasons.

In 2006, NIDA (the National Institute on Drug Abuse) reported that more than sixteen million Americans aged twelve years or older had taken one of several classes of drugs, including tranquillizers, stimulants, sedatives, and pain relievers, for nonmedical reasons (www.samhsa.gov/National Health Survey on Drug Use and Health (NHSDUH). In brief, the easy access to drugs plays a major role in fuelling substance abuse and addiction.

Alice teaches us many components of addiction and substance abuse by which the victim of these disorders attempts to hide his or her habits. Substance abuse and addiction creates emotional, mental, physical, and spiritual demise. The addicted person starts to lose his or her identity, but remorse often surfaces with a sense of loss of identity. This loss of self-awareness can end social relationships and result in isolation with feelings of despair. The addicted or established substance abuser will go to great lengths to fuel his or her habit. Sometimes they engage in pathological lying, obsequious behavior, and any other actions that can hide their habituation.

Marijuana use in young people is far from innocuous. Researchers have likened the effects of marijuana consumption to a short-term acute brain syndrome. This syndrome is composed of several adverse effects, including deficiencies in attention span, lack of ability to concentrate, learning disabilities, problems with short-term memory, and an inability to engage in mental processing or organization (Nahas, G. G., *Cannabis Physiopathology Epidemiology Detection* [CRC Press, 1992], 315).

The ability of cannabis to affect motor skills and judgment is well documented, and these problems interfere with an ability to operate computers, machinery, and driving. Added to these disabilities is a lingering (about twenty-four hours' duration) poor reaction time, and auditory or visual memory deficits can be protracted up to six weeks following cessation of cannabis smoking. Recent research has implied that heavy cannabis use with potent sources of THC (sinsemilla and skunk forms of cannabis) may be particularly damaging to cognitive skills in the short term and result in a higher prevalence of mental disorders, especially psychotic reactions (Nahas, G. G., *Cannabis Physiopathology Epidemiology Detection* [CRC Press, 1992], 315).

Detecting Cannabis Use

There are several unobtrusive questions that may be asked in a medical history that may alert the physician to the presence of a substance-abuse problem (Nahas, G. G., ibid. 1992). These items involve questioning about (1) daily cigarette use, (2) timing and occurrences of episodes of drunkenness, (3) poor performance on school tests, and (4) a tendency to engage in partying. The more the positive responses present to these items, the more likely that the young individual has a substance-abuse problem. Factors such as a family history of drug abuse add to the diagnostic strength of the aforementioned questions. It is valuable often to perform a toxicological screen for drugs on urine samples in these circumstances (Nahas, G. G., ibid. 1992).

There are many other circumstances of the patient that may

prompt drug screening for alcohol or marijuana or other drugs (e.g., cocaine or heroin). These circumstances include accidents, suicidal behavior, seizures, toxic psychosis, inebriation, violent outbursts, antisocial behavior, sexually transmitted diseases, unwanted pregnancy, and symptoms of mental disorders (e.g., manic-depressive behavior) (Nahas, G. G., ibid. 1992). Again, these problems may be elucidated by toxicological testing on blood or urine.

Holistic Approaches to Substance Abuse and Addiction

The transition from substance abuse to addiction is not an abrupt event. The rewards experienced from substance use seem to merge imperceptibly with the progression to addiction with its characteristic components of craving, drug-seeking behavior, and prominent symptoms of withdrawal. These processes of the establishment of addiction involve psychological processes, but they also disturb balance of mind and spirit. Hence, addiction or substance-abuse management is a holistic process that is best managed by a holistic approach.

A typical approach to treatment involves a twenty-eight- to thirty-day program, which is often a process of intense education for the drug user with planning to quit the substance in question. A modified and summarized process for a thirty-day quit regiment is presented earlier in this book in chapter 4.

While there is no consensus on guidelines for the management of the chronic heavy cannabis user or addict, programs have emerged to restore body and mind to a state of balance. This balance is lost in the drug-dependent individual (Giordano, J., *How to Beat Your Addiction and Live a Quality Life* (Tate Publishing, 2013), ISBN: 978-1-62295-669-2). Several factors are involved in the restoration of normal body and mind function together with recapture of spiritual well-being. Table 122 summarizes life changes that can be used to beat down addictive or self-destructive and abusive behavior (modified from Giordano, J., ibid. 2013).

Table 122. Life changes to combat addiction

Life Change	Comment
Define values and principles	In order, consider honesty, hope, faith, courage, integrity, willingness, humility, brotherly love, self-discipline, perseverance, spirituality, and service.
Keep a diary	Observe how patterns of thought determine actions. Learn new ways of thinking and behaving with abolition of negative influences or thoughts.
Meditate	Meditation assists in identification of subconscious thoughts. Consider guided meditation and use further techniques from books or tapes (CDs).
Extinction of obsessions	Success can bring obsessions with money and the ability to engage in expensive habits of which drug consumption is a prime example. Accelerated success can come with notable behavioral changes such as self-absorption, self-centered behavior, and the exaggerated consideration of the importance of "me and mine." Honesty and humility are good antidotes to those circumstances.
Meetings	Regular meetings or social activities permits emergence from self-isolation. Self-help groups such as Narcotics Anonymous (NA) or other meeting forums must occur frequently and in a sustained manner to obtain optimal benefits. Seek the company of winners in life and work with a sponsor who has demonstrated recovery success.
Set goals	Take manageable steps to achieve useful goals in the short and long term.

Develop internal dialogue	Talk yourself up! React against negative self-statements. Be kind to yourself and others. Take charge of feelings that are precipitated by your thoughts.
Denial, projection, and rationalization	Fight your denial that you have a problem. It is not someone else that has caused your problem even if they have encouraged you to use drugs. Drug-taking is a voluntary phenomenon. Stop rationalizing your actions, accept them for what they are, and deal with them.
Positive affirmations	Think positive thoughts and set aside time at least three times a day to write down these positive thoughts. For example, maintain focus, be kind to yourself and others. Be grateful to a higher power for your existence in greater comfort when you quit drugs.
Relationships	Avoid the drug crowd. Seek warm and friendly relationships. In relationships, control jealousy, anger, and possessive feelings.
Make amends	Consider the harm you have done to many people in your life. Consider the harm you have done to yourself. Turn it around and strive to make it right.
Evoke trust	If you relapse, take steps forward. Understand the negative effects of going back to habituation and the loss of trust it creates.
Restore your spirit	Spirituality involves the development of beliefs (e.g., a higher power). Do not lie, cheat, or steal. Perfection may not be an achievable goal, but positive results come from progress in the battle against addictions.

Miscellaneous positive changes	Avoid boredom, get up and move, do not act to create drama, seek proper help, act vigorously against sensations of loneliness or empty feelings, understand that you are not alone in your fight to get clean, live in the present and develop future plans (set goals), change your body language (smile and avoid slouching), fight against anger, blaming, and resentment, try fellowshipping among groups, engage in a good diet and use dietary supplements for health (e.g., vitamins, minerals and fish oil, etc.).

Notes on Addiction Treatments

This book is not intended to be a comprehensive guide to the treatment of addictions, but some basic principles of therapy are highly relevant. In order for therapy to be holistic, the previous guides of life changes that are responsible for recovery should be followed (table 122). Treatment has no single intervention that can be considered to be successful. Recovery programs should be holistic with a multifactorial approach.

Of pivotal importance is the selection of a therapist that is highly trained with demonstrated success in managing addiction or substance recovery. The therapist must have experience with multiple disorders, including concomitant drug use with mental disorder or chemical imbalances, which often require some kind of pharmaceutical intervention (drug prescription).

Several mental or physical disorders can be associated with substance abuse or addiction. Such disorders include heavy metal toxicity, nutritional disabilities, obsessive-compulsive disorders, bipolar disorder, attention-deficit hyperactivity disorder (ADHD), schizophrenia, and depression. It is sometimes seen that when a person becomes clear of substance abuse or addiction, an underlying psychiatric disorder or complementary problem surfaces.

The accomplished addiction counselor or therapist makes the client feel comfortable with him or herself and assists in goal orientation for future well-being. The therapist must show confidence with compassion and genuine qualities. The counselor should be ideally familiar with a variety of treatment modalities, such as biofeedback, neurolinguistic programming (NLP), dietary guidance, and the skilled use of dietary supplements (nutraceuticals).

Diagnostic evaluations and appropriate testing are an integral part of substance abuse or addiction management. A detailed medical history includes aspects of the use of substances, which must be documented to direct further investigation or treatment.

A popular approach to addiction treatment is psychotherapy, individualized or part of a group session and, of course, the twelve-step program of quitting. This latter program is notoriously unsuccessful in a large proportion of patients (up to 95 percent in some instances), and combined or preparatory therapies may improve the effectiveness of the twelve-step program. Table 123 summarizes certain treatment strategies that may complement each other in the management of addictions.

Table 123. A review of some principal therapies that can complement a twelve-step program, constituting an approach toward holistic care (modified from Giodarno, J., ibid. 2013)

Modality	Comment
Definition of intention	Individuals entering recovery programs are doomed to fail unless they are committed to getting better. The keeping of a list of priorities and acts to stay sober are important, and logging progress in a journal is quite valuable.

Assessment of drug or nutraceutical needs	Expert evaluation by a psychiatrist with neuropharmacological knowledge is advisable, and overt problems with mental disorders may require prescription medication (e.g., depression). Vitamin and other dietary supplements may be valuable (e.g., multivitamins, mineral supplements, fish oil, detoxifying herbs, sleeping supplements, liver or metabolic support, natural mood stabilizers, or specific agents known to have beneficial effects in substance abuse and addiction, such as kudzu for alcohol abuse).
Exercise	Exercise is an underestimated antidote to addictions. Aerobic exercise has been shown in many studies to help relieve anxiety or depression and relieve stress. Adequate exercise can result in the release of endorphins in the brain and assist in the restoration of healthy sleep patters. Sleep problems are very common in the substance abuser.
Meditation	Meditation can be used alone or combined with sound technology ranging from calming music to subliminal messaging. Binaural therapy with headphones has been applied to assist in meditation. In general, studies imply that these therapies can result in stress reduction, control of anxiety, sleep disorders, fatigue, and pain syndromes.

Massage therapy

Manipulation of the musculoskeletal system is an age-old approach to a variety of diseases, and it forms the basis of chiropractic and to a lesser degree osteopathic medicine. Simple massage is adequate for treatment, and bone or joint manipulation should be reserved for the medical expert. Massage improves circulation of both blood and lymph, and it has been defined as complementary to detoxification methods.

Spa therapies

A wide range of cleansing, detoxification strategies are used in a variety of spa treatments. One evidence based approach is the twenty-eight-day detoxification program that involves daily sauna treatments, exercise, and vitamin supplementation (the L. Ron Hubbard Method). Detoxification is a lengthy treatment, and single sittings with supplements or occasional sauna exposure is not adequate. Examples of spa therapies include Turkish baths, heated whirlpool baths, steam treatments, and infrared sauna therapy. Colon hydrotherapy is adjunctive in the process of detoxification.

Acupuncture

There is a group called the National Acupuncture Detoxification Association (NADA), which has a membership that claims with confidence that acupuncture restores balance to the body and effectively detoxifies an individual. Some studies have shown the value of acupuncture (at one point on the ear) to relieve symptoms during opiate withdrawal, but further research is required.

HBOT, color, sound, and image therapy

Each of these modalities has found a role in addiction treatments. So-called mild hyperbaric oxygen therapy (HBOT) has grown in popularity with a belief that it can assist in healing of brain damage from drug-induced toxicity. Harmonial color, sound, and image therapy causes beneficial effects on feeling and mood. These techniques may be complemented by the use of aromatherapy with essential oils. It has been suggested that harmonial therapy may produce a natural high in some people.

Neuro-linguistic programming, (NLP), eye-movement desensitization (EMD), and trauma relief therapy (TRT)

NLP is used to assist individuals in building goals. It is the study of the structure of subjective experience. This programming may help to change a client's belief systems and behaviors. Giodarno, J., (ibid. 2013) states that "it teaches you how to model success." EMDR is a type of psychotherapy that uses eye movements to stimulate information-processing in the brain. An advanced form of this therapy is known as TRT, which may produce much faster results than EMDR (Giodarno, J., ibid. 2013).

Social Aspects of Cannabis Use

There is no doubt that marijuana use in young people is increasing. In the early 1990s, cannabis use increased by a factor of 5 percent in youths in school grades six through eight, but a small decline in use of 2.2 percent was noted in 1998. It has been assumed that these trends in marijuana use were influenced by general perceptions of the safety of cannabis. These days, recreational marijuana legalization in several states and medical cannabis, with an attendant continuing and sustained rise in its use in the young.

Convinced that many people held a perception of marijuana as safe, the Partnership for a Drug-Free America commenced a widespread advertising campaign to highlight the opinion that cannabis caused harm and impacted good quality of life. It is known that more than four million people on an annual basis start using cannabis. Comparisons of new users of substances of abuse show that cannabis is the most commonly abused illicit drug behind the use of alcohol and tobacco.

It would appear that young people gain most information about cannabis from their teachers and not from parents and guardians. This finding suggests that there is a widespread need to educate parents on the use of marijuana and its advantages or limitations. Household surveys show a lack of understanding about marijuana in many adults, which interferes with an ability to impart frank, objective, and honest information to minors.

There tends to be a widespread rationalization of marijuana use in young people where parents or guardians have different motives to withhold information (e.g., attempts for parents to hide their own past use of drugs, lack of appreciation of the very common use of marijuana in youngsters, and unfounded beliefs that it cannot happen to their children or cannabis use is just a passing phase). Some of these issues contribute to denial by parents that their children have a cannabis problem. These circumstances assist in the retention of the identity of the problem and reinforce the behavior of the hidden potaholic. A striking statistic is that the average age of first marijuana use is 13.5 years old! Drug warnings to youngsters most often occur in school and not from parents.

Society pays a high price for its combat against cannabis use in young people. Studies in the midnineties and more recently have highlighted the multibillion-dollar cost of drug addiction for health and disability care. It is estimated that marijuana users are responsible for at least one-quarter to one-third of these costs to the federal government. It is argued that cannabis may be a major threat to society, but I believe that any threat to well-being is most apparent in young cannabis users. Studies imply that public safety is at risk from cannabis users who operate machinery or drive under the influence of this drug. Furthermore, cannabis may impart a false sense of confidence to an individual or sometimes precipitate impulsive behavior. While crime and drug addiction go hand in hand, it is sometimes argued that the relationship between marijuana use and excessive crime rates does not exist. In fact, data derived from several studies of this association are conflicting. That said, many criminal lifestyles are associated with drug abuse or addiction.

Cannabis and Teenagers

Curiosity, a sense of communal bonding with friends, and thoughts of appearing sophisticated may contribute to drug use in teens. There are many other reasons why young individuals may choose to use marijuana, including peer pressure, a desire for relaxation, rebellion, risk-taking behavior, and a need to feel mature.

Surveys of cannabis use have produced wide-ranging statistics, perhaps due to lack of disclosure (the hidden potaholics). In a back-to-school survey in 1997, it was reported that half of all a group of students' friends used drugs on at least a monthly basis. Moreover, in this study, about 8 percent of participants aged thirteen years had classmates who had died from drug-related illness. These statistics persist today in studies by the Center on Addiction and Substance Abuse (CASA).

There is a series of symptoms that are suggestive of an individual with a marijuana problem that needs help. These indicators are modified from information provided by Somdahl, G. L. (*Marijuana Drug Dangers* [Enslow Publishers Inc., 1999], ISBN 0-7660-1214-X).

Table 124. Features displayed by an individual with marijuana problems who needs help or intervention

- avoidance of friends who don't do cannabis
- a belief that cannabis is the only way to have fun
- feeling tired, anxious, depressed, or suicidal
- problems with authorities or the law
- suspended from school or dropped out
- giving up constructive activities (e.g., reading, sports, music, etc.)
- lying about cannabis use
- pressuring others to use marijuana
- taking risks (e.g., casual sex)
- obsessed with getting high

There are many myths in the minds of cannabis users, sometimes combined with the idea that no one else can understand the circumstances. It is very important to dispel many of these myths, which may on occasion interfere with an individual's chance of recovery. Several of these myths are summarized in table 125 with rational comments to counter the misunderstandings.

Table 125. Myths and facts about marijuana, modified from *Shapely, C., Marijuana: The Facts* [Irving, Texas: Drug Prevention Resources Inc., 1997], 2

Myth	Reality
Marijuana is not a gateway drug.	Research backs the notion that cannabis is a gateway drug. One switch may be to cocaine.
The effects of cannabis are short-lived for an hour or two.	Effects can be very protracted because components of marijuana are stored in fat and can be recycled in the body.
Creativity occurs with marijuana use.	Cannabis tends to cloud the mind and interfere with memory, performance, and logical thought.
Marijuana is safer than it used to be.	Exactly the opposite. Newer strains of cannabis contain greater amounts of the psychoactive substance (THC).
Marijuana is safe because it is natural.	Many dangerous and poisonous plants exist.
Cannabis counteracts stress.	Stress may be temporarily relieved by cannabis, but the drug often interferes with the resolution of issues that caused the stress.

Prevention and Treatment of Cannabis Abuse

A great deal of literature has been written about drug-abuse prevention programs in schools, but much remains to be accomplished. While society perceives drug education to be a primary responsibility of schools, arguments exist to the contrary (Schools and Drug Abuse Prevention Programming, Environmental

Resource Council, www.envrc.org, 2014). It is argued that schools need to define what resources it can provide and maintain their focus on education. We have noted earlier that schoolteachers are the most important source of education on drug abuse compared with parents, guardians, or peers. Against this background, there is a clear picture that funded resources to deal with drug problems in schools are quite inadequate.

It is recommended that school districts should not subordinate responsibilities for drug use or abuse to law enforcement agencies (ENVRC.org, ibid. 2014). Reaching out to drug users in schools may identify individuals with problems that can be readily dealt with by the educational system. Furthermore, the tendency to merely relate facts or technical information to students is unlikely to change drug habits (ENVRC.org, ibid. 2014). Education should be directed at sharing of information on drug-use patterns and associated lifestyles in a manner that exerts a positive influence on preventing drug abuse and harm.

In contrast, school districts may work to create drug policies that are age-appropriate. However, arguments that acceptance of drug behavior in youngsters is possible are to be rejected. Policies for drug prevention should have a proven track record and preferably involve third-party evaluations with close communication with students. The desired outcome is the abstinence from illicit drug use, but there is a question whether or not zero-tolerance policies actually work (cf. prohibition). The involvement of parents or guardians or family is important in harm prevention. There appears to be mounting evidence that family involvement may benefit prevention outcomes.

Drug-Education Programs

There is truth in the statement that the further back one goes the further forward one can progress (modified from Winston Churchill). In the 1970s, the Nixon administration declared a war on drugs that was accompanied by a 183-page federal report compiled by the National Committee on Marijuana Use and entitled "Marijuana: A Signal of Misunderstanding" (First Report of the National Commission on Marijuana and Drug Abuse, US government printing office, #5266-0001, 1972). This document uncovered findings that came as a surprise.

The report implied a negative correlation between marijuana use and violent crime (First Report of the National Commission on Marijuana and Drug Abuse, US government printing office, #5266-0001, 1972), and it warned of the importance of not creating an antagonistic law enforcement position that faced an impossible challenge of erasure of drug use. The report advised that school districts be reviewed by state governments concerning programs for drug abuse. It was argued that, at that time, many education programs on drug use were not of clear value, and some were quite irrelevant. Arguably, similar problems exist with many current drug-education programs in schools.

Arrests, prosecutions, and incarceration for cannabis possession have been reduced over time by acts of decriminalization. The possession of small amounts of marijuana has been handled in a variety of ways at the state level. These approaches save substantial amounts of money given the high cost of jail time or referral to residential penal institutions. However, among the possessors of small amounts of marijuana are the hidden potaholics who use the drug in a manner of substance abuse or frank addiction. Obviously, there is a major incentive to detect such individuals who are engaged in self-harm and harm to society in varying degrees. Against this background is the knowledge that approximately 50 percent of graduating high school students have used marijuana to a varying degree.

The Emergence of D.A.R.E.

The Drug Abuse Resistance Education Program (D.A.R.E.) emerged in 1983 as a consequence of proposals from the Los Angeles Police Department. This program was adopted as a national approach to drug abuse and addiction. D.A.R.E. was undertaken by police officers (out of uniform) who attended schools to provide information and educate students about resisting drug use.

The impact of D.A.R.E. on elementary students was successful, but the program generated far less effect on high school seniors. In fact, by the early 1990s, evaluations of the D.A.R.E. program showed relatively little effect on drug use and a negative impact in some circumstances in students who had graduated through the D.A.R.E. programs (School and Drug Abuse Programming, www. ercv.org, 2014).

A study performed by University of Maryland researchers implied that D.A.R.E. did not reduce substance abuse. However, the presence of D.A.R.E. did improve relationships between schools and law enforcement agencies. That said, further research on the role of D.A.R.E. in the reduction of substance in the late 1990s failed to show beneficial overall effects, with only occasional triumphs.

In 2007, a pivotal publication in the *American Psychological Journal* reported that D.A.R.E. could actually cause harm. This report triggered the need for D.A.R.E. to be focused on senior students with an expansion of its cultural diversity. Despite these findings, the D.A.R.E. program continues to be popular among many educators, parents, and children in elementary schools.

Despite the legalization of cannabis in certain states (Colorado, Washington state, Alaska, Oregon, and Washington, DC, at the time of writing), there is still a need to have programs to prevent the spread of illicit cannabis use. A major concern is the use of synthetic cannabis that has a serious toxicity profile. Synthetic cannabis has many pseudonyms (e.g., K-2, spice, black mamba, etc.), but it is not composed of naturally occurring cannabinoids such as Delta-9-tetrahydrocannabinol (THC) or Cannabidiol (CBD), and so forth. Synthetic cannabis is banned even in states where there is recreational legalization of marijuana. The serious consequences of synthetic cannabis include hallucinations, mental crises, kidney damage, convulsions, and possible permanent brain damage.

An evaluation of several drug education programs, including D.A.R.E., has been undertaken by several agencies. The School and Drug Abuse Prevention programming initiative has concluded several matters. The key findings of evaluations of drug education have been summarized at ERCV.org (ibid. 2014, www.ercv.org). These findings reiterate the fact that D.A.R.E. does not and did not exert favorable influences on high school seniors or early college-entry students. Finally, D.A.R.E. or similar programs should involve parents. In fact, a consensus has been reached that a principal determining factor in substance abuse was parental involvement with drug problems (www.ercv.org, 2014).

Identifying the Hidden Potaholic

The young pot user goes often to great efforts to hide his or her use of pot. A number of signs of pot use are listed in table 126. While these signs have a high diagnostic discrimination when combined, they are not foolproof for diagnosis of pot use or abuse. However, the more of the fifteen warnings signs that are present the more likely that one may be dealing with the hidden potaholic (Lee, J., 15 Signs of Marijuana Use Parents Need to Watch For. Accessed 4/4/2015. www.choosehelp.com/topics/teenagers/marijuana-use-15-signs-parents need to watch …).

Table 126. Behavior and signs of cannabis use that may assist in uncovering the hidden potaholic (modified from Lee, J., ibid. accessed at www.choosehelp.com on 4.4.15)

- Eyedrops to clear eyes (e.g., Visine). Cannabis smokers often have red eyes due to conjunctival vessel dilation.
- Rolling papers, pipes, a bong, roach clips, and other paraphernalia. The presence of paraphernalia signals passage through experimental stages to established use.
- Incense hides cannabis smells. Incense in a bedroom or sweet-smelling perfumed clothes or sickly-smelling odors on clothes are all telltale signs of cannabis use.
- Mouthwashes, strong toothpastes, and air fresheners are used for masking the scent of cannabis.
- Small burns on the thumb or forefinger indicate that a joint has been smoked to the end.
- Cannabis stickers or posters or T shirts. Teens identify with the cannabis culture and advertise their affiliation with posters or stickers (e.g., 420 on schoolbags).
- Talking in code or in a secretive manner.
- Sudden changes in friends, usually with groups who may do drugs.

- Poverty. A sudden need for money without much to show for it. Weed is expensive.
- Signs of depression or isolation. An unusual demand for isolation or reluctance to engage in family activities are warning signs.
- Reductions in academic performance. Threats to drop out of school may occur.
- Lack of participation in previously enjoyable and rewarding activities.
- Looking or acting stoned. The individual may be slow, lacking in energy, have a lack of expression, or exhibit fatuous behavior.
- Getaway excuses to smoke cannabis.
- Lack of motivation to achieve goals or rejection of activities.

There are several other "giveaway signs" that may help identify the surreptitious cannabis use. These include:

- hidden edibles (cannabis-infused food)
- blocking door cracks to hide smoke
- intermittent voracious appetite (munchies)
- finding cannabis plant parts
- a nagging, persistent cough
- cotton mouth (dry mouth)
- inappropriate emotional outbursts
- impulsive behavior
- risk-taking
- poor judgment
- loss of short-term memory
- poor work performance, academic or manual
- lying
- stealing
- other signs of intoxication

In this book, I have repeatedly expressed concern about the damaging effect of cannabis use in young people. There is no doubt that early identification of a cannabis problem with early intervention creates a better prognosis for recovery in youngsters.

This is a form of secondary prevention of cannabis use, which is relevant even in the presence of cannabis legalization. If chronic heavy cannabis use occurs in young people for a protracted period of time, then cannabis addiction can occur. Addiction to cannabis use or advanced cannabis abuse is particularly difficult to treat. Between one in nine or ten frequent cannabis users can be expected to become addicted (variable data).

There are several other compelling reasons to interrupt cannabis use in teenagers. These reasons are summarized below (adapted from Lee, J., ibid. 2014).

Outcomes of Heavy Cannabis Use

Cognitive problems	Reductions in short-term memory, impulse control, and thought speed. Brain processing, speed, attention, and executive functions are impaired.
Intelligence quotient	Lowered lifetime IQ may occur even if it is only modest.
Mental disorders	Cannabis use may result in schizophrenia, anxiety, and depression.

A Step-by-Step Approach to Cannabis Use in Young People

The parent or guardian of a cannabis-using student should precipitate the need for education on levels of care that are required. The first step is for the individual to move away from cannabis use. In most circumstances, it is wise to seek professional help, even if the assessment is thought to be a mild cannabis problem. Generally, students cannot be objective about their use of cannabis or any drugs. They may tend to continue to deny that they have a problem or project the problem onto other events in their life or even on to other family members. In addition, the mental dynamism of rationalization often enters the picture where self-talk may go like this: "I do smoke cannabis, but I can give up at any time, and therefore it is not a problem for me." This dangerous rationalization is a strong negative influence on recovery.

The strategy for cannabis abuse may start with low-key interventions with obvious advice to quit, but this is often unsuccessful. Further stages of recovery from cannabis abuse can involve intensive counseling, often best with involvement of parents, guardians, or other close family members. If problems persist, the recovery program should graduate from counseling to high-intensity outpatient treatments or even residential treatments. In this latter case, detailed evaluations and structured treatment programs can be applied with important follow-up (Lee, J., ibid. 2014).

Reasons Why Young People Do Drugs—A Review

There are many reasons why teenagers adopt drug habits. Factors that promote this activity include a desire to be popular with friends, parental use of drugs, peer pressure, to develop a sense of adulthood, and because their peers are actively using drugs (Novacek, J., et al., "Why Do Adolescents Use Drugs? Age, Sex, and User Differences," *Journal of Youth and Adolescence* 20, no. 5 [1991]: 476).

Youngsters who come from troubled families have a high risk of illicit drug use. This risk is compounded by use of addictive substances in the household, including alcohol, tobacco, and illicit drugs. Divorce within a family is a risk factor, as is ongoing conflict between divorced parents. Other factors that contribute to drug abuse among youngsters include sexual abuse, lack of a structured environment without rules, inadequate discipline, and mixed messages from parents or guardians (Ryan, S., *Drug Abuse and Teens* [Berkeley Heights, NJ: Enslow Publishers Inc., 2000]).

There are many other factors that can increase the risk of drug abuse, and these are summarized in table 127 (Ryan, S., ibid. 2000).

Table 127. Important factors that can increase the possibility of drug abuse in teenagers (adapted from Ryan, S., ibid. 2000)

Factor	Comment
Peer pressure	Adolescents cling to a group of friends, and this makes them likely to respond to peer pressure. If friends are drug users, a high risk of substance abuse presents itself.
Low self-esteem	Aggressive or impulsive character and low self-esteem may go hand in hand to form a major risk for drug abuse.
Adolescent challenges	Accelerated physical and emotional growth with stress can lead to drug use. Drug-using adolescents reach adulthood with less social skills and arrested emotional development.

Progression of Drug Use

There is often a common pattern of drug-use development in teenage years. Initiation to substance abuse starts often with alcohol and tobacco and often progresses to marijuana, sometimes combined with alcohol (dual substance abuse). Then comes the possibility of the continuum of the substance abuse pattern toward hard drugs, such as cocaine, LSD, heroin, and so forth. Sometimes drug use may develop into multisubstance abuse, with marijuana forming the background staple.

There are several recognized stages of marijuana use that are summarized below (Ryan, S., ibid. 2000).

- **Novice use.** The individual tries the drug a couple of times with or without progression to the next stage of use.
- **Social recreational use.** Often use may be a group phenomenon, but these habits may evolve into more substantial drug abuse.

- **Circumstantial use.** Individuals reach to use marijuana to cope with stressful life events or to open up for partying. This form of habituation may herald the onset of more frequent use.
- **Intensified use.** This is regular, habitual use of cannabis over a protracted period of time. Symptoms and signs of marijuana use emerge (e.g., weight loss, fatigue, poor short-term memory, academic decline, etc.).
- **Compulsive use.** This stage is addiction, which usually occurs as a consequence of chronic, heavy cannabis intake. Compulsive users are committed to propagate their habits and sociobehavioral consequences. Medical problems may emerge. Problems may occur with law enforcement. The objectives of maintaining habituation can lead to aggressive behavior, drug dealing, or theft.

More on How to Spot Cannabis Use—A Review

We have discussed several ways to spot cannabis use in a young person, but other data may be gathered to make an identification. Looking for physical evidence of cannabis use is important. The appearance of red eyes, pupillary dilatation, finger burns, poor dentition, bad breath, musty body odor, disheveled appearance, and shaking may be valuable signs of abuse. An analysis of arrest records, Internet history of cannabis pages, tracking of spending habits, missing household items, and lighters or apples and vegetables used as smoke filters can all be telling signs.

Odors from cannabis smoke can be present on bedding, drapery, carpets, and furniture may occur, with attempts at odor cover-up with incense, breath mints, and covered smoke detectors. Behavioral alterations can often be present in cannabis users with goofy behavior, gorging of snacks (the munchies), altered mental status, poor reaction times, memory impairments, poor work performance, and lack of motivation (www.wikihow.com/knowing if your teenage child is using marijuana).

Conclusion

While many people support the legalization of marijuana use for adults, the use of this drug mixture is increasing in young people. Smoking cannabis is quite common, but recent reports draw attention to the increasing use of vaporization delivery in young people.

Secondary prevention of marijuana use, involving early identification and intervention, are increasingly necessary in underage users of this drug concoction. This approach may reduce morbidity.

Education on the adverse effects of cannabis use in young people is required, with an increasing degree of intensity. The use of synthetic pot is a mounting public health danger in youngsters. The hidden potaholic is an increasing problem requiring structured interventions.

Chapter 19

THE FUTURE

The future of medicinal cannabis use seems promising, but its therapeutic role is far from clear in many circumstances. Recreational use of cannabis appears safe and often enjoyable in otherwise healthy adults. Throughout this book and in many other writings, a monotonous statement is made that "further research with cannabis is required." Beyond this obvious need for future research to clarify the science of marijuana is a need to develop monitoring methods for the study of the outcomes of the medical and recreational legalization of cannabis. There are no clear guidelines for the monitoring of cannabis use in humans. This situation casts a haze on the future of cannabis, use with its consumption increasing as a consequence of legalization and decriminalization strategies, together with improved marketing by suppliers of illicit drugs.

Cannabis research is now driven by economic prospects for both the pharmaceutical industry and the separate cannabis industry. There are conflicts of opinions about cannabis that are growing against and among these industries. Mixed approaches exist in the cannabis industry, where small pharmaceutical research and development corporations have emerged with serious or perhaps sham intent, because of perceived financial rewards. That said, some politicians and regulatory agencies have developed a jaded approach to some small cannabis business operations, such as independent dispensaries and cannabis-growing companies. Capitalistic tendencies are going to continue to govern the actions of pharmaceutical companies and the smaller cannabis industry players. It seems most likely that the pharmaceutical model will ultimately dominate the cannabis business as the treatment properties of cannabis and related drugs become more clear and lucrative. Consolidation of the cannabis industry is inevitable.

There is a long way to go for physicians, politicians, and others to define comprehensive guidelines for the responsible use of cannabis. The future dictates a need for further monitoring and regulatory interventions, and there will be a need for modification of current political legislation at the state level of government in the future. The crystal ball of marijuana use remains clouded, but meanwhile the cat has come out of the bag, and Pandora's half-open cannabis box leaves us with hope for the safe and responsible use of cannabis.

An important next step for society is widespread preparation for the many potential outcomes of widespread cannabis use. This involves an absolute need for good education about cannabis among health care staff and consumers. This education should be especially focused on youngsters to avoid early cannabis use. It is of some concern that society may not be ready for cannabis legalization, and victims of this inevitable situation are likely to be youngsters. What is the solution? While a pivotal factor in the optimum development of the responsible use of cannabis is public education, education of health care workers and effective controls of access to cannabis in youngsters are urgently required.

Several outcomes of cannabis use will occur with positive or negative effects on society, health, economics, and politics. Widespread use of cannabis will develop from further legalization strategies, but this early enthusiasm for cannabis use could be dampened by several issues. I have stressed the issue that major problems loom as a consequence of cannabis use by adolescents and teenagers who form a high-risk group for the development of mental, physical, and social disabilities in later life. Road traffic and work accidents will increase in prevalence, and methods to prevent DUI with cannabis will not be efficient, but they may occupy many courtrooms, thereby creating a legacy for the legal profession and further expense for society. Social services will require expansion for cannabis-related problems, and residual discrimination against cannabis users will persist to a variable degree, especially among elderly or mature individuals.

Cannabis use will increase mental-health problems, and certain physical disorders will develop in the heavy cannabis user. Addiction rates to cannabis and use of other drugs of addiction will increase (gateway phenomena). Treatment services and emergency rooms could be heavily challenged by health problems among cannabis users, especially circumstances of overdose. The use of synthetic pot will continue to be an increasing public health problem, and it will cause greater morbidity and mortality. Increased numbers of individuals will develop dependence on cannabis and the syndrome of cannabis use disorder.

Medical education about cannabis science and its effects on society will have to improve as use becomes more prevalent. Medical schools must provide structured training on cannabis from both a basic science perspective and its clinical use. Cannabis doctors have emerged without any evidence of formal training, and this trend will continue. Morbidity and occasional mortality will occur with cannabis consumption, and further political legislation must be developed to encourage the responsible use of cannabis.

The most common victims of adverse effects and outcomes of cannabis use will occur in those individuals who developed cannabis habits early in their lives. Harsh penalties should be applied to people who sell cannabis to children or encourage its use in youngsters without clear medical necessity. Well-defined and effective methods should be applied to eradicate the use of synthetic pot.

Productivity could fall in some sectors of industry as a consequence of cannabis use. Money from cannabis taxation will likely be subject to misdirection by political bureaucrats who will not adequately support cannabis research. The economics of cannabis purveyance will become of increasing interest as profits soar. The politics of cannabis will chop and change, and politicians will always have a job, even if it is to repeal legislation.

As revenue for overseas illegal drug cartels falls, there will be migration of cartel-sponsored business into the United States.

The illicit use of marijuana will rebound as a competitive market increases to avoid burdensome taxation. Moreover, drug cartels will see sense in participating in legal cannabis sales, but these groups will continue to operate their illegal businesses. While I have tried to predict future occurrences with expanding cannabis use in the United States, many aspects of the future of the anticipated widespread use of cannabis remain unclear!

A key issue of debate is how the cannabis industry will emerge in a fully organized manner. A keynote article in *The Economist,* November 8, 2014 (print edition) explores the topic "The Marlboro of marijuana," with a bold conclusion that "the legal cannabis industry is run by minnows. As liberalization spreads, that may not last." However, it should be remembered that most of the cannabis industry in the United States is still illegal.

Cannabis entrepreneurs have been described as competing with crime gangs for the control of cannabis commerce. It is recognized that a number of start-ups in cannabis production and sales has attracted management that is not a stranger to the illicit cannabis market.

While the cannabis boom is in sight of the nation and happening rapidly in states where recreational marijuana is approved, no dominant, controlling force has arisen (yet). Cannabis business is still locked into a cottage industry that enjoys relative freedom. I believe that the pharmaceutical model for cannabis will prevail.

There will be major research and development of cannabinoids, other than just THC or CBD. That said, CBD is emerging as an important dietary supplement that may have its wings clipped by the FDA. The FDA warning letters sent to companies purveying CBD as a supplement may be the start of more sanctions in the future. The FDA crocodile has shown its teeth, but dental conservation may be required.

Actions that move toward legalization of cannabis use have involved the cleaning-up of marijuana's medical and social identity. The overall perception of marijuana has been damaged over the greater part of the last century by systematic undermining for some good but many bad reasons. The future of cannabis use seems bright, but clouds and potholes exist on its pathway to more general use.

Reference List

Books

Armentano, Paul. *Emerging Clinical Applications for Cannabis and Cannabinoids. A Review of the Recent Scientific Literature,* 6th edition. Accessed 2/3/15. www.norml.org.

Backes, Michael. 2014. *Cannabis Pharmacy: The Practical Guide to Medical Marijuana.* Black Dog and Leventhal Publishers.

Bello, Joan. 2010. *The Benefits of Marijuana: Physical, Psychological and Spiritual.* CreateSpace Independent Publishing Platform.

Blesching, Uwe. 2013. *The Cannabis Health Index: How to Achieve Deep(er) Healing of 100 Chronic Symptoms and Diseases by Linking the Science of Medical Marijuana with the Art of Mind-Body Consciousness,* 2nd edition. Logos Publishing.

Boire, Richard Glen. 1996. *Marijuana Law.* Ronin Publishing.

Cantu, Aaron Miguel. Oct. 14, 2014. *Hemp Hustlers.* www.projectcbd.org.

Brownlee, Nick. 2010. *This Is Cannabis.* Music Sales Corp.

Carter, Gregory T., Dale Gieringer, PhD, and Ed Rosenthal. 2008. *Marijuana Medical Handbook: Practical Guide to Therapeutic Uses of Marijuana,* revised edition. Quick American Archives.

Caulkins, Jonathan P., Angela Hawken, Beau Kilmer, and Mark Kleimann. 2012. *Marijuana Legalization: What Everyone Needs to Know.* Oxford University Press.

Clarke, Robert and Mark D. Merlin. 2013. *Cannabis: Evolution and Ethnobotany.* University of California Press.

Conrad, Chris. 1997. *Hemp for Health: The Medicinal and Nutritional Uses of Cannabis.* Healing Arts Press.

Deal, Megan. 2014. *How to Get Medical Marijuana: A State-by-State Patient Guide.* Northstar Ink.

Earleywire, Mitch. 2002. *Understanding Marijuana: A New Look at the Scientific Evidence.* Oxford University Press.

Fankhauser, M. 2002. "History of cannabis in western medicine." In *Cannabis and Cannabinoids,* ed. F. Grotenhermen and E. Russo E, 37. New York: Haworth Integrative Healing Press.

Gerber, Rudolph J. 2004. *Legalizing Marijuana: Drug Policy Reform & Prohibition Politics.* Praeger.

Golub, Andrew, 2012. *The Cultural/Subcultural Contexts of Marijuana Use at the Turn of the Twenty-First Century.* Taylor and Francis.

Goode, Erich. 1969. *Marijuana.* Atherton.

Goode, Erich. 1970. *The Marijuana Smokers.* Basic Books.

Gottfried, Ted. 2005. *The Facts about Marijuana.* Marshall Cavendish Corp.

Gottfried, Ted. 2004. *The Facts about Marijuana.* Marshall Cavendish Corp.

Green, Greg. 2009. *The Cannabis Grow Bible.* Green Candy Press.

Grinspoon, L. 1971. *Marihuana Reconsidered.* Cambridge, MA: Harvard University Press.

Holland, Julie, MD. 2010. *The Pot Book: A complete Guide to Cannabis.* Park Street Press.

Jonathan, Green and Howard Sooley. 2013. *Cannabis: The Hip History of Hemp*. Running Press Book Publishers.

King, Jason and Robert Clarke. 2001. *The Cannabible*. Ten Speed Press.

McDonough, Elise. 2014. *Marijuana for Everybody: The Definitive Guide to Getting High, Feeling Good and Having Fun*. Chronicle Books, LLC.

Robbins, James. 2014. *Cannabis Oil: The Ultimate Guide to Using Cannabis Oil for Disease Prevention, Skin Conditions, and Many More Powerful Health Benefits*. CreateSpace Independent Publishing Platform.

Rosenthal, Ed and David Downs. 2014. *Beyond Buds: Marijuana Extracts—Hash, Vaping, Dabbing, Edibles, and Medicines*. Quick Trading Company.

Ruschmann, Paul, JD. 2004. *Legalizing Marijuana*. Infobase Publishing.

Ryder Management, Inc. 2014. *Cannabinoids and Terpenes: The Medicinal Benefits of Cannabis*. CreateSpace Independent Publishing Platform.

Walker, John. *After Legalization: Understanding the Future of Marijuana Policy*, Jan. 12, 2014, ISBN 0991239717.

Weiner, Richard S. et al. 2002. *Pain Management*. CRC Press.

Werner, Clint. 2011. *Marijuana Gateway to Health: How Cannabis Protects Us from Cancer and Alzheimer's Disease*. Dachstar Press.

Chapter 1: The Cannabis Revolution

British Medical Association. 1997. *Therapeutic Uses of Cannabis*. Amsterdam: Harwood Academic Publishers.

Institute of Medicine. 1999. *First, Do No Harm: Consequences of Marijuana Use and Abuse. Marijuana and Medicine: Assessing the*

Science Base, edited by Joy, J. E., S. J. Watson, and J. A. Benson. Washington, DC: National Academy Press.

Institute of Medicine. 1999. *The Medical Value of Marijuana and Related Substances. Marijuana and Medicine: Assessing the Science Base,* edited by Joy, J. E., S. J. Watson, and J. A. Benson. Washington, DC: National Academy Press.

Lichtman, A. H., and Martin, B. R. 2005. "Cannabinoid tolerance and dependence." *Handb. Exp. Pharmacol:* 691–717.

Musty, R. E. 2004. "Natural cannabinoids: interactions and effects." In *The Medicinal Uses of Cannabis and Cannabinoids,* edited by Guy, G. W., Whittle, B. A., and Robson, P. J. London: Pharmaceutical Press.

Office of Medicinal Cannabis, The Netherlands Ministry of Health Welfare and Sports. 2008. *Medicinal Cannabis, Information for Health Care Professionals.*

Robson, P. 2001. "Therapeutic aspects of cannabis and cannabinoids." *Br. J. Psychiatry* 178: 107–115.

Russo, E. B., and J. M. McPartland. 2003. "Cannabis is more than simply delta(9)-tetrahydrocannabinol." *Psychopharmacology* (Berl) 165: 431–432.

Russo, E. 2004. "History of cannabis as a medicine." In *The Medicinal Uses of Cannabis and Cannabinoids,* edited by Guy, G. W., Whittle, B. A., and Robson, P. J. London: Pharmaceutical Press.

Chapter 2: Different Modes of Delivery of Cannabis

Abrams, D. I., Vizoso, H. P., Shade, S. B., Jay, C., and others. 2007. "Vaporization as a Smokeless Cannabis Delivery System: A Pilot Study." *Clin. Pharmacol. Ther.* 82: 572–578.

Agrawal, A., Scherrer, J. F., Lynskey, M. T., Sartor, C. E., and others. 2011. "Patterns of use, sequence of onsets and correlates of tobacco and cannabis." *Addict. Behav.* 36: 1141–1147.

Ashton, C. H. 1999. "Adverse effects of cannabis and cannabinoids." *Br. J. Anaesth.* 83: 637–649.

Bramness, J. G., Khiabani, H. Z., and Morland, J. 2010. "Impairment due to cannabis and ethanol: clinical signs and additive effects." *Addiction* 105: 1080–1087.

Carter, G. T., Weydt, P., Kyashna-Tocha, M., and Abrams, D. I. 2004. "Medicinal cannabis: rational guidelines for dosing." *IDrugs* 7: 464–470.

Gieringer, D. H. 1988. "Marijuana, driving, and accident safety." *J. Psychoactive Drugs* 20: 93–101.

Gonzalez, S., Cebeira, M., and Fernandez-Ruiz, J. 2005. "Cannabinoid tolerance and dependence: a review of studies in laboratory animals." *Pharmacol. Biochem. Behav.* 81: 300–318.

Grotenhermen, F. 2003. "Pharmacokinetics and pharmacodynamics of cannabinoids." *Clin. Pharmacokinet.* 42: 327–360.

Guy, G. W., and Stott, C. G. 2005. "The development of Sativex—a natural cannabis-based medicine." In *Cannabinoids as Therapeutics*, edited by R. Mechoulam. Basel: Birkhäuser Verlag.

Hall, W., and Solowij, N. 1998. "Adverse effects of cannabis." *Lancet.* 352: 1611–1616.

Huestis, M. A. 2005. "Pharmacokinetics and metabolism of the plant cannabinoids, delta-9-tetrahydrocannabinol, cannabidiol and cannabinol." *Handb. Exp. Pharmacol.* 657–690.

Institute of Medicine. 1999. *Cannabinoids and Animal Physiology. Marijuana and Medicine: Assessing the Science Base*, edited by Joy, J. E., Watson, S. J., and Benson, J. A., Washington, DC: National Academy Press.

Izzo, A. A., Borrelli, F., Capasso, R., Di, Marzo, V., and others. 2009. "Non-psychotropic plant cannabinoids: new therapeutic opportunities from an ancient herb." *Trends Pharmacol. Sci.* 30: 515–527.

Kalant, H. 2001. "Medicinal use of cannabis: history and current status." *Pain Res. Manag.* 6: 80–91.

Kalant, H. 2004. "Adverse effects of cannabis on health: an update of the literature since 1996." *Prog. Neuropsychopharmacol. Biol. Psychiatry.* 28: 849–863.

Mehmedic, Z., Chandra, S., Slade, D., Denham, H., and others. 2010. "Potency Trends of Delta(9)-THC and Other Cannabinoids in Confiscated Cannabis Preparations from 1993 to 2008." *J. Forensic Sci.* 55: 1209–1217.

Pertwee, R. G. 2008. "The diverse CB1 and CB2 receptor pharmacology of three plant cannabinoids: delta9-tetrahydrocannabinol, cannabidiol and delta9-tetrahydrocannabivarin." *Br. J. Pharmacol.* 153: 199–215.

Rouzer, C. A., and L. J. Marnett. 2011. "Endocannabinoid oxygenation by cyclooxygenases, lipoxygenases, and cytochromes P450: cross-talk between the eicosanoid and endocannabinoid signaling pathways." *Chem. Rev.* 111: 5899–5921.

Sewell, R. A., Poling, J., and Sofuoglu, M. 2009. "The effect of cannabis compared with alcohol on driving." *Am. J. Addict.* 18: 185–193.

Chapter 3: The Expanding Use of Cannabis

Budney, A. J., and J. R. Hughes. 2006. "The cannabis withdrawal syndrome." *Curr. Opin. Psychiatry* 19: 233–238.

Davison, S. N., and J. S. Davison. 2011. "Is there a legitimate role for the therapeutic use of cannabinoids for symptom management in chronic kidney disease?" *J. Pain Symptom. Manage.* 41: 768–778.

Grotenhermen, F. 2007. "The toxicology of cannabis and cannabis prohibition." *Chem. Biodivers.* 4: 1744–1769.

Gunasekaran, N., Long, L. E., Dawson, B. L., Hansen, G. H., and others. 2009. "Reintoxication: the release of fat-stored delta(9)-tetrahydrocannabinol (THC) into blood is enhanced by food deprivation or ACTH exposure." *Br. J. Pharmacol.* 158: 1330–1337.

Holt S, Skinner HA, Israel Y. 1981. "Identification of alcohol abuse. II. Clinical and laboratory indicators." *Canadian Medical Association Journal* 124, no. 10: 1279–94.

Holt, S., and Skinner, HA, 1990. "Confronting Alcoholism." *Canadian Medical Association Journal* 51: 8–9.

Holt, S. 1989. "Tackling the alcohol problem: the case for secondary prevention." *Journal of the South Carolina Medical Association* 85, no. 12: 582–4.

Reiman, A. 2009. "Cannabis as a substitute for alcohol and other drugs." *Harm. Reduct. J.* 6: 35–39.

Whittle, B. A., and G. W. Guy. 2004. "Development of cannabis-based medicines: risk, benefit and serendipity." In *The Medicinal Uses of Cannabis and Cannabinoids*, edited by Guy, G. W., Whittle, B. A., and Robson, P. J. London: Pharmaceutical Press.

Zuardi, A. W. 2006. "History of cannabis as a medicine: a review." *Rev. Bras. Psiquiatr.* 28: 153–157.

Zuardi, A. W., Hallak, J. E., and Crippa, J. A. 2012. "Interaction between cannabidiol (CBD) and (9)- tetrahydrocannabinol (THC): influence of administration interval and dose ratio between the cannabinoids." *Psychopharmacology* (Berl.) 219: 247–249.

Chapter 4: Medical Cannabis

Edwards, D.A., Kim, J., and Alger, B. E. 2006. "Multiple mechanisms of endocannabinoid response initiation in hippocampus." *Journal of Neurophysiology*, vol. 95, no. 1: 67–75.

Howlett, A. C., Barth, F., Bonner, T. I., Cabral, G., and others. 2002. "International Union of Pharmacology. XXVII. Classification of cannabinoid receptors." *Pharmacol. Rev.* 54: 161–202.

King, LA, Carpentier, C, Griffiths, P. 2005. "Cannabis potency in Europe." *Addiction* 100: 884–886. doi: 10.1111/j. 1360-0443.2005.001137.

Kumar, R. N., Chambers, W. A., and Pertwee, R. G. 2001. "Pharmacological actions and therapeutic uses of cannabis and cannabinoids." *Anesthesia.* 56: 1059–1068.

Mikuriya, T., 1969. "Marijuana in medicine: Past, present and future." *Calif Med.* 110, no. 1: 34–40.

Munro, S., Thomas, K. L., and Abu-Shaar, M. 1993. "Molecular characterization of a peripheral receptor for cannabis." *Nature,* 365, no. 6441: 61–65.

Pertwee, R. G. 2005. "Pharmacological actions of cannabinoids." *Handb. Exp. Pharmacol.* 1–51.

Pertwee, R. G. 2009. "Emerging strategies for exploiting cannabinoid receptor agonists as medicines." *Br. J. Pharmacol.* 156: 397–411.

Russo, E. B. 2011. "Taming THC: potential cannabis synergy and phytocannabinoid-terpenoid entourage effects." *Br J Pharmacol* 163: 1344–1364. doi: 10.1111/j. 1476-5381.2011.01238.

Stafford, J., and L. Burns. 2012. *Australian Drug Trends 2011: Findings from the Illicit Drug Reporting System (IDRS).* Sydney: National Drug and Alcohol Research Center, University of New South Wales.

Sugiura, T. 2008. "Biosyntheses of anandamide and 2-arachidonoylglycerol." In *Cannabioids and the Brain.* 15–30.

Swift, W, Gates, P, Dillon, P. 2005. "Survey of Australians using cannabis for medical purposes." *Harm Reduct J* 2: 18. doi: 10.1186/1477-7517-2-18.

Turner, CE, Elsohly, MA, Boeren, EG. 1980."Constituents of Cannabis sativa L. XVII. A review of the natural constituents." *J Nat Prod* 43: 169–234. doi: 10.1021/np50008a001.

Ware, M. A., Adams, H., and Guy, G. W. 2005. "The medicinal use of cannabis in the UK: results of a nationwide survey." *Int. J. Clin. Pract.* 59: 291–295.

Chapter 5: Hemp

Al-Khalifa, A, Maddaford, TG, Chahine, MN, Austria, JA, et al. 2007. "Effect of dietary hempseed intake on cardiac ischemia-reperfusion injury." *Am J Physiol Regul Integr Comp Physiol.* 292: R1198–203.

Callaway, J, Schwab, U, Harvima, I, Halonen, P, et al. 2005. "Efficacy of dietary hempseed oil in patients with atopic dermatitis." *J Dermatolog Treat.* 16: 87–94. doi: 10.1080/09546630510035832.

Callaway, J.C. 2002. "Hemp as food at high latitudes." *J Ind Hemp* 7, no. 1: 105–117.

Callaway, J.C. 2004. "Hempseed as a nutritional resource: An overview." *Euphytica.* 140: 65–72. doi: 10.1007/s10681-004-4811-6.

Callaway, J.C., T. Tennila, and D.W. Pate. 1997. "Occurrence of 'omega-3' stearidonic acid (*cis*-6,9,12,15-octadecatetraenoic acid) in hemp (*Cannabis sativa* L.) seed." *J Int Hemp Assoc* 3: 61–63.

Callaway, J.C., and T. T. Laakkonen. 1996. "Cultivation of *Cannabis* oil seed varieties in Finland." *J Int Hemp Assoc* 3, no. 1: 32–34.

Darshan, S.K., and I.L. Rudolph. 2000. "Effects of fatty acids of w-6 and w-3 type on human immune status and role of eicosanoids." *Nutrition* 16: 143–145.

Deferne, J.L., and D.W. Pate. 1996. "Hemp seed oil: A source of valuable essential fatty acids." *J Int Hemp Assoc* 3, no. 1: 1–7.

Dupasquier, CMC, Weber, AM, Ander, BP, Rampersad, PP, et al. 2006. "The effects of dietary flaxseed on vascular contractile function and atherosclerosis in rabbits during prolonged hypercholesterolemia." *Am J Physiol.* 291: H2987–H2996.

Goyens, PL, Spilker, ME, Zock, PL, Katan, MB, Mensink, RP. 2006. "Conversion of alpha-linolenic acid in humans is influenced by the absolute amounts of alpha-linolenic acid and linoleic acid in the diet and not by their ratio." *Am J Clin Nutr.* 84: 44–53.

Grigoriev, O.V. 2002. "Application of hempseed (*Cannabis sativa* L.) oil in the treatment of the ear, nose and throat (ENT) disorders." *J Ind Hemp 7*, no. 2: 5–15.

Hampson, A.J., M. Grimaldi, M. Lolic, D. Wink, R. Rosenthal, J. Axelrod. 2000. "Neuroprotective antioxidants from marijuana." *ANN N Y Acad Sci* 899: 274–282.

Holler, JM, Bosy, TZ, Dunkley, CS, Levine, B, Past, MR, Jacobs, A. 2008. "Delta9-tetrahydrocannabinol content of commercially available hemp products." *J Anal Toxicol.* 32: 428–32.

Horia, E, and BA Watkins. 2005. "Comparison of stearidonic acid and alpha-linolenic acid on PGE2 production and COX-2 protein levels in MDA-MB-231 breast cancer cell cultures." *J Nutr Biochem.* 16: 184–92. doi: 10.1016/j.jnutbio.2004.11.001.

Horrobin, D. F. 2000. "Essential fatty acid metabolism and its modification in atopic eczema." *Am J Clin Nutr* 71, no. 1: 367–72S.

Kaul, N, Kreml, R, Austria, JA, Richard, MN, Edel, AL, Dibrov, E, Hirono, S, Zettler, ME, Pierce, GN. 2008. "A comparison of fish oil, flaxseed oil and hempseed oil supplementation on selected parameters of cardiovascular health in healthy volunteers." *J Am Coll Nutr.* 27: 51–8.

Kinosian, B, Glick, H, Preiss, L, Puder, KL. 1995. "Cholesterol and coronary heart disease: predicting risks in men by changes in levels and ratios." *J Investig Med.* 43: 443–450.

Kriese, U., E. Schumann, W.E. Weber, M. Beyer, L. Bruhl, and B. Matthaus, 2004. "Oil content, tocopherol composition, and fatty acid patterns of the seeds of 51 *Cannabis sativa* L. genotypes." *Euphytica* 137: 339–351.

Laakkonen, T. T., and J. C. Callaway. 1998. "Update on FIN-314." *J Int Hemp Assoc* 5, no. 1: 34–35.

Leson, G., P. Pless, and J. W. Roulac (eds.). 1999. *Hemp Foods & Oils for Health*, 2nd edn. Sebastopol: Hemptech, Ltd.

Leson, G., P. Pless, F. Grotenhermen, H. Kalant, and M. A. ElSohly. 2001. "Evaluating the impact of hemp food consumption on workplace drug tests." *J Anal Toxicol* 25, no. 8: 691–698.

McPartland, M. J., and G. Geoffrey. 2004. "Random queries concerning the evolution of *Cannabis* and coevolution with the cannabinoid receptor." In *The Medicinal Use of Cannabis,* edited by G. Guy, R. Robson, K. Strong, and B. Whittle. London: Royal Society of Pharmacists. 71–102.

Mechoulam, R. 1986. *Cannabinoids as Therapeutic Agents*. Boca Raton: CRC Press. 1–20.

Mechoulam, R., D. Panikashvili, and E. Shohami, 2002. "Cannabinoids and brain injury: Therapeutic implications." *Trends Mol Med* 8, no. 2: 58–61.

Mensink, RP, Zock, PL, Kester, AD, Katan, MB. 2003. "Effects of dietary fatty acids and carbohydrates on the ratio of serum total to HDL cholesterol and on serum lipids and apolipoproteins: a meta-analysis of 60 controlled trials." *Am J Clin Nutr.* 77: 1146–55.

Mustafa, A. F., J. J. McKinnon, and D.A. Christensen. 1999. "The nutritive value of hemp meal for ruminants." *Can J Anim Sci* 79, no. 1: 91–95.

Odani, S., and S. Odani, 1998. "Isolation and primary structure of a methionine and cystine-rich seed protein of Cannabis sativa L." *Biosci Biotechnol Biochem*, 62: 650–654.

Prociuk, M, Edel, A, Gavel, N, Deniset, J, Ganguly, R, Austria, J, Ander, B, Lukas, A, Pierce, G. 2006. "The effects of dietary hempseed on cardiac ischemia/reperfusion injury in hypercholesterolemic rabbits." *Exp Clin Cardiol.* 11: 198–205.

Prociuk, MA, Edel, AL, Richard, MN, Gavel, NT, Ander, BP, Dupasquier, CM, Pierce, GN. 2008. "Cholesterol-induced stimulation of platelet aggregation is prevented by a hempseed-enriched diet." *Can J Physiol Pharmacol.* 86: 153–9. doi: 10.1139/Y08-011.

Richard, MN, Ganguly, R, Steigerwald, SN, Al-Khalifa, A, Pierce, GN. 2007. "Dietary hempseed reduces platelet aggregation." *J Thromb Haemost.* 5: 424–5. doi: 10.1111/j.1538-7836.2007.02327.x.

Ross, SA, Mehmedic, Z, Murphy, TP, Elsohly, MA. 2000. "GC-MS analysis of the total 9-THC content of both drug-and fiber-type cannabis seeds." *J Anal Toxicol.* 24: 715–717.

Salonen, JT, Salonen, R, Ihanainen, M, Parviainen, M, Seppänen, R, Kantola, M, Seppänen, K, Rauramaa, R. 1998. "Blood pressure, dietary fats, and antioxidants." *Am J Clin Nutr.* 48: 1226–1232.

Schwab, US, Callaway, JC, Erkkilä, AT, Gynther, J, Uusitupa, MI, Järvinen, T. 2006. "Effects of hempseed and flaxseed oils on the profile of serum lipids, serum total, and lipoprotein lipid concentrations and haemostatic factors." *Eur J Nutr.* 45: 470–7. doi: 10.1007/s00394-006-0621-z.

Simopoulos, A. P. 1999. "Essential fatty acids in health and chronic disease." *Am J Clin Nutr* 70: 560–569.

Small, E., and D. Marcus. 2003. "Tetrahydrocannabinol levels in hemp (*Cannabis sativa*) germplasm resources." *Econ Bot* 57, no. 4: 545–558.

West, DP. 1998. *Hemp and Marijuana: Myths & Realities.* North American Industrial Hemp Council, Inc. April 8, 2009. http://www.votehemp.com/PDF/myths_facts.pdf.

Xiaozhai, L., and R. C. Clarke. 1995. "The cultivation and use of hemp (*Cannabis sativa* L.) in ancient China." *J Int Hemp Assoc* 2, no. 1: 26–33.

Zias, J., H. Stark, J. Sellgman, R. Levy, et al. 1993. "Early medicinal use of cannabis." *Nature* 363, no. 6426: 215.

Chapter 6: Cannabinoids and the Endocannabinoid System

Alger, B. E. 2004. "Endocannabinoids: getting the message across." *Proc. Natl. Acad. Sci. USA* 101: 8512–8513.

Battista, N., Di, Tommaso M., Bari, M., and Maccarrone, M. 2012. "The endocannabinoid system: an overview." *Front. Behav. Neurosci.* 6: 9.

Maccarrone, M., Gasperi, V., Catani, M. V., Diep, T. A., and others. 2010. "The endocannabinoid system and its relevance for nutrition." *Annu. Rev. Nutr.* 30: 423–440.

Bisogno, T. 2008. "Endogenous cannabinoids: structure and metabolism." *J. Neuroendocrinol.* 20 Suppl 1: 1–9.

Bradshaw, H. B., and Walker, J. M. 2005. "The expanding field of cannabimimetic and related lipid mediators." *Br. J. Pharmacol.* 144: 459–465.

Brown, A. J. 2007. "Novel cannabinoid receptors." *Br. J. Pharmacol.* 152: 567–575.

De Petrocellis, L., and Di Marzo, V. 2009. "An introduction to the endocannabinoid system: from the early to the latest concepts." *Best. Pract. Res. Clin. Endocrinol. Metab.* 23: 1–15.

De Petrocellis, L. and Di, Marzo, V. 2010. "Non-CB1, non-CB2 receptors for endocannabinoids, plant cannabinoids, and synthetic cannabimimetics: focus on G-protein-coupled receptors and transient receptor potential channels." *J. Neuroimmune. Pharmacol.* 5: 103–121.

Huestis, M. A. 2007. "Human cannabinoid pharmacokinetics." *Chem. Biodivers.* 4: 1770–1804.

Karniol, I. G., Shirakawa, I., Kasinski, N., Pfeferman, A., and others. 1974. "Cannabidiol interferes with the effects of delta 9-tetrahydrocannabinol in man." *Eur. J. Pharmacol.* 28: 172–177.

Martin, B. R. and Cone, E. J. 1999. "Chemistry and pharmacology of cannabis." In *The Health Effects of Cannabis,* edited by Kalant, H., Corrigall, W., Hall, W., and Smart, R. Toronto, Canada: Centre of Addiction and Mental Health.

Pava, M. J., and Woodward, J. J. 2012. "A review of the interactions between alcohol and the endocannabinoid system: implications for alcohol dependence and future directions for research." *Alcohol.* 46: 185–204.

Pertwee, R. G., Howlett, A. C., Abood, M. E., Alexander, S. P. and others. 2010. "International Union of Basic and Clinical Pharmacology. LXXIX. Cannabinoid receptors and their ligands: beyond CB and CB." *Pharmacol. Rev.* 62: 588–631.

Pertwee, R. G. 2010. "Receptors and channels targeted by synthetic cannabinoid receptor agonists and antagonists." *Curr. Med. Chem.* 17: 1360–1381.

Russo, E. B. 2011. "Taming THC: potential cannabis synergy and phytocannabinoid-terpenoid entourage effects." *Br. J. Pharmacol.* 163: 1344–1364.

Wang, T., Collet, J. P., Shapiro, S., and Ware, M. A. 2008. "Adverse effects of medical cannabinoids: a systematic review." *CMAJ.* 178: 1669–1678.

Zhu, H. J., Wang, J. S., Markowitz, J. S., Donovan, J. L., and others. 2006. "Characterization of P-glycoprotein inhibition by major cannabinoids from marijuana." *J. Pharmacol. Exp. Ther.* 317: 850–857.

Chapter 7: Cancer

Abrahamov, A., Abrahamov, A., and Mechoulam, R. 1995. "An efficient new cannabinoid antiemetic in pediatric oncology." *Life Sci.* 56: 2097–2102.

Alexander, A., Smith, P. F., and Rosengren, R. J. 2009. "Cannabinoids in the treatment of cancer." *Cancer Lett.* 285: 6–12.

Caffarel, M. M., Sarrio, D., Palacios, J., Guzman, M., and others. 2006. "Delta 9-tetrahydrocannabinol inhibits cell cycle progression in human breast cancer cells through Cdc2 regulation." *Cancer Res.* 66: 6615–6621.

Carracedo, A., Lorente, M., Egia, A., Blazquez, C., and others. 2006. "The stress-regulated protein p8 mediates cannabinoid-induced apoptosis of tumor cells." *Cancer Cell.* 9: 301–312.

Guzman, M. 2003. "Cannabinoids: potential anticancer agents." *Nat. Rev. Cancer.* 3: 745–755.

Guzman, M., Duarte, M. J., Blazquez, C., Ravina, J., and others. "A pilot clinical study of Delta9-tetrahydrocannabinol in patients with recurrent glioblastoma multiforme." *Br. J. Cancer.* 95: 197–203.

Hermanson, D. J., and Marnett, L. J. 2011. "Cannabinoids, endocannabinoids, and cancer." *Cancer Metastasis Rev.* 30: 599–612.

Johnson, J. R., Burnell-Nugent, M., Lossignol, D., Ganae-Motan, E. D., and others. 2010. "Multicenter, double-blind, randomized, placebo-controlled, parallel-group study of the efficacy, safety, and tolerability of THC:CBD extract and THC extract in patients with intractable cancer-related pain." *J. Pain Symptom. Manage.* 39: 167–179.

Ligresti, A., Bisogno, T., Matias, I., De, Petrocellis, L., and others. 2003. "Possible endocannabinoid control of colorectal cancer growth." *Gastroenterology.* 125: 677–687.

Ligresti, A., Moriello, A. S., Starowicz, K., Matias, I., and others. 2006. "Antitumor activity of plant cannabinoids with emphasis on the effect of cannabidiol on human breast carcinoma." *J. Pharmacol. Exp. Ther.* 318: 1375–1387.

Machado Rocha, F. C., Stefano, S. C., De Cassia, Haiek R., Rosa Oliveira, L. M., and others. 2008. "Therapeutic use of Cannabis sativa on chemotherapy-induced nausea and vomiting among cancer patients: systematic review and meta-analysis." *Eur. J. Cancer Care* (Engl.) 17: 431–443.

Malfitano, A. M., Ciaglia, E., Gangemi, G., Gazzerro, P., and others. 2011. "Update on the endocannabinoid system as an anticancer target." *Expert. Opin. Ther. Targets.* 15: 297–308.

Strasser, F., Luftner, D., Possinger, K., Ernst, G., and others. 2006. "Comparison of orally administered cannabis extract and delta-9-tetrahydrocannabinol in treating patients with cancer-related anorexia-cachexia syndrome: a multicenter, phase III, randomized, double-blind, placebo-controlled clinical trial from the Cannabis-In-Cachexia-Study-Group." *J. Clin. Oncol.* 24: 3394–3400.

Torres, S., Lorente, M., Rodriguez-Fornes, F., Hernandez-Tiedra, S., and others. 2011. A combined preclinical therapy of cannabinoids and temozolomide against glioma. Mol. Cancer Ther. 10: 90–103.

Walsh, D., Nelson, K. A., and Mahmoud, F. A. 2003. "Established and potential therapeutic applications of cannabinoids in oncology." *Support. Care Cancer* 11: 137–143.

Chapter 8: Mental Disorders

Asbridge, M., Hayden, J. A., and Cartwright, J. L. 2012. "Acute cannabis consumption and motor vehicle collision risk: systematic review of observational studies and meta-analysis." *BMJ* 344: e536.

Ashton, C. H. 2001. "Pharmacology and effects of cannabis: a brief review." *Br. J. Psychiatry* 178: 101–106.

Bhattacharyya, S., Morrison, P. D., Fusar-Poli, P., Martin-Santos, R., and others. 2010. "Opposite effects of delta-9-tetrahydrocannabinol and cannabidiol on human brain function and psychopathology." *Neuropsychopharmacology* 35: 764–774.

Bolla, K. I., Brown, K., Eldreth, D., Tate, K., and others. 2002. "Dose-related neurocognitive effects of marijuana use." *Neurology* 59: 1337–1343.

Caspi, A., Moffitt, T. E., Cannon, M., McClay, J., and others. 2005. "Moderation of the effect of adolescent-onset cannabis use on adult psychosis by a functional polymorphism in the catechol-O-methyltransferase gene: longitudinal evidence of a gene X environment interaction." *Biol. Psychiatry*. 57: 1117–1127.

Crean, R. D., Crane, N. A., and Mason, B. J. 2011. "An Evidence Based Review of Acute and Long-Term Effects of Cannabis Use on Executive Cognitive Functions." *J. Addict. Med.* 5: 1–8.

Crippa, J. A., Zuardi, A. W., Martin-Santos, R., Bhattacharyya, S., and others. 2009. "Cannabis and anxiety: a critical review of the evidence." *Hum. Psychopharmacol.* 24: 515–523.

Denson, T. F., and Earleywine, M. 2006. "Decreased depression in marijuana users." *Addict. Behav.* 31: 738–742.

Drake, R. E., C. Mercer McFadden, 1995. edited by Lehman, A. F., and Dixon, L. B. New York: Harwood Academic.

D'Souza, D. C., Abi-Saab, W. M., Madonick, S., Forselius-Bielen, K., and others. 2005. "Delta-9-tetrahydrocannabinol effects in schizophrenia: implications for cognition, psychosis, and addiction." *Biol. Psychiatry*. 57: 594–608.

Fernandez-Espejo, E., Viveros, M. P., Nunez, L., Ellenbroek, B. A., and others. 2009. Role of cannabis and endocannabinoids in the genesis of schizophrenia." *Psychopharmacology* (Berl.) 206: 531–549.

Henquet, C., van, Os J., Kuepper, R., Delespaul, P., and others. 2010. "Psychosis reactivity to cannabis use in daily life: an experience sampling study." *Br. J. Psychiatry* 196: 447–453.

Henquet, C., Krabbendam, L., Spauwen, J., Kaplan, C., and others. 2005. "Prospective cohort study of cannabis use, predisposition for psychosis, and psychotic symptoms in young people." *BMJ* 330: 11–15.

Henquet, C., Rosa, A., Delespaul, P., Papiol, S. and others. 2009. "COMT ValMet moderation of cannabis-induced psychosis: a momentary assessment study of 'switching on' hallucinations in the flow of daily life." *Acta Psychiatr. Scand.* 119: 156–160.

Johns, A. 2001. "Psychiatric effects of cannabis." *Br. J. Psychiatry* 178: 116–122.

Marsicano, G., Wotjak, C. T., Azad, S. C., Bisogno, T. and others. 2002. "The endogenous cannabinoid system controls extinction of aversive memories." *Nature* 418: 530–534.

Messinis, L., Kyprianidou, A., Malefaki, S., and Papathanasopoulos, P. 2006. "Neuropsychological deficits in longterm frequent cannabis users." *Neurology* 66: 737–739.

Moore, T. H., Zammit, S., Lingford-Hughes, A., Barnes, T. R., and others. 2007. "Cannabis use and risk of psychotic or affective mental health outcomes: a systematic review." *Lancet.* 370: 319–328.

Mueser, K. T., et al. 1992. "Comorbidity of Schizophrenia and substance abuse: implications for treatment," *Journal of Consulting and Clinical Psychology* 60: 845–856.

Musty, R. 2005. "Cannabinoids and anxiety." In *Cannabinoids as Therapeutics*, edited by R. Mechoulam. Basel: Birkhaüser.

Passmore, M. J. 2008. "The cannabinoid receptor agonist nabilone for the treatment of dementia-related agitation." *Int. J. Geriatr. Psychiatry* 23: 116–117.

Pelayo-Teran, J. M., Perez-Iglesias, R., Mata, I., Carrasco-Marin, E., and others. 2010. "Catechol-O-Methyltransferase (COMT) Val158Met variations and cannabis use in first-episode non-affective psychosis: clinical-onset implications." *Psychiatry Res.* 179: 291–296.

Rach Beisel, J., et al. "Co-occurring Severe Mental Illness and Substance Abuse: A Review of Recent Research. Accessed 2/17/15. ps.psychiatryonine.org/doi/abs/10.11176/ps.50.11.1427.

van Os, J., Bak, M., Hanssen, M., Bijl, R. V., and others. 2002. "Cannabis use and psychosis: a longitudinal population-based study." *Am. J. Epidemiol.* 156: 319–327.

van Rossum, I., Boomsma, M., Tenback, D., Reed, C., and others. 2009. "Does cannabis use affect treatment outcome in bipolar disorder? A longitudinal analysis." *J. Nerv. Ment. Dis.* 197: 35–40.

Witkin, J. M., Tzavara, E. T., and Nomikos, G. G. 2005. "A role for cannabinoid CB1 receptors in mood and anxiety disorders." *Behav. Pharmacol.* 16: 315–331.

Zuardi, A. W., Shirakawa, I., Finkelfarb, E., and Karniol, I. G. 1982. "Action of cannabidiol on the anxiety and other effects produced by delta 9-THC in normal subjects." *Psychopharmacology* (Berl.) 76: 245–250.

Chapter 9: The Gastrointestinal Tract

Batkai, S., Mukhopadhyay, P., Horvath, B., Rajesh, M., and others. 2012. "Delta8-Tetrahydrocannabivarin prevents hepatic ischaemia/reperfusion injury by decreasing oxidative stress and inflammatory responses through cannabinoid CB2 receptors." *Br. J. Pharmacol.* 165: 2450–2461.

Bermudez-Silva, F. J., Suarez, J., Baixeras, E., Cobo, N., and others. 2008. "Presence of functional cannabinoid receptors in human endocrine pancreas." *Diabetologia*. 51: 476–487.

Brusberg, M., Arvidsson, S., Kang, D., Larsson, H., and others. 2009. "CB1 receptors mediate the analgesic effects of cannabinoids on colorectal distension-induced visceral pain in rodents." *J. Neurosci*. 29: 1554–1564.

Chen, J., Matias, I., Dinh, T., Lu, T. and others. 2005. "Finding of endocannabinoids in human eye tissues: implications for glaucoma." *Biochem. Biophys. Res. Commun*. 330: 1062–1067.

Cianchi, F., Papucci, L., Schiavone, N., Lulli, M., and others. 2008. "Cannabinoid receptor activation induces apoptosis through tumor necrosis factor alpha-mediated ceramide de novo synthesis in colon cancer cells." *Clin. Cancer Res*. 14: 7691–7700.

Esfandyari, T., Camilleri, M., Ferber, I., Burton, D., and others. 2006. "Effect of a cannabinoid agonist on gastrointestinal transit and postprandial satiation in healthy human subjects: a randomized, placebo-controlled study." *Neurogastroenterol. Motil*. 18: 831–838.

Fouad, A. A., and Jresat, I. 2011. "Therapeutic potential of cannabidiol against ischemia/reperfusion liver injury in rats." *Eur. J. Pharmacol*. 670: 216–223.

Grimaldi, C., and Capasso, A. 2011. "The endocannabinoid system in the cancer therapy: an overview." *Curr. Med. Chem*. 18: 1575–1583.

Herrstedt, J., and Dombernowsky, P. 2007. "Anti-emetic therapy in cancer chemotherapy: current status." *Basic Clin. Pharmacol. Toxicol*. 101: 143–150.

Hezode, C., Roudot-Thoraval, F., Nguyen, S., Grenard, P., and others. 2005. "Daily cannabis smoking as a risk factor for progression of fibrosis in chronic hepatitis C." *Hepatology* 42: 63–71.

Hezode, C., Zafrani, E. S., Roudot-Thoraval, F., Costentin, C., and others. 2008. "Daily cannabis use: a novel risk factor of steatosis severity in patients with chronic hepatitis C." *Gastroenterology* 134: 432–439.

Ishida, J. H., Peters, M. G., Jin, C., Louie, K., and others. 2008. "Influence of cannabis use on severity of hepatitis C disease." *Clin. Gastroenterol. Hepatol.* 6: 69–75.

Izzo, A. A., and Sharkey, K. A. 2010. "Cannabinoids and the gut: new developments and emerging concepts." *Pharmacol. Ther.* 126: 21–38.

Jarvinen, T., Pate, D. W., and Laine, K. 2002. "Cannabinoids in the treatment of glaucoma." *Pharmacol. Ther.* 95: 203–220.

Kennedy, P. J., Clarke, G., Quigley, E. M., Groeger, J. A., and others. 2012. "Gut memories: towards a cognitive neurobiology of irritable bowel syndrome." *Neurosci. Biobehav. Rev.* 36: 310–340.

Lal, S., Prasad, N., Ryan, M., Tangri, S., and others. 2011. "Cannabis use amongst patients with inflammatory bowel disease." *Eur. J. Gastroenterol. Hepatol.* 23: 891–896.

Linari, G., Agostini, S., Amadoro, G., Ciotti, M. T., and others. 2009. "Involvement of cannabinoid CB1- and CB2-receptors in the modulation of exocrine pancreatic secretion." *Pharmacol. Res.* 59: 207–214.

Mallat, A., Teixeira-Clerc, F., Deveaux, V., Manin, S., and others. 2011. "The endocannabinoid system as a key mediator during liver diseases: new insights and therapeutic openings." *Br. J. Pharmacol.* 163: 1432–1440.

Marquez, L., Suarez, J., Iglesias, M., Bermudez-Silva, F. J., and others. 2009. "Ulcerative colitis induces changes on the expression of the endocannabinoid system in the human colonic tissue." *PLoS. One.* 4: e6893.

Massa, F., Marsicano, G., Hermann, H., Cannich, A., and others. 2004. "The endogenous cannabinoid system protects against colonic inflammation." *J. Clin. Invest.* 113: 1202–1209.

Matias, I., Bisogno, T., and Di, Marzo, V. 2006. "Endogenous cannabinoids in the brain and peripheral tissues: regulation of their levels and control of food intake." *Int. J. Obes.* (Lond.) 30 Suppl 1: S7–S12.

Mattes, R. D., Engelman, K., Shaw, L. M., and Elsohly, M. A. 1994. "Cannabinoids and appetite stimulation." *Pharmacol. Biochem. Behav.* 49: 187–195.

Naftali, T., Lev, L. B., Yablecovitch, D., Half, E., and others. 2011. "Treatment of Crohn's disease with cannabis: an observational study." *Isr. Med. Assoc. J.* 13: 455–458.

Parker, L. A., Rock, E., and Limebeer, C. 2010. "Regulation of nausea and vomiting by cannabinoids." *Br. J. Pharmacol.* 163: 1411–1422.

Patterson, D. A., Smith, E., Monahan, M., Medvecz, A., and others. 2010. "Cannabinoid hyperemesis and compulsive bathing: a case series and paradoxical pathophysiological explanation." *J. Am. Board Fam. Med.* 23: 790–793.

Purohit, V., Rapaka, R., and Shurtleff, D. 2010. "Role of cannabinoids in the development of fatty liver (steatosis)." *AAPS. J.* 12: 233–237.

Sannarangappa, V., and Tan, C. 2009. "Cannabinoid hyperemesis." *Intern. Med. J.* 39: 777–778.

Siegmund, S. V., and Schwabe, R. F. 2008. "Endocannabinoids and liver disease. II. Endocannabinoids in the pathogenesis and treatment of liver fibrosis." *Am. J. Physiol Gastrointest. Liver Physiol.* 294, no. 2: G357–G362.

Smit, E., and Crespo, C. J. 2001. "Dietary intake and nutritional status of US adult marijuana users: results from the Third National Health and Nutrition Examination Survey." *Public Health Nutr.* 4: 781–786.

Storr, M. A., Keenan, C. M., Zhang, H., Patel, K. D., and others. 2009. "Activation of the cannabinoid 2 receptor (CB2) protects against experimental colitis." *Inflamm. Bowel. Dis.* 15: 1678–1685.

Storr, M. A., Yuce, B., Andrews, C. N., and Sharkey, K. A. 2008. "The role of the endocannabinoid system in the pathophysiology and treatment of irritable bowel syndrome." *Neurogastroenterol. Motil.* 20: 857–868.

Sullivan, S. 2010. "Cannabinoid hyperemesis." *Can. J. Gastroenterol.* 24: 284-285.

Tam, J., Liu, J., Mukhopadhyay, B., Cinar, R., and others. 2011. "Endocannabinoids in liver disease." *Hepatology* 53: 346–355.

Tibirica, E. 2010. "The multiple functions of the endocannabinoid system: a focus on the regulation of food intake." *Diabetol. Metab Syndr.* 2: 5–10.

Tramer, M. R., Carroll, D., Campbell, F. A., Reynolds, D. J., and others. 2001. "Cannabinoids for control of chemotherapy induced nausea and vomiting: quantitative systematic review." *BMJ* 323: 16–21.

Wallace, E. A., Andrews, S. E., Garmany, C. L., and Jelley, M. J. 2011. "Cannabinoid hyperemesis syndrome: literature review and proposed diagnosis and treatment algorithm." *South. Med. J.* 104: 659–664.

Wargo, K. A., Geveden, B. N., and McConnell, V. J. 2007. "Cannabinoid-induced pancreatitis: a case series." *JOP* 8: 579-583.

Wright, K., Rooney, N., Feeney, M., Tate, J., and others. 2005. "Differential expression of cannabinoid receptors in the human colon: cannabinoids promote epithelial wound healing." *Gastroenterology* 129: 437–453.

Zyromski, N. J., Mathur, A., Pitt, H. A., Wade, T. E., and others. 2009. "Cannabinoid receptor-1 blockade attenuates acute

pancreatitis in obesity by an adiponectin mediated mechanism."
J. Gastrointest. Surg. 13: 831–838.

Chapter 10: Bones and Joints

Bab, I., and Zimmer, A. 2008. "Cannabinoid receptors and the regulation of bone mass." *Br. J. Pharmacol.* 153: 182–188.

Clauw, D. J., Arnold, L. M., and McCarberg, B. H. 2011. "The science of fibromyalgia." *Mayo Clin. Proc.* 86: 907–911.

Dunkley, L and Tattersall, R. 2012. "Osteoarthritis and the inflammatory arthritides." *Surgery* 30: 67–71.

Fiz, J., Duran, M., Capella, D., Carbonell, J., and others. 2011. "Cannabis use in patients with fibromyalgia: effect on symptoms relief and health-related quality of life." *PLoS. One* 6: e18440.

Idris, A. I. and Ralston, S. H. 2010. "Cannabinoids and bone: friend or foe?" *Calcif. Tissue Int.* 8 : 285–297.

Idris, A. I., van 't Hof, R. J., Greig, I. R., Ridge, S. A., and others. 2005. "Regulation of bone mass, bone loss and osteoclast activity by cannabinoid receptors." *Nat. Med.* 11: 774–779.

Nogueira-Filho, Gda R., Cadide, T., Rosa, B. T., Neiva, T. G., and others. 2008. "Cannabis sativa smoke inhalation decreases bone filling around titanium implants: a histomorphometric study in rats." *Implant. Dent.* 17: 461–470.

Ofek, O., Karsak, M., Leclerc, N., Fogel, M., and others. 2006. "Peripheral cannabinoid receptor, CB2, regulates bone mass." *Proc. Natl. Acad. Sci. U.S.A.* 103: 696–701.

Richardson, D., Pearson, R. G., Kurian, N., Latif, M. L., and others. 2008. "Characterisation of the cannabinoid receptor system in synovial tissue and fluid in patients with osteoarthritis and rheumatoid arthritis." *Arthritis Res. Ther.* 10: R43.

Ruhaak, L. R., Felth, J., Karlsson, P. C., Rafter, J. J., and others. 2011. "Evaluation of the cyclooxygenase inhibiting effects of six major cannabinoids isolated from Cannabis sativa." *Biol. Pharm. Bull.* 34: 774–778.

Russo, E. B. 2004. "Clinical endocannabinoid deficiency (CECD): can this concept explain therapeutic benefits of cannabis in migraine, fibromyalgia, irritable bowel syndrome and other treatment-resistant conditions?" *Neuro. Endocrinol. Lett.* 25: 31–39.

Skrabek, R. Q., Galimova, L., Ethans, K., and Perry, D. 2008. "Nabilone for the treatment of pain in fibromyalgia." *J. Pain* 9: 164–173.

Tam, J., Trembovler, V., Di, Marzo, V, Petrosino, S., and others. 2008. "The cannabinoid CB1 receptor regulates bone formation by modulating adrenergic signaling." *FASEB J.* 22: 285–294.

Tomida, I., Azuara-Blanco, A., House, H., Flint, M., and others. 2006. "Effect of sublingual application of cannabinoids on intraocular pressure: a pilot study." *J. Glaucoma.* 15: 349–353.

Tomida, I., Pertwee, R. G., and zuara-Blanco, A. 2004. "Cannabinoids and glaucoma." *Br. J. Ophthalmol.* 88: 708–713.

Chapter 11: Cardiorespiratory Disorders

Abboud, R. T., and Sanders, H. D. 1976. "Effect of oral administration of delta-tetrahydrocannabinol on airway mechanics in normal and asthmatic subjects." *Chest* 70: 480–485.

Aryana, A., and Williams, M. A. 2007. "Marijuana as a trigger of cardiovascular events: speculation or scientific certainty?" *Int. J. Cardiol.* 118: 141–144.

Beaconsfield, P., Ginsburg, J., and Rainsbury, R. 1972. "Marihuana smoking. Cardiovascular effects in man and possible mechanisms." *N. Engl. J. Med.* 287: 209–212.

Calignano, A., Katona, I., Desarnaud, F., Giuffrida, A., and others. 2000. "Bidirectional control of airway responsiveness by endogenous cannabinoids." *Nature* 408: 96–101.

Clark, S. C., Greene, C., Karr, G. W., MacCannell, K. L., and others. 1974. "Cardiovascular effects of marihuana in man." *Can. J. Physiol Pharmacol.* 52: 706–719.

Cottencin, O., Karila, L., Lambert, M., Arveiller, C., and others. 2010. "Cannabis arteritis: review of the literature." *J. Addict. Med.* 4: 191–196.

Fligiel, S. E., Roth, M. D., Kleerup, E. C., Barsky, S. H., and others. 1997. "Tracheobronchial histopathology in habitual smokers of cocaine, marijuana, and/or tobacco." *Chest* 112: 319–326.

Jones, R. T. 2002. "Cardiovascular system effects of marijuana." *J. Clin. Pharmacol.* 42: 58S–63S.

Lindsay, A. C., Foale, R. A., Warren, O., and Henry, J. A. 2005. "Cannabis as a precipitant of cardiovascular emergencies." *Int. J. Cardiol.* 104: 230–232.

Mittleman, M. A., and Mostofsky, E. 2011. "Physical, psychological and chemical triggers of acute cardiovascular events: preventive strategies." *Circulation* 124: 346–354.

Moore, B. A., Augustson, E. M., Moser, R. P., and Budney, A. J. 2005. "Respiratory effects of marijuana and tobacco use in a U.S. sample." *J. Gen. Intern. Med.* 20: 33–37.

Pacher, P., Batkai, S., and Kunos, G. 2005. "Cardiovascular pharmacology of cannabinoids." *Handb. Exp. Pharmacol.* 599–625.

Pletcher, M. J., Vittinghoff, E., Kalhan, R., Richman, J., and others. 2012. "Association between marijuana exposure and pulmonary function over 20 years." *JAMA* 307: 173–181.

Roth, M. D., Arora, A., Barsky, S. H., Kleerup, E. C., and others. 1998. "Airway inflammation in young marijuana and tobacco smokers." *Am. J. Respir. Crit Care Med.* 157: 928–937.

Shmist, Y. A., Goncharov, I., Eichler, M., Shneyvays, V., and others. 2006. "Delta-9-tetrahydrocannabinol protects cardiac cells from hypoxia via CB2 receptor activation and nitric oxide production." *Mol. Cell Biochem.* 283: 75–83.

Singla, S., Sachdeva, R., and Mehta, J. L. 2012. "Cannabinoids and atherosclerotic coronary heart disease." *Clin. Cardiol.* 35: 329–335.

Steffens, S., Veillard, N. R., Arnaud, C., Pelli, G., and others. 2005. "Low dose oral cannabinoid therapy reduces progression of atherosclerosis in mice." *Nature* 434: 782–786.

Steffens, S., and Pacher, P. 2012. "Targeting cannabinoid receptor CB(2) in cardiovascular disorders: promises and controversies." *Br. J. Pharmacol.* 167: 313–323.

Sugamura, K., Sugiyama, S., Nozaki, T., Matsuzawa, Y., and others. 2009. "Activated endocannabinoid system in coronary artery disease and antiinflammatory effects of cannabinoid 1 receptor blockade on macrophages." *Circulation* 119: 28–36.

Sidney, S. 2002. "Cardiovascular consequences of marijuana use." *J. Clin. Pharmacol.* 42: 64S–70S.

Tashkin, D. P., Coulson, A. H., Clark, V. A., Simmons, M., and others. 1987. "Respiratory symptoms and lung function in habitual heavy smokers of marijuana alone, smokers of marijuana and tobacco, smokers of tobacco alone, and nonsmokers." *Am. Rev. Respir. Dis.* 135: 209–216.

Tashkin, D. P. 2001. "Airway effects of marijuana, cocaine, and other inhaled illicit agents." *Curr. Opin. Pulm. Med.* 7: 43–61.

Taylor, D. R., Poulton, R., Moffitt, T. E., Ramankutty, P., and others. 2000. "The respiratory effects of cannabis dependence in young adults." *Addiction* 95: 1669–1677.

Tetrault, J. M., Crothers, K., Moore, B. A., Mehra, R., and others. 2007. "Effects of marijuana smoking on pulmonary function and respiratory complications: a systematic review." *Arch. Intern. Med.* 167: 221–228.

Williams, S. J., Hartley, J. P., and Graham, J. D. 1976. "Bronchodilator effect of delta1-tetrahydrocannabinol administered by aerosol of asthmatic patients." *Thorax* 31: 720–723.

Chapter 12: Neurological Disorders

Abrams, D. I., Couey, P., Shade, S. B., Kelly, M. E., and others. 2011. "Cannabinoid-opioid interaction in chronic pain." *Clin. Pharmacol. Ther.* 90: 844–851.

Agrawal, A., Nurnberger, J. I., Jr., and Lynskey, M. T. 2011. "Cannabis involvement in individuals with bipolar disorder." *Psychiatry Res.* 185: 459–461.

Ameri, A. 1999. "The effects of cannabinoids on the brain." *Prog. Neurobiol.* 58: 315–348.

Amtmann, D., Weydt, P., Johnson, K. L., Jensen, M. P., and others. 2004. "Survey of cannabis use in patients with amyotrophic lateral sclerosis." *Am. J. Hosp. Palliat. Care* 21: 95–104.

Baker, D., Pryce, G., Croxford, J. L., Brown, P., and others. 2000. "Cannabinoids control spasticity and tremor in a multiple sclerosis model." *Nature* 404: 84–87.

Benito, C., Nunez, E., Pazos, M. R., Tolon, R. M., and others. 2007. "The endocannabinoid system and Alzheimer's disease." *Mol. Neurobiol.* 36: 75–81.

Bolla, K. I., Lesage, S. R., Gamaldo, C. E., Neubauer, D. N., and others. 2008. "Sleep disturbance in heavy marijuana users." *Sleep* 31: 901–908.

Centonze, D., Rossi, S., Finazzi-Agro, A., Bernardi, G., and others. 2007. "The (endo)cannabinoid system in multiple sclerosis and amyotrophic lateral sclerosis." *Int. Rev. Neurobiol.* 82: 171–186.

Cichewicz, D. L. 2004. "Synergistic interactions between cannabinoid and opioid analgesics." *Life Sci.* 74: 1317–1324.

Clark, A. J., Ware, M. A., Yazer, E., Murray, T. J., and others. 2004. "Patterns of cannabis use among patients with multiple sclerosis." *Neurology* 62: 2098–2100.

Consroe, P., and Sandyk, R. 1986. "Therapeutic potential of cannabinoids in neurological disorders." In *Marijuana/ Cannabinoids as Therapeutic Agents*, edited by Mechoulam, R. Boca Raton, FL: CRC Press.

Corey-Bloom, J., Wolfson, T., Gamst, A., Jin, S., and others. 2012. "Smoked cannabis for spasticity in multiple sclerosis: a randomized, placebo-controlled trial." *CMAJ* 184: 1143–1150.

Esposito, G., Scuderi, C., Savani, C., Steardo, L., Jr., and others. 2007. "Cannabidiol in vivo blunts beta-amyloid induced neuroinflammation by suppressing IL-1beta and iNOS expression." *Br. J. Pharmacol.* 151: 1272–1279.

Fernandez-Ruiz, J. 2009. "The endocannabinoid system as a target for the treatment of motor dysfunction." *Br. J. Pharmacol.* 156: 1029–1040.

Fraser, G. A. 2009. "The use of a synthetic cannabinoid in the management of treatment-resistant nightmares in posttraumatic stress disorder (PTSD)." *CNS. Neurosci. Ther.* 15: 84–88.

Fridberg, D. J., Vollmer, J. M., O'Donnell, B. F., and Skosnik, P. D. 2011. "Cannabis users differ from non-users on measures of personality and schizotypy." *Psychiatry Res.* 186: 46–52.

Gonzalez, R., Carey, C., and Grant, I. 2002. "Nonacute (residual) neuropsychological effects of cannabis use: a qualitative analysis and systematic review." *J. Clin. Pharmacol.* 42: 48S–57S.

Gowran, A., Noonan, J., and Campbell, V. A. 2011. "The multiplicity of action of cannabinoids: implications for treating neurodegeneration." *CNS. Neurosci. Ther.* 17: 637–644.

Greco, R., Gasperi, V., Maccarrone, M., and Tassorelli, C. 2010. "The endocannabinoid system and migraine." *Exp. Neurol.* 224: 85–91.

Hagenbach, U., Luz, S., Ghafoor, N., Berger, J. M., and others. 2007. "The treatment of spasticity with delta-9-tetrahydrocannabinol in persons with spinal cord injury." *Spinal Cord* 45: 551–562.

Hemming, M. and Yellowlees, P. M. 1993. "Effective treatment of Tourette's syndrome with marijuana." *Journal of Psychopharmacology* 7: 389–391.

Hill, A. J., Weston, S. E., Jones, N. A., Smith, I. and others. 2010. "Delta-Tetrahydrocannabivarin suppresses in vitro epileptiform and in vivo seizure activity in adult rats." *Epilepsia* 51: 1522–1532.

Honarmand, K., Tierney, M. C., O'Connor, P., and Feinstein, A. 2011. "Effects of cannabis on cognitive function in patients with multiple sclerosis." *Neurology* 76: 1153–1160.

Jean-Gilles, L., Gran, B., and Constantinescu, C. S. 2010. "Interaction between cytokines, cannabinoids and the nervous system." *Immunobiology* 215: 606–610.

Kalliomaki, J., Philipp, A., Baxendale, J., Annas, P., and others. 2012. "Lack of effect of central nervous system-active doses of nabilone on capsaicin-induced pain and hyperalgesia." *Clin. Exp. Pharmacol. Physiol.* 39: 336–342.

Karst, M., Wippermann, S., and Ahrens, J. 2010. "Role of cannabinoids in the treatment of pain and (painful) spasticity." *Drugs* 70: 2409–2438.

Koppel, J. and Davies, P. 2008. "Targeting the endocannabinoid system in Alzheimer's disease." *J. Alzheimers. Dis.* 15: 495–504.

Kraft, B., Frickey, N. A., Kaufmann, R. M., Reif, M., and others. 2008. "Lack of analgesia by oral standardized cannabis extract on acute inflammatory pain and hyperalgesia in volunteers." *Anesthesiology* 109: 101–110.

Krishnan, S., Cairns, R., and Howard, R. 2009. "Cannabinoids for the treatment of dementia." *Cochrane. Database. Syst. Rev.* CD007204.

Lynch, M. E. and Campbell, F. 2011. "Cannabinoids for Treatment of Chronic Non-Cancer Pain; a Systematic Review of Randomized Trials." *Br. J. Clin. Pharmacol.* 72: 735–744.

Lyketsos, C. G., Garrett, E., Liang, K. Y., and Anthony, J. C. 1999. "Cannabis use and cognitive decline in persons under sixty-five years of age." *Am. J. Epidemiol.* 149: 794–800.

Marsicano, G., Moosmann, B., Hermann, H., Lutz, B., and others. 2002. "Neuroprotective properties of cannabinoids against oxidative stress: role of the cannabinoid receptor CB1." *J. Neurochem.* 80: 448–456.

Martin-Sanchez, E., Furukawa, T. A., Taylor, J., and Martin, J. L. 2009. "Systematic review and meta-analysis of cannabis treatment for chronic pain." *Pain Med.* 10: 1353–1368.

Mechoulam, R., Panikashvili, D., and Shohami, E. 2002. "Cannabinoids and brain injury: therapeutic implications." *Trends Mol. Med.* 8: 58–61.

Meier, M. H., Caspi, A., Ambler, A., Harrington, H., and others. 2012. "Persistent cannabis users show neuropsychological decline from childhood to midlife." *Proc. Natl. Acad. Sci. U.S.A.* 109: E2657–E2664.

Miller, L. L. 1999. "Marihuana: Acute effects on human memory." In *Marihuana and Medicine*, edited by Nahas, C. G., Sutin, K. M., Harvey, D. J., and Agurell, S. Totowa, New Jersey: Humana Press.

Page, S. A., Verhoef, M. J., Stebbins, R. A., Metz, L. M., and others. 2003. "Cannabis use as described by people with multiple sclerosis." *Can. J. Neurol. Sci.* 30: 201–205.

Panikashvili, D., Simeonidou, C., Ben-Shabat, S., Hanus, L., and others. 2001. "An endogenous cannabinoid (2-AG) is neuroprotective after brain injury." *Nature* 413: 527–531.

Papa, S. M. 2008. "The cannabinoid system in Parkinson's disease: multiple targets to motor effects." *Exp. Neurol.* 211: 334–338.

Pazos, M. R., Sagredo, O., and Fernandez-Ruiz, J. 2008. "The endocannabinoid system in Huntington's disease." *Curr. Pharm. Des.* 14: 2317–2325.

Pertwee, R. G. 2007. "Cannabinoids and multiple sclerosis." *Mol. Neurobiol.* 36: 45–59.

Pisani, A., Fezza, F., Galati, S., Battista, N., and others. 2005. "High endogenous cannabinoid levels in the cerebrospinal fluid of untreated Parkinson's disease patients." *Ann. Neurol.* 57: 777–779.

Pope, H. G., Jr., Gruber, A. J., and Yurgelun-Todd, D. 1995. "The residual neuropsychological effects of cannabis: the current status of research." *Drug Alcohol Depend.* 38: 25–34.

Rahn, E. J., and Hohmann, A. G. 2009. "Cannabinoids as pharmacotherapies for neuropathic pain: from the bench to the bedside." *Neurotherapeutics* 6: 713–737.

Ramaekers, J. G., Kauert, G., van, Ruitenbeek P., Theunissen, E. L., and others. 2006. "High-potency marijuana impairs executive function and inhibitory motor control." *Neuropsychopharmacology* 31: 2296–2303.

Rios, C., Gomes, I., and Devi, L. A. 2006. "Mu opioid and CB1 cannabinoid receptor interactions: reciprocal inhibition of receptor signaling and neuritogenesis." *Br. J. Pharmacol.* 148: 387–395.

Robbins, M. S., Tarshish, S., Solomon, S., and Grosberg, B. M. 2009. "Cluster attacks responsive to recreational cannabis and dronabinol." *Headache* 49: 914–916.

Romigi, A., Bari, M., Placidi, F., Marciani, M. G., and others. 2010. "Cerebrospinal fluid levels of the endocannabinoid anandamide are reduced in patients with untreated newly diagnosed temporal lobe epilepsy." *Epilepsia* 51: 768–772.

Rossi, S., Bernardi, G., and Centonze, D. 2010. "The endocannabinoid system in the inflammatory and neurodegenerative processes of multiple sclerosis and of amyotrophic lateral sclerosis." *Exp. Neurol.* 224: 92–102.

Russo, E. B., and Hohmann, A. G. 2012. "Role of cannabinoids in pain management." In *Comprehensive Treatment of Chronic Pain by Medical, Interventional, and Behavioral Approaches: The American Academy of Pain Medicine Textbook on Patient Management*, edited by Deer, T. R., and Leong, M. S. New York: Springer.

Sanchez, A. J., and Garcia-Merino, A. 2011. "Neuroprotective agents: Cannabinoids." *Clin. Immunol.* 142: 57–67.

Scotter, E. L., Abood, M. E., and Glass, M. 2010. "The endocannabinoid system as a target for the treatment of neurodegenerative disease." *Br. J. Pharmacol.* 160: 480–498.

Serpell, M. G., Notcutt, W., and Collin, C. 2012. "Sativex long-term use: an open-label trial in patients with spasticity due to multiple sclerosis." *J. Neurol.* 260: 285–295.

Singh, N. N., Pan, Y., Muengtaweeponsa, S., Geller, T. J., and others. 2012. "Cannabis-related stroke: case series and review of literature." *J. Stroke Cerebrovasc. Dis*. 21: 555–560.

Smith, PF. 2005. "Cannabinoids as potential anti-epileptic drugs," *Curr Opin Investig Drugs* 6, no. 7: 680–685.

Svendsen, K. B., Jensen, T. S., and Bach, F. W. 2004. "Does the cannabinoid dronabinol reduce central pain in multiple sclerosis? Randomised double blind placebo controlled crossover trial." *BMJ* 329: 253–260.

Van Laere K., Casteels, C., Dhollander, I., Goffin, K., and others. 2010. "Widespread decrease of type 1 cannabinoid receptor availability in Huntington disease in vivo." *J. Nucl. Med.* 51: 1413–1417.

Wade, D. T., Makela, P., Robson, P., House, H., and others. 2004. "Do cannabis-based medicinal extracts have general or specific effects on symptoms in multiple sclerosis? A double-blind, randomized, placebo-controlled study on 160 patients." *Mult. Scler.* 10: 434–441.

Wallace, M., Schulteis, G., Atkinson, J. H., Wolfson, T., and others. 2007. "Dose-dependent effects of smoked cannabis on capsaicin-induced pain and hyperalgesia in healthy volunteers." *Anesthesiology* 107: 785–796.

Ware, M. A., Wang, T., Shapiro, S., Robinson, A., and others. 2010. "Smoked cannabis for chronic neuropathic pain: a randomized controlled trial." *CMAJ* 182: E694–E701.

Weber, M., Goldman, B., and Truniger, S. 2010. "Tetrahydrocannabinol (THC) for cramps in amyotrophic lateral sclerosis: a randomised, double-blind crossover trial." *J. Neurol. Neurosurg. Psychiatry.* 81: 1135–1140.

Wilsey, B., Marcotte, T., Tsodikov, A., Millman, J., and others. 2008. "A randomized, placebo-controlled, crossover trial of cannabis cigarettes in neuropathic pain." *J. Pain* 9: 506–521.

Wilsey, B., Marcotte, T., Deutsch, R., Gouaux, B., and others. 2012. "Low-Dose Vaporized Cannabis Significantly Improves Neuropathic Pain." *J. Pain* 14: 136–148.

Wolff, V., Lauer, V., Rouyer, O., Sellal, F., and others. 2011. "Cannabis use, ischemic stroke, and multifocal intracranial vasoconstriction: a prospective study in 48 consecutive young patients." *Stroke* 42: 1778–1780.

Zajicek, J., Fox, P., Sanders, H., Wright, D., and others. 2003. "Cannabinoids for treatment of spasticity and other symptoms related to multiple sclerosis (CAMS study): multicentre randomised placebo-controlled trial." *Lancet.* 362: 1517–1526.

Chapter 13: Diabetes Mellitus

Bermudez-Siva, F. J., Serrano, A., Diaz-Molina, F. J., Sanchez, Vera, I., and others. 2006. "Activation of cannabinoid CB1 receptors induces glucose intolerance in rats." *Eur. J. Pharmacol.* 531: 282–284.

Cardinal, P., Bellocchio, L., Clark, S., Cannich, A., and others. 2012. "Hypothalamic CB1 cannabinoid receptors regulate energy balance in mice." *Endocrinology* 153: 4136–4143.

Christensen, R., Kristensen, P. K., Bartels, E. M., Bliddal, H., and others. 2007. "Efficacy and safety of the weight-loss drug rimonabant: a meta-analysis of randomised trials." *Lancet.* 370: 1706–1713.

Cota, D., Marsicano, G., Tschop, M., Grubler, Y., and others. 2003. "The endogenous cannabinoid system affects energy balance via central orexigenic drive and peripheral lipogenesis." *J. Clin. Invest.* 112: 423–431.

Deveaux, V., Cadoudal, T., Ichigotani, Y., Teixeira-Clerc, F., and others. 2009. "Cannabinoid CB2 receptor potentiates obesity-associated inflammation, insulin resistance and hepatic steatosis." *PLoS. One* 4: e5844.

Di Marzo, V., Piscitelli, F., and Mechoulam, R. 2011. "Cannabinoids and endocannabinoids in metabolic disorders with focus on diabetes." *Handb. Exp. Pharmacol.* 75–104.

El-Remessy, A. B., Al-Shabrawey, M., Khalifa, Y., Tsai, N. T., and others. 2006. "Neuroprotective and blood-retinal barrier-preserving effects of cannabidiol in experimental diabetes." *Am. J. Pathol.* 168: 235–244.

Engeli, S. 2012. "Central and peripheral cannabinoid receptors as therapeutic targets in the control of food intake and body weight." *Handb. Exp. Pharmacol.* 357–381.

Hayatbakhsh, M. R., O'Callaghan, M. J., Mamun, A. A., Williams, G. M., and others. 2010. "Cannabis use and obesity and young adults." *Am. J. Drug Alcohol Abuse* 36: 350–356.

Hollister, L. E., and Reaven, G. M. 1974. "Delta-9-tetrahydrocannabinol and glucose tolerance." *Clin. Pharmacol. Ther.* 16: 297–302.

Jourdan, T., Djaouti, L., Demizieux, L., Gresti, J., and others. 2010. "CB1 antagonism exerts specific molecular effects on visceral and subcutaneous fat and reverses liver steatosis in diet-induced obese mice." *Diabetes.* 59: 926–934.

Le Strat, Y., and Le Foll, B. 2011. "Obesity and cannabis use: results from 2 representative national surveys." *Am. J. Epidemiol.* 174: 929–933.

Hayatbakhsh, M. R., O'Callaghan, M. J., Mamun, A. A., Williams, G. M., and others. 2010. "Cannabis use and obesity and young adults." *Am. J. Drug Alcohol Abuse.* 36: 350–356.

Le Strat, Y., and Le Foll, B. 2011. "Obesity and cannabis use: results from 2 representative national surveys." *Am. J. Epidemiol.* 174: 929–933.

Li, C., Jones, P. M., and Persaud, S. J. 2011. "Role of the endocannabinoid system in food intake, energy homeostasis and regulation of the endocrine pancreas." *Pharmacol. Ther.* 129: 307–320.

Liu, J., Zhou, L., Xiong, K., Godlewski, G., and others. 2012. "Hepatic cannabinoid receptor-1 mediates diet-induced insulin resistance via inhibition of insulin signaling and clearance in mice." *Gastroenterology.* 142: 1218–1228.

Novotna, A., Mares, J., Ratcliffe, S., Novakova, I., and others. 2011. "A randomized, double-blind, placebo-controlled, parallel-group, enriched-design study of nabiximols* (Sativex), as add-on therapy, in subjects with refractory spasticity caused by multiple sclerosis." *Eur. J. Neurol.* 18: 1122–1131.

O'Hare, J. D., Zielinski, E., Cheng, B., Scherer, T., and others. 2011. "Central endocannabinoid signaling regulates hepatic glucose production and systemic lipolysis." *Diabetes* 60: 1055–1062.

Osei-Hyiaman, D., Depetrillo, M., Pacher, P., Liu, J., and others. 2005. "Endocannabinoid activation at hepatic CB1 receptors stimulates fatty acid synthesis and contributes to diet-induced obesity." *J. Clin. Invest.* 115: 1298–1305.

Osei-Hyiaman, D., Liu, J., Zhou, L., Godlewski, G., and others. 2008. "Hepatic CB1 receptor is required for development of diet-induced steatosis, dyslipidemia, and insulin and leptin resistance in mice." *J. Clin. Invest.* 118: 3160–3169.

Silvestri, C., Ligresti, A., and Di, Marzo, V. 2011. "Peripheral effects of the endocannabinoid system in energy homeostasis: adipose tissue, liver and skeletal muscle." *Rev. Endocr. Metab Disord.* 12: 153–162.

Selvarajah, D., Gandhi, R., Emery, C. J., and Tesfaye, S. 2010. "Randomized placebo-controlled double-blind clinical trial of cannabis-based medicinal product (Sativex) in painful diabetic neuropathy: depression is a major confounding factor." *Diabetes Care* 33: 128–130.

Teixeira, D., Pestana, D., Faria, A., Calhau, C., and others. 2010. "Modulation of adipocyte biology by delta(9)-tetrahydrocannabinol." *Obesity* (Silver. Spring) 18: 2077–2085.

Toth, C., Mawani, S., Brady, S., Chan, C., and others. 2012. "An enriched-enrolment, randomized withdrawal, flexible-dose, double-blind, placebo-controlled, parallel assignment efficacy study of nabilone as adjuvant in the treatment of diabetic peripheral neuropathic pain." *Pain.* 153: 2073–2082.

Chapter 14: Infections, HIV Disease, and Inflammation

Abrams, D. I., Jay, C. A., Shade, S. B., Vizoso, H., and others. 2007. "Cannabis in painful HIV-associated sensory neuropathy: a randomized placebo-controlled trial." *Neurology* 68: 515–521.

Bolognini, D., Costa, B., Maione, S., Comelli, F., and others. 2010. "The plant cannabinoid Delta9-tetrahydrocannabivarin can decrease signs of inflammation and inflammatory pain in mice." *Br. J. Pharmacol.* 160: 677–687.

Cabral, G. A. 1999. "Marihuana and the immune system." In *Marihuana and Medicine*, edited by Nahas, G. G., Sutin, K. M., Harvey, D. J., and Agurell, S. Totowa: Humana Press.

Di Franco, M. J., Sheppard, H. W., Hunter, D. J., Tosteson, T. D., and others. 1996. "The lack of association of marijuana and other recreational drugs with progression to AIDS in the San Francisco Men's Health Study." *Ann. Epidemiol.* 6: 283–289.

Nagarkatti, P., Pandey, R., Rieder, S. A., Hegde, V. L., and others. 2009. "Cannabinoids as novel anti-inflammatory drugs." *Future. Med. Chem.* 1: 1333–1349.

Quarta, C., Mazza, R., Obici, S., Pasquali, R., and others. 2011. "Energy balance regulation by endocannabinoids at central and peripheral levels." *Trends Mol. Med.* 17: 518–526.

Reiss, C. S. 2010. "Cannabinoids and viral infections." *Pharmaceuticals* (Basel) 3: 1873–1886.

Roth, M. D., Baldwin, G. C., and Tashkin, D. P. 2002. "Effects of delta-9-tetrahydrocannabinol on human immune function and host defense." *Chem. Phys. Lipids.* 121: 229–239.

Rukwied, R., Watkinson, A., McGlone, F., and Dvorak, M. 2003. "Cannabinoid agonists attenuate capsaicin-induced responses in human skin." *Pain* 102: 283–288.

Sallan, S. E., Cronin, C., Zelen, M., and Zinberg, N. E. 1980. "Antiemetics in patients receiving chemotherapy for cancer: a randomized comparison of delta-9-tetrahydrocannabinol and prochlorperazine." *N. Engl. J. Med.* 302: 135–138.

Sylvestre, D. L., Clements, B. J., and Malibu, Y. 2006. "Cannabis use improves retention and virological outcomes in patients treated for hepatitis C." *Eur. J. Gastroenterol. Hepatol.* 18: 1057–1063.

Tanasescu, R., and Constantinescu, C. S. 2010. "Cannabinoids and the immune system: an overview." *Immunobiology* 215: 588–597.

Watson, E. S., Murphy, J. C., and Turner, C. E. 1983. "Allergenic properties of naturally occurring cannabinoids." *J. Pharm. Sci.* 72: 954–955.

Woolridge, E., Barton, S., Samuel, J., Osorio, J., and others. 2005. "Cannabis use in HIV for pain and other medical symptoms." *J. Pain Symptom. Manage.* 29: 358–367.

Zhang, X., Wang, J. F., Kunos, G., and Groopman, J. E. 2007. "Cannabinoid modulation of Kaposi's sarcoma-associated herpesvirus infection and transformation." *Cancer Res.* 67: 7230–7237.

Chapter 15: Skin Disease and Reproductive Health

Battista, N., Pasquariello, N., Di, Tommaso M., and Maccarrone, M. 2008. "Interplay between endocannabinoids, steroids and cytokines in the control of human reproduction." *J. Neuroendocrinol.* 20 Suppl 1: 82–89.

Biro, T., Toth, B. I., Hasko, G., Paus, R., and others. 2009. "The endocannabinoid system of the skin in health and disease: novel perspectives and therapeutic opportunities." *Trends Pharmacol. Sci.* 30: 411–420.

Brown, T. T. and Dobs, A. S. 2002. "Endocrine effects of marijuana." *J. Clin. Pharmacol.* 42: 90S–96S.

Garry, A., Rigourd, V., Amirouche, A., Fauroux, V., and others. 2009. "Cannabis and breastfeeding." *J. Toxicol.* 2009: 596149.

Gorzalka, B. B., Hill, M. N., and Chang, S. C. 2010. "Male-female differences in the effects of cannabinoids on sexual behavior and gonadal hormone function." *Horm. Behav.* 58: 91–99.

Hembree, W. C., Nahas, G. G., Zeidenberg, P., and Huang, H. F. S. 1999. "Changes in human spermatozoa associated with high-dose marihuana smoking." In *Marihuana and Medicine*, edited by Nahas, G. G., Sutin, K. M., Harvey, D. J., and Agurell, S. Totowa: Humana Press.

Karasu, T., Marczylo, T. H., Maccarrone, M., and Konje, J. C. 2011. "The role of sex steroid hormones, cytokines and the endocannabinoid system in female fertility." *Hum. Reprod. Update.* 17: 347–361.

Lacson, J. C., Carroll, J. D., Tuazon, E., Castelao, E. J., and others. 2012. "Population-based case-control study of recreational drug use and testis cancer risk confirms an association between marijuana use and nonseminoma risk." *Cancer.* 118: 5374–5383.

Maccarrone, M., Di Rienzo M., Battista, N., Gasperi, V., and others. 2003. "The endocannabinoid system in human keratinocytes. Evidence that anandamide inhibits epidermal differentiation through CB1 receptor-dependent inhibition of protein kinase C, activation protein-1, and transglutaminase." *J. Biol. Chem.* 278: 33896–33903.

O'Sullivan, S. E., and Kendall, D. A. 2010. "Cannabinoid activation of peroxisome proliferator-activated receptors: potential for modulation of inflammatory disease." *Immunobiology* 215: 611–616.

Perez-Reyes, M. and Wall, M. E. 1982. "Presence of delta9-tetrahydrocannabinol in human milk." *N. Engl. J. Med.* 307: 819–820.

Rossato, M., Pagano, C., and Vettor, R. 2008. "The cannabinoid system and male reproductive functions." *J. Neuroendocrinol.* 20 Suppl 1: 90–93.

Scragg, R. K., Mitchell, E. A., Ford, R. P., Thompson, J. M., and others. 2001. "Maternal cannabis use in the sudden death syndrome." *Acta Paediatr.* 90: 57–60.

Shamloul, R., and Bella, A. J. 2011. "Impact of cannabis use on male sexual health." *J. Sex Med.* 8: 971–975.

Stinchcomb, A. L., Valiveti, S., Hammell, D. C., and Ramsey, D. R. 2004. "Human skin permeation of Delta8-tetrahydrocannabinol, cannabidiol and cannabinol." *J. Pharm. Pharmacol.* 56: 291–297.

Toth, B. I., Dobrosi, N., Dajnoki, A., Czifra, G., and others. 2011. "Endocannabinoids modulate human epidermal keratinocyte proliferation and survival via the sequential engagement of cannabinoid receptor-1 and transient receptor potential vanilloid-1." *J. Invest Dermatol.* 131: 1095–1104.

Wilkinson, J. D., and Williamson, E. M. 2007. "Cannabinoids inhibit human keratinocyte proliferation through a non-CB1/CB2 mechanism and have a potential therapeutic value in the treatment of psoriasis." *J. Dermatol. Sci.* 45: 87–92.

Zuckerman, B., Frank, D. A., Hingson, R., Amaro, H., and others. 1989. "Effects of maternal marijuana and cocaine use on fetal growth." *N. Engl. J. Med.* 320: 762–768.

Chapter 16: Miscellaneous Topics

Ashton, C. 2011. "Pharmacology and effects of cannabis: A brief review." *Br J Psychiatry.* 78: 101–6.

Bryson, E O, Frost, A M. 2011. "The Perioperative Implications of Tobacco, Marijuana and Other Inhaled Toxins." *International Anesthesiology Clinics* 49, no. 1: 103–18.

Feinberg, I., et al. 1975. "Effects of high dosage delta-9-tetrahydrocannabinol on sleep patters in man." *Clin. Pharmacol. Ther.* 17, no. 4: 458–66.

Sidney, S, Quesenberry, CJ, Friedman, G, Tekawa, I. 1997. "Marijuana use and cancer incidence (California, US)." *Cancer Causes Control* 8, no. 5:722–8.

Summa, K. C., and Turek F. W. Feb. 2015. "The Clocks within Us." *Scientific American.* 51–55.

Vaughn, L K, et al. June 2010. "Endocannabinoid Signaling: has it got rhythm?" *Br. J. Pharmacol* 160, no. 3: 538–43.

Williams, C. M., and Kirkham, T. C. 1999. "Anandamide induces overeating: mediation by central cabnabinoid (CB1) receptors." *Psychopharmacology* vol. 143, no. 3: 315–317.

Wu, TC, Tashkin, DP, Djahed, B, Rose, JE. 1988. "Pulmonary hazards of smoking marijuana as compared with tobacco." *N Engl J Med.* 318, no. 6: 347–51.

Zhang, LR, Morgenstern, H, Greenland, S, et al. 2014. "Cannabis smoking and lung cancer risk: Pooled analysis in the international lung cancer consortium." *Int J Cancer.*

www.researchgate.net.publications/51845657.

www.psychologytoday.com/blog/the teenage mind.

www.ncbi.nim.nih.gov/pmc/articles PMC 244 2418.

www.davidwolfe.com/invasion-of-the-cannabinoids.

www.critterology.com/marijuana_toxicity_ in/author S. M. Esneault.

www.skepvet.com/Blog/medical_use_of_marijuana_for_pets.

www.canorma.org/healthfacts/drugtestguide).

Chapter 17: Social Perspectives

Collins English Dictionary 2012, Digital Edition.

DSM-IV and recommendations.

Hotakainen, R. McClatchey Washington Bureau. May 23, 2013. www.mclatchey.com.

Pertwee, RG, Thomas, A, Stevenson, LA, Ross, RA, Vanel, SA, et al. 2007. "The psychoactive plant cannabinoid, Delta9-tetrahydrocannabinoid, is antagonized by Delta8- and Delta9-tetrahydrocannabivarin in mice in vivo." *Br J Pharmacol* 150: 586–594. doi: 10.1038/sj.bjp.0707124.

"Substance abuse and mental health services administration." 2013. *Results from the 2012 national survey on drug use and health: Summary of national findings.* NSDUH series H-46, HHS Publication no. (SMA) 13-4795. Rockville, MD: Substance abuse and mental Services Administration.

www.theweedblog.com/what-will-the-future-of-the-marijuana-industry-look-like.

www.dallasnews.com/news/local-news/2014-12-11.

www.azcentral.com/story/news/arizona/politics/2014/12/22.

oade.nd.edu/educate-yourself-drugs/marijuana.

www.marijuana-caregiver.com/ about_marijuana_caregivers.htm.

michiganmedicalmarijuana.org/page/articles/caregivers/what-cg-do.

www.pewresearch.org/fact-tank,2014/11/05/6-facts-about-marijuana.

Cannabis Quiz

These questions are to be answered as True and False. The answers are given after the quiz.

Chapter 1: Medical Cannabis

1. The federal government has denied any future possibility of cannabis legalization.

2. President Barack Obama (United States) has indicated that legislation and regulation for the use of cannabis should occur at the level of state government.

3. Prohibition of cannabis occurred under the 1937 Marijuana Tax Act.

4. Physicians are generally quite knowledgeable about cannabis.

5. Information produced online about cannabis is universally reliable.

6. The majority of people are in favor of the medical use of cannabis.

7. The Drug Enforcement Agency (DEA) of the United States does not enforce the Controlled Substances Act against cannabis.

8. The Cole Memorandum describes the focus of certain enforcement priorities that are considered to be important by the federal government.

9. The Cole Memorandum permits cannabis use on federal government properties.

10. The most common reason for most use of cannabis is to achieve a high.

11. Children or teenagers of the twelfth-grade level rarely use cannabis (less than 3 percent).

12. Cannabis use is completely safe without any incidence of addiction.

13. Cannabis works by specific receptor stimulation.

14. Terpenoids found in cannabis are physiologically inactive.

15. Cannabinoid receptors of type 1 are common only on immunologically competent tissues.

16. Cannabis use never causes death.

17. This book encourages people to smoke cannabis without concerns.

18. Recreational cannabis in Colorado and Washington State is sold without taxation (tax-free).

19. Cannabis from modern illicit sources may result in a stronger psychoactive effect than standardized cannabis used in medical treatment.

20. The main psychoactive component of cannabis is 9-delta-tetrahydrocannabinol (THC).

21. All vertebrate animals have an endocannabinoid control system.

22. Smoking or eating cannabis containing THC can cause a feeling of euphoria.

23. Synthetic pot is the safest form of cannabis to use.

24. Cannabis ruderalis has the highest content of THC.

25. Hemp can be derived from Cannabis sativa.

26. Religions or ceremonial use of cannabis is permitted in the United States.

27. Hash or hashish refers to the resinous secretions of the cannabis plant.

28. Cannabidiol CBD can work to reduce the psychoactive actions of cannabis.

29. Sativex is a drug that is a proprietary mixture of CBD and THC.

30. Anandamide is a phytocannabinoid.

Chapter 2: Different Modes of Delivery of Cannabis

31. Schedule I drugs have no potential for abuse.

32. The endocannabinoid system helps to maintain body homeostasis.

33. Alcohol is the most harmful drug overall.

34. Cannabis is metabolized at first pass through the liver.

35. Vaporizing cannabis for use is healthier than cigarette "joint" smoking.

36. Vaporizing involves complete combustion of cannabis.

37. Edible cannabis is a particular risk for use in children.

38. The onset of the psychoactive effect of edible cannabis is faster than smoking cannabis.

39. Dabbing involves the vaporization of high concentrations of cannabis.

40. Topical delivery of cannabinoids results in high blood levels of these compounds.

41. Rimonabant (SR141716A) was withdrawn from use because it caused depression and increased suicide.

42. Ajulemic acid (CT3) has cannabinoid receptor type-1 stimulating effects.

43. Bias of scientific investigators has sometimes been noted with investigators who oppose cannabis legalization.

44. Cannabis use can variably result in relief of muscle spasms.

45. Cannabis sativa is the main source of THC.

46. Most research on the effects of cannabis is derived from human experiments.

47. Cannabis edibles are often called jollies.

48. Rectal delivery of cannabis in humans may reduce the effects of first-pass metabolism by the human liver.

49. Distribution of cannabis to minors is not a serious federal offense.

50. State laws on cannabis in Washington state,Colorado, Oregon, Alaska, and Washington, DC, are in conflict with US federal law.

Chapter 3: The Expanding Use of Cannabis

51. Cannabis use probably first occurred several thousand years ago in Germany.

52. The LaGuardia Report in the United States in 1938 implied that the catastrophic reports of the effects of marijuana were not founded.

53. Harry Anslinger Jr. encouraged the Federal Bureau of Narcotics to prosecute three thousand doctors who were American Medical Association members, in the period 1937–9.

54. Dr. Ralph Mechoulam from Israel is regarded as the father of cannabis research.

55. THC and CBD were discovered in the 1960s.

56. Cannabis plants contain flavonoids.

57. Drugs, such as Marinol (dronabinol), do not usually have the same broad effects as whole herbal cannabis.

58. A cannabis high is associated with improved short-term memory.

59. Cannabis can cause music appreciation.

60. Cannabis often increases appetite and interest in food.

61. A whitey is a severe adverse reaction to cannabis.

62. Coffee drinking can result in the extension of a cannabis high.

63. Cannabis alters dopamine neurotransmitter functions.

64. Glutamate is a neurotransmitter involved in memory formation and learning.

65. Skunk-type cannabis is of low THC content.

66. Cardiovascular disease can be made worse by cannabis smoking.

67. A history of schizophrenia is a contraindication to cannabis use.

68. Cannabis has no drug interaction potential.

69. Cannabis is safe for use in pregnancy.

70. Cannabis use should be avoided in the presence of severe liver or kidney disease.

71. THC may cause significant anxiety.

72. Cannabinoids can be detected in maternal milk after cannabis use.

73. The gateway phenomenon refers to chest infections from cannabis smoking.

74. Medical school teaching is often focused on cannabis science and use.

75. Cannabis is sold always with federal warnings.

76. Cannabis can alter estrogen metabolism.

77. Cannabis smoking can reduce aspects of immune function.

78. Seizures may occur with marijuana use.

79. Marijuana smoking usually slows the rate of the heart after intake.

80. Cannabis smoking increases phlegm production and increases tendencies to lung infections.

81. Individuals with cannabis use disorder (CUD) often persist with cannabis use despite harmful consequences.

82. Adolescents and teenagers who use cannabis are at special risk for developmental disorders in later life.

83. About 40 percent of cannabis users may prefer illicit cannabis, even in states of approved recreational use.

84. Street cannabis may be contaminated with microbes that form exotoxins.

85. Cannabis use may permit a lowering of dosage of opioids in many people.

86. Plants other than cannabis contain compounds that can interact with cannabinoid receptors.

87. Smoking hashish often creates greater toxicity than whole herbal cannabis.

88. Illicit cannabis used thirty years ago was weaker than illicit cannabis used today.

89. Cannabis legalization in the United States is damaging the black market for cannabis sales from adjacent countries.

90. Cannabis may treat low intraocular pressure.

Chapter 4: Medical Cannabis

91. Physicians in many US states, Canada, Australia, and several European countries are permitted to prescribe or advise on the use of cannabis.

92. General guidelines for the use of cannabis as a medicine recommend the use of cannabis only after conventional treatments have been attempted and found to be ineffective. Physicians may exercise further discretion on cannabis use, especially when conventional therapy is not anticipated to be effective.

93. Cannabis is most often a first-line option in medical treatment.

94. An obligation rests with a physician to demonstrate that cannabis prescriptions constitute a medical necessity.

95. Cannabis is often used in an unapproved manner.

96. It is often not possible to make accurate statements about the potential effects of various cannabis products.

97. Synthetic pot is a safe option to substitute for illicit drug use of whole herbal cannabis.

98. Drugs or analogues of cannabis may not be overall as effective as whole herbal cannabis.

99. There is good evidence that cannabis administration is useful in the management of chronic pain.

100. Cannabis use may improve quality-of-life scores in palliative care.

101. Good evidence exists to support the use of cannabis in multiple sclerosis.

102. The act of decriminalization of cannabis is the same as legalization of the drug.

103. The current opinion of the federal government is that cannabis is a drug without currently accepted medical use.

104. Education about the outcome of cannabis use is now an important public health initiative.

105. Controlled clinical studies show the diverse functions of the endocannabinoid system.

106. Cannabis has been demonstrated to have potential value in the management of metabolic syndrome X.

107. Dietary supplements containing hemp with CBD content are universally approved without any question.

108. With cannabis smoking there are substantial differences often in the amount of active ingredients that are delivered into the body with different forms of cannabis.

109. The action of cannabinoids remains largely under explored.

110. Cannabinol (CBN) is an oxidation product often formed by poor herbal cannabis storage.

111. Herbal cannabis is most potent when derived from the root of the cannabis plant.

112. Dronabinol (Marinol) produces a greater euphoriant effect than smoking high-THC-content herbal marijuana.

113. Many hemp oil products are sold in health food stores.

114. According the National Institute on Drug Abuse (NIDA), there has been a steady increase in the use of cannabis in young people in recent times.

115. Cannabinoids have no characteristic smell.

116. The time of onset of cannabis edibles is later than the time of onset of effects from smoking cannabis.

117. The effects of consuming cannabis edibles are often shorter in time than the onset effects of smoking herbal cannabis.

118. The psychoactive effects of cannabinoids occur mainly by binding to type 2 cannabinoid receptors in the brain.

119. The context in which cannabis is smoked has a significant effect on the euphoriant effects of cannabis.

120. Cannabis users are known to often select drug-using friends.

121. Heavy and frequent cannabis use improves social relationships.

122. Cannabis use in large amounts can often lead to a high degree of motivation.

123. Daily heavy use of cannabis is often more associated with various disabilities.

124. Avoidance of boating or other recreational pursuits should be delayed for a period of at least twelve hours following cannabis use.

125. Individuals with established cardiovascular disease can use cannabis with safety.

126. About 18 percent of motor vehicle drivers may test positive for illicit drug use other than alcohol.

127. Some current studies demonstrate that there is about a 10 percent decrease in deaths due to traffic accidents in certain states that have legalization of medicinal or recreational cannabis use.

128. Cannabis may cause acute myocardial infarction in young people.

129. A lack of availability of cannabis in a regular cannabis user is often associated with excessive alcohol drinking.

130. Smoke from cannabis cigarettes contains carcinogens.

131. Long-term heavy cannabis use by smoking may cause compromise of lung function.

132. Cannabis can often cause the munchies.

133. Cannabis use has been associated with occasional hyperemesis.

134. Cannabis use sharpens mental cognition.

135. There is a difference of opinion on the effects of cannabis on memory and cognition in the long term.

136. The Centers for Disease Control and Prevention (CDC) have described an alarming increase in death from opioid overdoses.

137. Overdose of opioids is a rare event .

138. Recent research shows that the presence of medical marijuana legalization could reduce the prevalence of deaths from opioid overdosing.

139. THC may cause anxiety and act as an anxiolytic.

140. Cannabis may lower insulin needs in patients with diabetes mellitis.

141. Cannabis is generally perceived to be neurotoxic.

142. Ideal dosing of cannabis is often easy to predict.

143. There can be inconsistency in the effects of the same brand of whole herbal cannabis sold in a dispensary.

144. The National Institute On Drug Abuse (NIDA) has supplied standardized prescribed amounts of cannabis for individuals who are enrolled in the Compassionate Investigational New Drug (CIND) program.

145. The route of delivery of cannabis has a major effect on required dosages for medical use.

146. Low dosage of all forms of cannabis is advisable when an individual is starting to use cannabis.

147. Tolerance to cannabis can occur within a couple of weeks.

148. The self-titration dosing paradigm is always best avoided.

149. The largest tolerated dose of cannabis is always preferred at the initial time of prescription of medication.

150. Physicians are obliged to review all treatments mixed with cannabis and determine safety and efficacy.

151. Family-based therapies have been shown to be of value in circumstances of cannabis use.

152. Hashish use is usually safer than regular cannabis use.

153. About one in nine teenagers in twelfth-grade school are using synthetic pot.

154. The issuance of public health warnings about synthetic pot appears to have done little to interfere with the overall use of synthetic pot.

155. Black mamba is a safe form of cannabis to consider for initial use.

156. The number of types of synthetic pot has decreased in recent times.

157. Death from cannabis overdosing has occurred in children.

158. Synthetic pot has never been recorded to cause death.

159. Cannabis can complement opioid drugs in the management of chronic pain.

160. Cannabis has drug interaction potential with warfarin.

161. Cannabis is quite safe when mixed with the antidepressant Fluoxetine (Prozac).

162. Pregnenolone may reduce the occurrence of a cannabis high.

163. Cannabis generally improves work performance.

164. Cannabis users have a higher prevalence of job security.

165. Intrusive or obsessional thoughts about using cannabis may signal the occurrence of cannabis dependence.

Chapter 5: Hemp Nutrition

166. Hemp is only derived from Cannabis indica.

167. Hemp has no significant nutritional value.

168. Hemp usually contains less than 0.3 percent delta-9-tetrahydrocannabinol.

169. Oils constitute about 35–45 percent by weight of whole hemp seed.

170. Edestin is a highly active fatty acid.

171. Hemp oils usually have an essential fatty-acid content with a ratio of omega-6 to omega-3 of 20:1.

172. Whole hemp seed contains 80 percent carbohydrates by weight.

173. Hemp protein is a complete source of protein without any limiting amino acids.

174. Animal experiments indicate that hemp seed has positive benefit on memory and learning.

175. Hemp seed in high dosage can lower blood cholesterol.

176. Dietary studies in cannabis users have not shown large overall reduction in measured parameters of health, but marijuana users show differences in nutritional practices.

177. Cannabis users tend to eat more sodium in their diet.

178. The genome of cannabis has no role in defining the potential production of cannabis components.

179. More than 60 percent of hemp contents form groups of essential nutrients.

180. Whole hemp is a useful source of dietary fiber.

181. Hemp is a sustainable, disease-resistant crop.

182. The heart of the hemp seed is called the hemp nut.

183. Hemp tofu is a viable functional food.

184. Growing hemp in the United States has been forbidden under the 2014 Farm Bill.

185. Illicit cannabis is often contaminated with solvents or bacterial organisms.

186. Cannabis can be grown indoors and outdoors in the northern states of America.

187. Greater than three cannabis crops per year can be obtained by growing hemp outdoors in northern parts of the United States.

188. The recreational use of hemp is popular to obtain a euphoriant effect.

189. Hemp is often grown using genetic engineering technology.

190. Hemp contains vitamin E.

Chapter 6: Cannabinoids and the Endocannabinoid System

191. Phyto-cannabinoids are only present in hash.

192. Enzyme inhibitors can prevent the degradation of endocannabinoids.

193. Cannabinoid receptors play a role in newborn suckling.

194. CB-2 receptor agonists generally increase immune function.

195. Endocannabinoids are best described as lipid ligands.

196. Arachidonic acid is the precursor of Anandamide or AEA.

197. Endocannabinoids use a pathway of retrograde signaling across a synapse.

198. Endocannabinoids do not diffuse for long distances in body tissues.

199. The sum total of the effects of cannabinoids is due mainly to cannabinoid receptor interactions.

200. Failure of degradation of endocannabinoids results in their persistent actions.

201. Cannabinoid receptors are examples of T-carbohydrate receptors.

202. Cannabinoid receptors are located in both brain and body.

203. There is a cross communication between cannabinoid receptors and opioid receptors.

204. Type-2 cannabinoid receptors are present on immune tissues.

205. Cannabinoid receptors (type 2) appear to exert control over liver function.

206. Cannabinoid receptors (type 2) do not alter body metabolism.

207. Cannabinoid type-2 receptors are present in bone tissue.

208. Cannabinoid type-2 receptors are present on astrocytes in the central nervous system.

209. The receptor termed GPR55 is another putative cannabinoid receptor, in addition to cannabinoid type-1 and type-2 receptors.

210. Alteration in endocannabinoid functions can be altered by phytocannabinoids.

211. The density of cannabinoid receptors in the brain stem is quite low in comparison to other areas of the brain.

212. Cannabinoid type-2 receptor activity may balance certain aspect of type-1 cannabinoid receptor function.

213. Agonists of cannabinoid receptors type 2 tend to be proinflammatory.

214. THC acts via CB-1 receptors to increase appetite.

215. Cannabinoids have shown an ability to suppress noxious stimuli to the brain from traumatic injury.

216. There is no evidence that the endocannabinoid system works with tonic activity.

217. Entourage effects of cannabis have been well described by Ethan B. Russo, MD, who has described a state of endocannabinoid excess.

218. Ethan B. Russo has described the entourage effects in an accurate manner.

219. Terpenoids contribute to the entourage effect of cannabis.

220. Terpenoids have actions that influence cannabinoid receptors.

221. Cannabinol has psychoactive effects that are stronger than THC.

222. Cannabinol has no psychoactive actions.

223. Cannabigerol compounds are precursor molecules for cannabinoids, THC, and cannabidiol (CBD).

224. Overall, THC mimics the actions of anandamide.

225. Dronabinol (Marinol) is a schedule-I controlled drug.

226. Cannabis is a schedule III prescribed drug.

227. The potency of marijuana used in recreational activity can be gauged for its "high" effect based upon its THC content.

228. Smoking cannabis is the most rapid way of absorbing THC.

229. THC and other cannabinoids are known to produce paradoxical effects.

230. It is estimated that more cases of cannabis addiction will occur as a consequence of recreational legalization of cannabis.

231. THC tends to be stored in fat in the body.

232. Cannabis is often used to treat psychosis.

233. Cannabis may cause retention of urine.

234. Cannabis use in pregnancy has caused reductions in birth weight of the newborn.

235. Young people who have used cannabis in a persistent manner tend to have lower levels of educational achievement.

236. Cannabis users have a greater prevalence of lung infections than noncannabis users.

237. Chronic fatigue has been associated with marijuana use.

238. Cannabichromene (CBC) is present most often in cannabis grown in the tropics.

239. Tetrahydrocannabivarin (THCV) is referred to as the "sports car" of the cannabinoids because of its energizing and short-term effects.

240. Cannabidiol has been shown to act as 5-HT1A receptor antagonist.

241. CBD may be useful in reducing both social and anxiety disorders.

242. Arguments exist about the legality of CBD (cannabidiol).

243. Sativex is a solid dosage form of cannabis, a tablet.

244. A dietary supplement is a form of food.

245. Beta-caryophyllene is a newly discovered cannabinoid.

246. Rimonabant (SR141716) has been removed from the market as a treatment for obesity.

247. Popular or common names for herbal marijuana are often quite accurate in relationship to their content of cannabinoids.

248. Cannabis has potential for use in antiaging.

249. Cannabis has little effect on gastrointestinal function.

250. There is convincing evidence to support the use of cannabis for medical treatment in several hundred diseases.

251. Sativex is an oro-nucosal spray containing cannabinoids and ballast components.

252. Dronabinol (Marinol) is most often used for headaches.

253. Denbinobin is found in cannabis, and it exerts antiviral effects.

254. Allergy to cannabis is very common.

255. Homeopathic cannabis remains under-investigated.

256. Adolescent, chronic use of cannabis doubles the risk of schizophrenia or psychosis in adults.

257. Cannabis has been shown to be useful in the variable control of chronic neuropathic pain.

258. Spasticity is often quite responsive to THC or Nabilone or whole herbal cannabis.

259. Epilepsy is 100 percent responsive to cannabis or CBD administration.

260. Cannabis has shown promise in the treatment of autoimmune disease.

261. Suicide risk with cannabis use seems to be present in adults who started cannabis use in childhood.

Chapter 7: Cancer

262. Cannabis may reduce the blood supply to some types of cancer (antiangiogenic actions).

263. Current evidence shows that cannabis is a cancer cure.

264. Cannabis can interfere with the spread of breast cancer.

265. Both CBD and THC have antimetastatic effects.

266. Cannabis can be considered to belong to a novel category of anticancer drugs.

267. Patients are never prosecuted when they use cannabis for cancer on their own initiative.

268. Administration of cannabis drugs is compatible with driving.

269. Cannabis use can promote apoptosis in cancer cells.

270. Cannabis has been shown to kill certain cancer cells in laboratory experiments.

271. Sativex (THC:CBD in a 1:1 ratio) always results in significant decrease of pain scores caused by cancer.

272. Cannabis smoke contains a number of potent carcinogens and is a definite cause of lung cancer.

273. Cannabis administration may cause autophagy in cancer cells.

274. The brain tumor, glioblastoma multiforme, is consistently responsive to cannabis infusion directly into the brain.

275. Cannabis has not shown any benefit in the treatment of hematological malignancy.

276. Research has shown that synthetic agonists of type-1 and type-2 cannabinoid receptors may produce pain relief with an equivalent effect to that of morphine.

277. Claims of cancer cures with cannabis are misleading.

278. There is a lot of evidence that cannabis can cause cancer.

279. Cannabis can increase the risk of testicular cancer in some patients.

280. Endocannabinoid tone is believed to be a significant factor in controlling the malignant potential of several different tumors.

281. The biological effects of cannabis in malignancy are altered by many external and internal factors

Chapter 8: Mental Disorders

282. Cannabis smoking may cause anhedonia.

283. The use of cannabis in patients with mental disorders is quite common.

284. Cannabis use has been encouraged in recent times by a common reputation of being quite safe.

285. When the population perceives cannabis use to have side effects or adverse effects, the general use of cannabis tends to fall in the population.

286. Mental-health workers often express concern about the occurrence of common adverse effects of cannabis in individuals with mental disorders consuming marijuana.

287. Marijuana use can produce irritability and impulsive behavior.

288. Genetic or hereditary tendencies seem to operate to some degree in mental reactions to cannabis consumption.

289. Whole herbal cannabis may be valuable in the treatment of attention-deficit disorder in children, without any risk of addiction.

290. Cannabis may be valuable in certain types of neurodegenerative diseases.

291. Cannabis may cause or is sometimes useful in the management of depression.

292. Elevated levels of anandamide occur in the cerebrospinal fluid of schizophrenic patients.

293. Reports suggest that some schizophrenic symptoms may improve with the administration of cannabis.

294. The cannabinoid THC seems to be the principal component of cannabis that precipitates psychosis.

295. CBD has value in the treatment of schizophrenia when administered alone.

296. European studies (EMBLEM Study) have shown that cannabis users with bipolar disorder have increased levels of mania and general illness severity compared with controls who did not use cannabis.

297. ADHD is often associated with low levels dopamine in the central nervous system.

298. Recent studies show that the hyperactive-impulsive type of ADHD may be more responsive to cannabis use than inattentive types of this disorder.

299. The hippocampus and amygdala of the brain play a role in emotion, memory, and mood.

300. Sleep disorders do not tend to occur during cannabis withdrawal.

301. Addiction to or dependence on cannabis affects at least one in nine users or more, especially in young people.

302. Twin studies show that a member of the twins who uses cannabis may tend to have a greater tendency to develop problems in adulthood and use other drugs compared with a nonusing twin.

303. Marijuana use in teenagers has been shown to cause modest reductions in IQ, at least in the short term.

304. High school dropout rates are not increased by marijuana use.

305. The loss of memory in the long term with marijuana use is arguable.

306. Chronic alcohol use tends to result in shrinkage of the brain.

307. Cannabis seems to cause changes in the structure of the brain, but regional variations occur, and some arguments prevail.

308. Post-traumatic stress disorder (PTSD) seems to respond to cannabis smoking.

309. Only anecdotal information is available to support the use of cannabis in the treatment of autism.

310. Chronic cannabis use can be associated with poor motivation and impaired judgment (antimotivational syndrome).

311. Whether or not cannabis increases the prevalence of violent crime is arguable.

312. Recent studies show no benefit of cannabis treatment in brain injury.

Chapter 9: The Gastrointestinal Tract

313. Cannabinoids may play a role in the development of failure to thrive in infants.

314. Cannabinoids appear to exert effects on gastrointestinal hormone secretion.

315. Cannabinoid receptors in the brain may reduce gastric acid secretions.

316. Cannabinoids can reduce the production of saliva.

317. The density of cannabinoid receptors in the gut is highest in the stomach and upper parts of the large intestine.

318. Smoking marijuana often reduces vomiting caused by chemotherapy.

319. Dronabinol causes vomiting after chemotherapy.

320. Cannabis treatment may be valuable in reducing side effects of the anti-viral treatment used for hepatitis C and HIV virus infections.

321. Cannabis may affect ion transport in the bowel.

322. Cannabinoids often have anti-inflammatory effects in the bowel.

323. Cannabinoids may modulate transient receptor potential Vanilloid-1-receptors.

324. Cannabinoids do not interact with alpha-receptors in the gastrointestinal tract.

325. The munchies may be produced by the effects of THC on the nucleus acumbens.

326. Reduction of saliva secretion occurs with cannabis smoking to produce a "cotton mouth."

327. Cannabis has been shown to both relieve and cause constipation.

328. Bowel function is often unaffected in many people who use cannabis.

329. Cannabis worsens the effects of inflammation in the bowel.

330. Cannabis is valuable in the management of functional digestive disease.

331. Cannabis has no effect on secretory diarrhea.

332. Agents that block cannabis type-1 receptors promote intestinal water secretion.

333. Smoking cannabis is contraindicated in the management of cystic fibrosis.

334. The pancreas expresses only type-2 cannabinoid receptors.

335. Animal studies show reduction in pain responses following mechanical distention of the bowel after cannabis administration.

336. Cannabis can delay small bowel transit overall.

337. Alterations in endocannabinoid concentrations occur in inflammatory bowel disease.

338. Cannabis smoking may reduce nausea and improve appetite in individuals with Crohn's disease.

339. Cannabis can produce a hyperemesis syndrome.

Chapter 10: Bones and Joints

340. Cannabis has a role in altering immune function in autoimmune types of arthritis.

341. Cannabis may reduce morning stiffness of joints and increase joint mobility in rheumatoid disease.

342. CT-3 (dimethylheptyl-THC-11-oic acid) promotes joint inflammation and has painkilling actions in animals.

343. Cannabis (CBD) can reduce the secretion of inflammatory cytokines.

344. Ajumelic acid can relieve experimentally induced arthritis in laboratory animals.

345. Some medical review articles do not provide good support for the effectiveness of cannabis use in rheumatoid disease.

346. Ananamide (2-AG concentrations) is elevated in humans with degenerative osteoarthritis.

347. The endocannabinoid system plays a role in modulating bone deposition, resorption, and growth.

348. Cannabis may reduce bone tissue in young animals and increase bone mass in elderly animals.

349. A significant number of patients with fibromyalgia self-medicate with cannabis.

350. Nabilone makes sleep disturbances worse in patients with fibromyalgia.

Chapter 11: Cardiorespiratory Disorders

351. Cannabis does not affect lung structure.

352. Cannabis smoking is a clear cause of lung cancer.

353. Literature supports the opinion that cannabis may cause heart attack to a degree greater than reported.

354. Research implies that cannabinoid type-1 and type-2 receptors play opposite roles in the cause and progression of hardening of the arteries (arteriosclerosis).

355. Cannabidiol interferes with the enzyme lipoxygenase, which plays a role in the development of atheroma.

356. Cannabis smoking can precipitate angina.

357. Cannabis has been associated with transient cerebral ischemic attacks.

358. Cannabis has been associated with inflammation of blood vessels (angitis).

359. Immediately following cannabis smoking, heart rate most often declines, and blood pressure is lowered.

360. THC can contribute to poor oxygen supply to heart muscle.

361. Cannabis smoking may precipitate cardiac arrhythmias.

362. Cannabis may cause malignant hypertension.

363. Alterations in pain perception following cannabis use can result in a delay of patients seeking acute medical care for heart attack.

364. Cardiovascular events with cannabis use in animals may be different from those in humans.

365. Cannabis can precipitate heart attacks in young people who do not have coronary artery disease.

366. Cannabis related reports of cardiovascular problems are much more common in elderly women.

367. Higher levels of apolipoprotein-C111 occur in cannabis users.

368. Cannabis smoking can cause premalignant changes in the lining of the respiratory tract.

369. Smoking cannabis increases the occurrence of euphoria.

370. Extreme smoking conditions deliver lesser amounts of toxic chemicals into the body.

371. Vaporization of cannabis for inhalation occurs at temperatures equivalent to burning.

372. Cannabis smoking can cause changes in respiratory function tests.

Chapter 12: Neurological Disorders

373. The endocannabinoid system plays a role in neuroprotection.

374. Endocannabinoids cause oxidative stress.

375. Impaired control of the endocannabinoid system is often encountered in neurodegenerative diseases.

376. The key enzymes involve in degradation of endocannabinoids are fatty acid amide hydrolase (FAAH) and monoglyceride lipase (MAGL).

377. Cannabinoid receptors type-2 are more common on nervous tissue than on immune tissue.

378. Most cases of epilepsy are of unknown cause.

379. Cannabidiol has received orphan drug status for the treatment of severe childhood epilepsy in many states of the United States.

380. Cannabis shows universal benefit in the reduction of epileptic fits.

381. Cannabidivarin (CBDV) has powerful antiepileptic effects in rats.

382. Cannabis may precipitate epilepsy.

383. The type of cannabis called Charlotte's Web is high in its THC content and very low in its CBD content.

384. Endocannabinoids are often disturbed in circumstances of altered motor function in the nervous system.

385. Cannabis is of no value in the management of Tourette's syndrome.

386. Cannabinoid type-1 and type-2 receptor agonists delay the progression of all Alzheimers disease.

387. Cannabis may improve tremor at rest and rigidity in Parkinson's disease.

388. Cannabis is of no value in the management of L-Dopa-induced dyskinesia, in Parkinson's disease.

389. Nabilone has shown little benefit in the treatment of Huntington's disease.

390. Animal studies show that cannabinoids can reduce chemokine secretion in amyotrophic lateral sclerosis (ALS).

391. Cannabis alters glutamine uptake in the central nervous system.

392. The neuroprotective effects of CBD appear to exceed those of THC in patients with ALS.

393. Activation of both types of cannabinoid receptors (CB-1 and CB-2) may reduce symptoms in patients with multiple sclerosis.

394. Vaping (vaporization) of cannabis may cause symptom relief in patients with multiple sclerosis.

395. The CUPID study of multiple sclerosis found no overall evidence to support a benefit of THC on the progression of the course of multiple sclerosis.

396. Nabiximols and whole herbal cannabis have been shown to exert positive benefit in multiple sclerosis.

397. Alzheimer's disease is not influenced in any positive way by cannabis administration.

398. Clinical trials demonstrate the ability of marijuana smoking to ease neuropathic pain.

399. Cannabis may reduce pain in some subjects who do not respond to other pain therapies.

400. Migraine has been described as a syndrome of excess endocannabinoid presence.

401. Cannabinoids interact with opioid systems in the brain and may spare the need for opioid drug use.

402. Cannabis usually produces a state of awakening.

403. Cannabis has a potential beneficial effect in sleep apnea management.

Chapter 13: Diabetes Mellitus

404. Data from surveys show a lower occurrence of disturbed carbohydrate metabolism with cannabis use.

405. The human pancreas islet cells have both CB-1 and CB-2 receptors.

406. Energy balance as a consequence of hypothalamic control is mediated in part by endocannabinoid receptors.

407. Impaired controls of the endocannabinoid system are associated with obesity in humans.

408. It is postulated that increased endocannabinoid tone exists in several tissues in obese humans.

409. Cannabis administration increases the effects and production of stress hormones, resulting in common loss of consciousness.

410. Endocannabinoid receptor inhibition with Rimonabant causes severe depression with increased suicide risk, and it has been withdrawn from use.

411. Cannabidiol (CBD) can exert benefit in the management of neurological complications from diabetes mellitus.

412. Cannabis use in diabetic subjects tends to improve blood-glucose control and improve regional blood flow to several organs.

413. It is estimated that about eighteen million Americans use marijuana on a regular or semiregular basis.

414. Diet and weight control are factors that can modulate the function of the endocannabinoid control systems in the body.

415. Cannabis may cause poor memory, which can influence behavior and sugar control in diabetics.

416. Cannabis can relieve muscle cramps in the presence of diabetes mellitus.

417.Research in animals demonstrates the ability of endocannabinoids to activate macrophages in a manner that is associated with loss of beta cells in the pancreas.

418. Sativex produces uniform control of pain in diabetic peripheral neuropathy.

419. Cannabidiol (CBD) reduces the blood level of VEGF (vascular endothelial growth factor), which is a promoter of new blood vessel growth in body tissues.

Chapter 14: Infections, HIV Disease, and Inflammation

420. Illicit drug use may often be associated with a number of different lung infections.

421. Contaminants in illicit cannabis may become opportunistic infections in patients with AIDS.

422. Cannabis tends to impair lymphocyte blastogenic transformation by mitogens.

423. THC can reduce monocyte function in a dose-related manner.

424. Both CB-1 and CB-2 receptors are present on immune-competent cells.

425. CB-2 receptor stimulation tends to promote immune function overall.

426. Both THC and CBD alter cell-mediated immunity.

427. Individuals with HIV infection who smoke cannabis are more prone to infection with herpes virus.

428. Cannabidiol has been shown to inhibit prion accumulation in animal studies.

429. Cannabis may have antiviral actions.

430. Infections with Ebola virus are not known to be responsive to cannabis administration.

431. Cannabinoid use in AIDS or HIV infection may cause apoptosis in immune cells with a resulting decrease in inflammatory responses.

432. Cannabis is used by approximately 60 percent of patients with AIDS or HIV infection.

433. Cannabis is of no value in pain relief in patients with AIDS.

434. Cannabis use can improve the treatment tolerance of patients taking antiretroviral therapy for AIDS.

435. Cannabis can play a valuable role in the terminal AIDS patients.

436. Cannabis can improve sleep in patients with AIDS.

Chapter 15: Skin Disease and Reproductive Health

437. Topical applied cannabinoids are well absorbed and produce high blood levels.

438. Cannabidiol can act as a repressor of transcription.

439. Cannabis has been proposed as a treatment for acne.

440. Cannabis smoking may make acne worse.

441. Rosacea may often be responsive to cannabis use.

442. Cannabis smoking is the preferred mode of delivery for individuals with skin diseases.

443. Cannabis may decrease skin itching.

444. There is a general perception that cannabis use promotes sexual behavior in women.

445. Regular cannabis use has been associated with erectile dysfunction.

446. Cannabis administered to women may result in some increase in testosterone secretion.

447. Endocannabinoids control implantation of the embryo.

448. Cannabis may decrease the motility of sperm.

449. Cannabis may interfere with fetal development.

450. Some studies suggest that cannabis can result in babies with low birth weight.

451. Cannabis is the most frequently used illicit drug in pregnancy.

452. Heavy and chronic use of cannabis is linked to increased fertility in men and women.

453. Cannabis use may improve symptoms in the menopausal transition.

454. Cannabis has been described to increase symptoms in women with premenstrual syndrome (PMS).

Chapter 16: Miscellaneous Topics

455. Cannabis use can result in misperceptions of an increased or distorted intensity.

456. Cannabis dependence is more likely to occur with chronic heavy use.

457. Following acute intake of cannabis blood flow to the brain increases.

458. Smoking cannabis can open the airways or sometimes constrict the airways in the lungs.

459. Cannabis is very valuable in the control of several types of pain.

460. Cannabis increases the pressure within the eyeball.

461. Cannabis has an overall depressant effect on immune function.

462. Cannabis has been shown to be useful in the treatment of an overactive bladder.

463. Cannabis may improve symptoms of urinary retention.

464. Cannabis has shown value in the treatment of interstitial cystitis.

465. Whole herbal cannabis smoking is a cause of renal failure.

466. Synthetic pot can cause acute renal failure.

467. Synthetic pot is considered toxic and dangerous.

468. Synthetic pot is illegal in Colorado.

469. Cannabis can cause alterations in hormonal controls of the adrenal and thyroid glands.

Chapter 17: Social Perspectives

470. Cannabis legalization will tend to increase cannabis consumption in young people.

471. Cannabis smoking is allowed in public in Washington State and Colorado.

472. The cannabis industry is predicted to undergo major consolidation over the next few years.

473. American Indian tribes are allowed to grow cannabis on their lands.

474. A spot blood test after cannabis consumption can readily define the time at which cannabis was taken.

475. Cannabis use is allowed in the United States for religious purposes.

476. The sale of cannabis in the United States is likely to decrease substantially.

Chapter 18: The Hidden Potaholic

477. Adolescent use of cannabis is associated with adult disability.

478. Urine testing is advisable with any suspicion of cannabis use in youngsters.

479. Hidden potaholics share symptoms encountered among hidden alcoholics.

Chapter 19: The Future

480. Cannabis legalization presents insignificant medical, political, and legal implications for society.

Answer Sheet

To Be Detached and Mailed with Your Score and

1. F	26. F	51. F	76. T
2. T	27. T	52. T	77. T
3. T	28. T	53. T	78. T
4. F	29. T	54. T	79. F
5. F	30. F	55. T	80. T
6. T	31. F	56. T	81. T
7. F	32. T	57. T	82. T
8. T	33. T	58. F	83. T
9. F	34. T	59. T	84. T
10. T	35. T	60. T	85. T
11. F	36. F	61. T	86. T
12. F	37. T	62. T	87. T
13. T	38. F	63. T	88. T
14. F	39. T	64. T	89. T
15. F	40. F	65. F	90. F
16. F	41. T	66. T	91. T
17. F	42. T	67. T	92. T
18. F	43. T	68. F	93. F
19. T	44. T	69. F	94. T
20. T	45. T	70. T	95. T
21 T	46. F	71. T	96. T
22. T	47. T	72. T	97. F
23. F	48. T	73. F	98. T
24. F	49. F	74. F	99. T
25. T	50. T	75. F	100. F

101. T	139. T	177. T	215. T
102. F	140. T	178. F	216. F
103. T	141. T	179. T	217. F
104. T	142. F	180. T	218. T
105. T	143. T	181. T	219. T
106. T	144. T	182. T	220. T
107. F	145. T	183. T	221. F
108. T	146. T	184. F	222. F
109. T	147. T	185. T	223. T
110. T	148. F	186. T	224. T
111. F	149. F	187. F	225. F
112. F	150. T	188. F	226. F
113. T	151. T	189. F	227. T
114. T	152. F	190. T	228. T
115. T	153. T	191. F	229. T
116. T	154. T	192. T	230. T
117. F	155. F	193. T	231. T
118. F	156. F	194. F	232. F
119. T	157. F	195. T	233. T
120. T	158. F	196. T	234. T
121. F	159. T	197. T	235. T
122. F	160. T	198. T	236. T
123. T	161. F	199. T	237. T
124. T	162. T	200. T	238. T
125. F	163. F	201. F	239. T
126. T	164. F	202. T	240. F
127. T	165. T	203. T	241. T
128. T	166. F	204. T	242. T
129. T	167. F	205. T	243. F
130. T	168. T	206. F	244. F
131. F	169. T	207. T	245. F
132. T	170. F	208. T	246. T
133. T	171. F	209. T	247. F
134. F	172. F	210. T	248. T
135. T	173. F	211. T	249. F
136. T	174. T	212. T	250. F
137. F	175. T	213. F	251. T
138. T	176. T	214. T	252. F

253. T	291. T	329. F	367. T
254. F	292. T	330. T	368. T
255. T	293. T	331. F	369. T
256. T	294. T	332. T	370. F
257. T	295. T	333. T	371. F
258. T	296. T	334. F	372. T
259. F	297. T	335. T	373. T
260. T	298. T	336. F	374. F
261. T	299. T	337. T	375. T
262. T	300. F	338. T	376. T
263. F	301. T	339. T	377. F
264. T	302. T	340. T	378. T
265. T	303. T	341. T	379. T
266. T	304. F	342. F	380. F
267. F	305. T	343. T	381. T
268. F	306. T	344. T	382. T
269. T	307. T	345. T	383. F
270. T	308. T	346. T	384. T
271. F	309. T	347. T	385. F
272. F	310. T	348. T	386. F
273. T	311. T	349. T	387. T
274. F	312. F	350. F	388. F
275. F	313. T	351. F	389. T
276. T	314. T	352. F	390. T
277. T	315. T	353. T	391. T
278. F	316. T	354. T	392. T
279. T	317. T	355. T	393. T
280. T	318. T	356. T	394. T
281. T	319. F	357. T	395. T
282. T	320. T	358. T	396. T
283. T	321. T	359. F	397. F
284. T	322. T	360. T	398. T
285. T	323. T	361. T	399. T
286. T	324. F	362. F	400. F
287. T	325. T	363. T	401. T
288. T	326. T	364. T	402. F
289. F	327. T	365. T	403. T
290. T	328. T	366. F	404. T

405. T	424. T	443. T	462. T
406. T	425. F	444. T	463. T
407. T	426. T	445. T	464. T
408. T	427. T	446. T	465. F
409. F	428. T	447. T	466. T
410. T	429. T	448. T	467. T
411. T	430. T	449. T	468. T
412. T	431. T	450. T	469. T
413. T	432. T	451. T	470. T
414. T	433. F	452. F	471. F
415. T	434. T	453. T	472. T
416. T	435. T	454. F	473. T
417. T	436. T	455. T	474. F
418. F	437. F	456. T	475. F
419. T	438. T	457. T	476. F
420. T	439. T	458. T	477. T
421. T	440. T	459. T	478. T
422. T	441. T	460. F	479. T
423. T	442. F	461. T	480. F

Signature_____Your self-score on the exam (number of questions answered correctly out of 480 questions)

I certify that I have read this book and answered the questions in good faith.

Sign Here

Mail your score out 480 and $50. (Fee to obtain your diploma.)

Other Books By The Author

(available for purchase at www.stephenholtmd.com)

Skinner, HA, Holt, S. 1993. *The Alcohol Clinical Index*. Toronto: Addiction Research Foundation.

Holt, S. 1996. *Soya for Health*. Larchmont, NY: Mary Ann Liebert Publishers.

Holt, S, and Comac, L. 1997. *Miracle Herbs*. Secaucus, NJ: Carol Publishing.

Holt, S, and Barilla, J. 1998. *The Power of Cartilage*, NY, NY: Kensington Publishers.

Holt, S. 1999. *The Sexual Revolution*. San Diego, California: ProMotion Publishing.

Holt, S. 1999 (second printing 2002). *The Natural Way to a Healthy Heart*. NY, NY: M. Evans Inc.

Holt, S. 1999 (third printing 2002). *The Soy Revolution*. NY, NY: Dell Publishing, Random House.

Holt, S. 2000 (second printing 2002). *Natural Ways to Digestive Health*. NY, NY: M. Evans Inc.

Holt, S, and Bader, D. 2001. *Natures Benefit for Pets*. Newark, NJ: Wellness Publishing.

Holt, S. 2002. *The Antiporosis Plan*. Newark, NJ: Wellness Publishing.

Holt, S. 2002. *Combat Syndrome X, Y, and Z*. Newark, NJ: Wellness Publishing.

Holt, S, and Wright, J. 2003. *Syndrome X Nutritional Factors*. Newark, NJ: Wellness Publishing.

Holt, S. 2004. *Enhancing Low Carb Diets*. Newark, NJ: Wellness Publishing.

Holt, S. 2003. *Sleep Naturally*. Newark, NJ: Wellness Publishing.

Holt, S. 2005. *Supreme Properties of Hoodia*. Newark, NJ: Wellness Publishing.

Holt, S. 2011. *The HCG Diet Revolution*. Indiana: Authorhouse (www.authorhouse.com).

Holt, S. 2011. *The Antiaging Triad*. Indiana: Authorhouse (www.authorhouse.com).

Holt, S. 2009. *A Primer of Natural Therapeutics*. Holt Institute of Medicine (www.stephenholtmd.com).

Holt, S. 2012. *Holt on: Sex The Natural Way*. Indiana: Authorhouse

(www.authorhouse.com).

Holt, S. 2013. *The Definitive Guide to Colon Hydrotherapy*. Holt Institute of Medicine.

Holt, S, Carroll, C, Nwosu, U. 2014. *The Topical Pain Relief Revolution: Principles and Practice of Compounding Pharmacy*. Holt Institute of Medicine, Creative Publishing Platform.

About The Author

Dr. Stephen Holt is a best-selling author, medical practitioner in New York, and distinguished professor of medicine (emeritus). He has been described as a visionary and a pioneer of integrative medicine, and he is world renowned for his work on therapeutics with nutrition and dietary supplements. He is a frequent guest lecturer at medical and scientific conferences.

For many years Dr. Holt has developed management pathways for several public health initiatives, with an emphasis on lifestyle changes and nutritional interventions. He believes that health care should be portable, widely available, and free for children and the elderly. Dr. Holt has been described as the "doctor's doctor" because many of his patients are medical practitioners. Given the major pressure on Dr. Holt's time as an international lecturer and so forth, he restricts his patient care in New York to referrals only from other doctors.

Dr. Holt's principal training has been in allopathic medicine, but he has charted new treatment paradigms using natural medicines. He believes in the concept of medical pluralism, where many different medical disciplines come together to provide holistic health care. Dr. Holt supports the practice of many forms of medicine, including chiropractic medicine, naturopathic medicine, podiatric medicine, homeopathic medicine, as well as traditional medical disciplines that offer many alternative strategies for health maintenance.

He is an author of more than twenty books in the popular health care field, and he has also contributed chapters and many articles to peer-reviewed medical textbooks and journals. As well as publishing several hundred scientific articles in leading medical journals, Dr. Holt has been cited thousands of times in the medical and lay press.

An honors graduate in medicine from Liverpool University Medical School, in England, UK, Dr. Holt holds subspecialty qualifications in gastroenterology and internal medicine in the United States, Canada, and Europe. He has practiced clinical nutrition medicine for four decades. Dr. Holt has held the rank of full professor of medicine and bioengineering adjunct for many years, and he has received awards for medical teaching and research in the United States, China, Indonesia, Great Britain, Malaysia, Thailand, Taiwan, South Korea, and other countries, where he has served as a visiting professor. He now holds the highest academic rank as a distinguished professor of medicine (emeritus).

Index

t denotes table

breast cancer, 145, 179, 227, 235*t*,
241, 400
Brunet, L., 289
Bryson, E. O., 395
buds, as synonym for cannabis,
23, 25, 26, 167

C

caffeinated energy drinks,
cannabis use with, 57–58
California Board for
Physicians, 118
California Department of Social
Services, 421
California Environmental
Protection Agency, 232
Callaway, J. C., 139, 140, 141
Canada
acceptance of vaping devices
in, 39
permission for physicians
to advise/prescribe
cannabis for medical
use in, 89
cancer. *See also specific cancers*
advocacy for cannabis use
in? 239
anticancer effects of
cannabinoids: revision,
242–244
anticancer observations,
more, 240–242
applying medical cannabis,
228–232
brief overview of and
its responses to
cannabinoids, 234–237
cancer pain and
cannabinoids, 237–238
cannabinoids and malignancy
of immune origin, 237

carcinogenicity of cannabis
smoke, 232–233
does marijuana cause?
239–240
Guzman's classic cancer
studies, 234
laboratory and clinical
research in, 233
major effects of cannabis in,
227–228
use of cannabis for treatment
of, 24
Cancer Research UK, 228
candies, as intake/delivery mode,
37, 40, 124, 398
Cannabaceae, 68*t*, 137
cannabichromene (CBC), 55*t*, 98*t*,
163, 165*t*, 177–178, 184–185*t*,
224*t*, 285, 364, 399
cannabichromevarin (CBCV), 165*t*
cannabicyclol (CBL), 55*t*, 165*t*,
224*t*
cannabidiol (CBD)
as acting to reduce
psychoactive effects of
THC, 24
as antiemetic in AIDS
patients, 363
benefits of in cancer
management, 111, 145,
235–236*t*
in cascade of cannabinoid
synthesis, 176*t*
content of in hemp versus
marijuana, 137
as counteracting some
psychoactive effects of
THC, 80, 138
as dietary supplement (or
not), xxvii, xxxv, 24,
25, 35–36, 49*t*, 96, 150,

cannabis knowledge, milestones
in, 51–54
cannabis laws
costs of enforcement of, 413
history of, 53*t*
repealing of? 418
cannabis legalization. *See also*
Alaska; Arizona; Colorado;
Oregon; Washington
(state); Washington, DC
author's opinion of, xxiii, xxix,
xxx–xxxi, xxxiii, 18
and black market, 81
compared to
decriminalization, 93–
94, 95*t*
decisions about, 1
driving quest for, 150
impacts of on economic
issues, 416–417
for medical use, xxiii–xxiv, xxv
Pew Research Center survey
on public support
for medical cannabis
legalization, 3
for recreational use, xxv
support for in US, 49*t*, 418
cannabis literature, 220
cannabis products
drugs based on cannabis in
use or in development,
205–206*t*
quality of, 75
range of, 203
safety of, 19–20
cannabis quiz, 503–536
cannabis receptors. *See*
cannabinoid receptor
agonists; cannabinoid
receptor antagonists;
cannabinoid receptors;

endocannabinoid receptor
system/endocannabinoid
system (ECS)
cannabis research
Colorado Department of
Public Health funding
for, 223–224
as driven by economic
prospects, 455
expansion of clinical studies
on, 95, 96
further research as
required, 455
history of, 2
limited knowledge from, 95
problems with, 85–87, 305
Cannabis Revolution, emergence
of, 29
Cannabis ruderalis (C. ruderalis),
23, 26, 49*t*, 137, 149, 191, 193
Cannabis sativa (C. sativa), xx,
xxiii, 4, 22–23, 25, 26, 27*t*,
49*t*, 80, 97, 98, 137, 139,
147, 149, 163, 167, 191, 192,
193, 206
cannabis science
area of dispute in, 265
concern about lack of
knowledge about, 3
contributors to, xxii
key principles in, 167
key to understanding of, 156
teaching of, xxx, 17, 66, 457
Cannabis Science Inc., 403
cannabis soda, 43*t*, 202–203, 229
cannabis tea, 43*t*, 202–203, 229
cannabis therapy, 90, 117, 199–201,
223, 234, 258, 345, 406
cannabis use
adverse effects of, 86*t*

adverse outcomes of,
  summary, 173–174*t*
and attendances at
  hospital emergency
  departments, 15–16
in ceremonial and religious
  activity, 23
compared to alcohol and
  tobacco use, 126
dearth of definitive data
  on, 19
detection of, 431–432
diet and nutritional status in
  adult users, 146
early physiological effects
  of, 101
estimated frequency of in
  adults in US, 248
future of, 455–458
how to spot: review, 452
key characteristics, 48–49
lack of information on long-
  term effects of, 65
links between mental illness
  and cannabis, 245–247
long-term effects of, 100,
  212–216
medical conditions that may
  respond to, 195–199*t*
monitoring of, 455, 456
need for secondary
  prevention of? 174–175
outcomes of heavy cannabis
  use, 449
as part of antiaging
  strategy, 194
physical and psychological
  effects of, summary,
  208–209*t*
precautions and warnings
  for, 61

reasons for, 14*t*
reducing problems with,
  102–103
responsible use of, 16, 59–65
by schoolchildren in 2011, 15*t*
self-identification of
  problems with, 135
short-term effects of, 100
signs/symptoms that may
  form eclectic side-
  effect profile of, 172*t*
social aspects of, 440–441
sociobehavioral factors
  associated with
  increased risks of, 101*t*
testing for, 105, 135, 217, 218,
  305, 406, 414–415, 417
WHO estimates of, 423
and work performance,
  134–135
by young people. *See* young
  people
cannabis use disorder (CUD), 71–
  74, 99, 172, 214, 402, 428, 457
cannabis withdrawal, 132*t*, 133,
  249, 261, 336. *See also*
  marijuana withdrawal
cannabis-derived products, 16,
  71*t*, 199, 203, 336
cannabis-like products
  (synthetic pot), 3. *See also*
  synthetic pot
cannabis-related drugs, 45, 89,
  225, 349, 365
cannabitriol (CBT), 55*t*, 98*t*, 225*t*
cannabivarin (CBV), 165*t*
cannaceutical, 25
Cannador, 99, 204, 329*t*
cantheism, 415

373, 390. *See also* nabiximols (Sativex)

Schachter (on epilepsy.com), 316

Schedule 1 drugs, 33, 49*t*, 53*t*, 125, 167, 183

Schedule III drugs, 167

Schicho, R., 287

schizophrenia, 62, 93*t*, 99, 104, 116*t*, 179, 201*t*, 202, 209*t*, 211, 212, 214, 215, 221, 249, 250, 251, 252–256, 260, 400, 429, 435, 449

Schneider, M., 429

Science Daily, 48

Scientific Reports, 126

Scott, E., 223

secondary prevention programs, 174–175

secretory diarrhea, 275*t*, 282*t*, 284

self-titration dosing paradigm, 64*t*, 117, 169

Sensi Kush (cannabis strain), 193

SERENADE study, 344

set and setting circumstances, 56

sexual health and function, 374–376

Shabat, S. Ben, 164

Shafer, (on epilepsy.com), 316

Shafer Report, 53*t*

Shen, K., 388

Shinyo, N., 400

shit, as synonym for cannabis, 25

short-term acute brain syndrome, marijuana use and, 430

side effects, 38, 65, 67, 69*t*, 118, 184, 192, 229–230, 238, 245, 259, 266, 267, 270, 285, 289, 292, 317, 318, 321, 322, 331*t*, 332*t*, 334, 362, 364, 380, 382, 395

sinsemilla, 25, 80, 428, 431

skin, cannabis effects on, 370

skin cancer, 236*t*, 369*t*

skin disease, 179, 367–369, 370

skin esthetics, 373

Skinner, H. A., 60

skunk
   as THC content, 23, 80, 168
   use of term, 25, 100

skunk-like cannabis/skunk-like strains, xxiv, 20, 22, 46, 59, 253, 254, 428–429, 431. *See also* Made in England

sleep, cannabis and, 338

sleep apnea, 201*t*, 339

sleep disorders, 201*t*, 211, 250*t*, 259, 293, 295*t*, 296, 338–339, 394, 437

Smith, C. K., 371

Smith, E., 146*t*

Smith, Owen, 188, 189

smoking
   carcinogenicity of cannabis smoke, 232–233
   impact of, 38
   as intake/delivery mode, 37, 41, 42*t*, 49*t*, 97, 114, 169, 308–311

social aspects, of cannabis use, 440–441

social perspectives
   African Americans and cannabis, 413–414
   American Indian tribes and marijuana, 411–413
   cannabis, violence, and crime, 417–418
   cannabis and economics, 416–417
   cannabis and religion, 415–416
   cannabis industry, 410–411

"What Will the Future of the Marijuana Industry Look Like?" (Green), 410

whitey (bad trip) (negative ride), 57

withdrawal
from cannabis. *See* cannabis withdrawal
from marijuana. *See* marijuana withdrawal
symptoms of, 249*t*, 429
value of cannabis in alcohol and opioid withdrawal, 268

Wolff, V., 315

work performance, cannabis and, 134–135, 260, 448, 452

World Health Organization (WHO)
description of cannabis dependence syndrome, 71
estimates of cannabis use, 423

Wozniaka, G., 411

Wyatt, Kristen, 221

Y

yangonin, 79

young people. *See also* children; teens/teenagers
early onset of cannabis use in as predictor of later life problems, 18, 456
importance of preventing use of cannabis among, 112
and information about cannabis, 440–441
need for control of use of cannabis by, 61
prevalence of dependence on cannabis use of, 429
reasons why they do drugs: review, 450–451
step-by-step approach to cannabis use in, 449–450
thoughts and behavior of towards cannabis use, 102
use of cannabis among, 15*t*, 99, 150, 429–431
use of synthetic pot by, 125, 398, 453, 457

Yucatan weed, as synonym for synthetic pot, 31

Printed in the United States
By Bookmasters